浙江省『十三五』重点出版物出版规划项目

歷代名方精要

连建伟　主　编

沈淑华　朱文佩　副主编

浙江大学出版社·杭州

ZHEJIANG UNIVERSITY PRESS

图书在版编目（CIP）数据

历代名方精要 = Essential Famous Formula of
Past Dynasties（Chinese and English Versions） :
汉英对照 / 连建伟主编. -- 杭州 ： 浙江大学出版社，
2023.6
　ISBN 978-7-308-23389-7

　Ⅰ. ①历… Ⅱ. ①连… Ⅲ. ①方剂－汇编－汉、英
Ⅳ. ①R289.2

中国版本图书馆CIP数据核字(2022)第239106号

历代名方精要：汉英对照

连建伟　主编

沈淑华　朱文佩　副主编

策划编辑	殷晓彤
责任编辑	殷晓彤
责任校对	徐　瑾
封面设计	续设计—黄晓意
出版发行	浙江大学出版社
	（杭州市天目山路148号　　邮政编码310007）
	（网址：http://www.zjupress.com）
排　　版	杭州林智广告有限公司
印　　刷	杭州高腾印务有限公司
开　　本	710mm×1000mm　1/16
印　　张	35
字　　数	710千
版 印 次	2023年6月第1版　2023年6月第1次印刷
书　　号	ISBN 978-7-308-23389-7
定　　价	178.00元

版权所有　侵权必究　　印装差错　负责调换

浙江大学出版社市场运营中心联系方式：0571-88925591；http://zjdxcbs.tmall.com

内容提要

　　《历代名方精要》收载了目前临床较为常用、疗效确切，具有代表性的中医历代名方175首。全书分18章，系统介绍了每首方剂的组成、用法、功效、主治、方解、临床运用等6项。全书既便于掌握，又裨于实用，从而使中外读者更好地熟悉、掌握中医历代名方的临床运用规律，以满足当前临床实际的需要。

　　本书可供中外医务工作者、医药院校师生及中医爱好者阅读，以作临床及学习参考之用。

编写说明

中医药学是一个伟大的宝库，应当努力发掘、加以提高、传承精华、守正创新，故编著《历代名方精要》一书，以弘扬中医药学、造福世界人民。

一、本书旨在阐明中医历代名方的临床运用规律。共精选历代名方175首，均为现代临床常用而又疗效确切、具有代表性的历代名方。根据治法、功效的不同，将方剂分为解表、涌吐、泻下、和解、温里、清热、开窍、补益、固涩、安神、治风、治燥、消导化积、理气、理血、祛湿、祛痰、驱虫等18章。

二、每章均有概说，其内容包括方剂的概念、分类等。并在每节之首介绍该类方剂的适应证、常用药物、配伍特点、代表方等，有助于学者对每类方剂有一个总的认识。

三、每方内容分组成、用法、功效、主治、方解、临床运用等6项。

四、为保持历代名方的原貌，每方的组成、用法两项均标明原方剂量及用法，并注出现代剂量及用法。其中，现代剂量一般按原方剂量的比例折算而成，如原方剂量与现代临床实际不符，则剂量一律以现代中药常用量为依据加以拟定。现代剂量均以"克"为单位。若原方剂量为"各等分"者，则一般不注出现代剂量，读者可根据病情灵活掌握。

五、主治一项以叙述原方主治证为主，并增入古今医案比较成熟的治疗经验。

六、方解一项就各个方剂的君、臣、佐、使组方原则做了深入浅出的分析解释，说明组方用药的特点，以指导临床实践。

七、临床运用一项着重联系临床实际，阐明古今医家对该方剂的应用经验、主编的临床心得、使用注意及禁忌等。

八、方名索引、注释附于书末，以供读者查阅。

连建伟于浙江中医药大学

二〇二二年九月一日

目录

1

第一章

解表剂

凡用解表药为主组成，具有发汗、解肌、透疹等作用，用以疏散外邪、解除表证的方剂，统称解表剂，属于"八法"中的"汗法"。

第一节　辛温解表

辛温解表剂，适用于外感风寒的表证。症见恶寒发热，头项强痛，肢体酸痛，口不渴，无汗或汗出，舌苔薄白，脉浮紧或浮缓等。盖辛以发散，温以祛寒，故常用辛温解表药如麻黄、桂枝、苏叶、葱白等为主组成方剂。根据病情的需要，辛温药有时也可适当配合辛凉药或清热药，但辛温药在方剂中仍占有主要地位，不改变其辛温解表的性质。辛温解表的代表方有麻黄汤、桂枝汤、大青龙汤、小青龙汤、葱豉汤、香苏散、香薷散等。

麻黄汤《伤寒论》[1]

[组成]　麻黄三两，去节（9克）　桂枝二两，去皮（6克）　杏仁七十枚，去皮、尖（9克）　甘草一两，炙（3克）

[用法]　原方四味，以水九升，先煮麻黄，减二升，去上沫，内诸药，煮取二升半，去滓，温服八合，覆取微似汗，不须啜粥，余如桂枝法将息。

现代用法：水煎服，服后盖被取微汗。

[功效]　发汗解表，宣肺平喘。

[主治]　外感风寒表实证。症见恶寒发热，头痛，身疼，腰痛，骨节疼痛，无汗而喘，舌苔薄白，脉浮紧。

[方解]

本方证乃风寒束表所致。方中重用麻黄味辛性温，发汗解表以散风寒，宣利肺气以平喘逆，《神农本草经》[2]谓其"发表出汗，去邪热气，止咳逆上气"，故为君药；桂枝辛温发散，配伍麻黄宣卫阳，透营气，两药相须为用，增强发汗散邪之力，故为臣药；杏仁苦温，宣降肺气，助主药平喘，为佐药；炙甘草调和诸药，使入卫分的麻黄与入营分的桂枝、升散的麻黄与苦降的杏仁更好地配合，且能缓和麻、桂峻猛之性，使无过汗伤正之弊，为使药。四药配伍，以解除在表之寒邪，开泄闭郁之肺气，使表邪解散，肺气宣通，诸症自愈。

[临床运用]

本方为辛温解表峻剂，《伤寒论》以本方治太阳伤寒。所谓太阳伤寒，实为外感风寒表实证，故《医宗金鉴》[3]说："此方为仲景开表逐邪发汗第一峻药也。"

桂枝汤《伤寒论》

[组成] 桂枝三两，去皮（9克） 芍药三两（9克） 甘草二两，炙（6克） 生姜三两，切（9克） 大枣十二枚，擘（4枚）

[用法] 原方五味㕮咀，以水七升，微火煮取三升，去滓，适寒温，服一升。服已须臾，啜热稀粥一升余，以助药力，温覆令一时许，遍身漐漐微似有汗者益佳，不可令如水流漓，病必不除。若一服汗出病差，停后服，不必尽剂；若不汗，更服，依前法；又不汗，后服小促其间，半日许，令三服尽；若病重者，一日一夜服，周时观之。服一剂尽，病证犹在者，更作服；若汗不出者，乃服至二三剂。禁生冷、黏滑、肉面、五辛、臭恶等物。

现代用法：水煎服，服后进少量热稀粥，覆被取微汗。

[功效] 解肌发表，调和营卫。

[主治] 外感风邪，发热头痛，汗出恶风，鼻鸣干呕，舌苔薄白，脉浮缓。

[方解]

本方证乃外感风邪，营卫不和所致。方中桂枝辛温，温经散寒，解肌发表，能入营透卫，故为君药；芍药酸苦微寒，收敛阴气，补养营阴，为臣药；桂、芍相配，一散一收，解肌发表而不致营阴外泄，调和营卫，使表邪得解，里气以和。炙甘草配桂枝，辛甘发散为阳，以增强发汗解肌作用，配芍药，酸甘化合为阴，以增强敛液益阴作用，故为佐药；生姜、大枣补益脾胃，调和营卫，《伤寒明理论》[4]说"姜、枣之用，专行脾之津液而和营卫者也"，故为使药。盖汗为水谷之精气所化，汗生于谷，补益脾胃则能为发汗之资。

[临床运用]

1.《伤寒论》以本方治太阳中风。所谓太阳中风，实为外感风寒表虚证，"太阳病，发热，汗出，恶风，脉缓者，名曰中风"是也。此外，临床还用于杂病及病后、产后因营卫不和以致时而微恶风寒，时而发热，汗出，脉缓等症。

2.外感风寒，表实无汗，或表郁里热，不汗出而烦躁，或温病初起，即见里热口渴，舌红脉数，以及酒客湿热内蕴者，均不可使用本方。王叔和[5]所谓"桂枝下咽，阳盛则毙"，李时珍[6]说"无汗不得用桂枝"，确有临床参考价值。

大青龙汤《伤寒论》

[组成] 麻黄六两，去节（18克） 桂枝二两，去皮（6克） 甘草二两，炙（6克） 杏仁四十枚，去皮、尖（6克） 生姜三两，切（9克） 大枣十二枚，擘（4枚） 石膏如鸡子大，碎（30克）

[用法] 原方七味，以水九升，先煮麻黄，减二升，去上沫，内诸药，煮取三升，去滓，温服一升，取微似汗。汗出多者，温粉扑之。一服汗者，停后服。汗多亡阳，遂虚，恶风烦躁，不得眠也。

现代用法：水煎服。

[功效] 发汗解表，清热除烦。

[主治] 外感风寒，发热恶寒，寒热俱重，脉浮紧，身疼痛，不汗出而烦躁者。

[方解]

脉浮而紧，浮则为风，紧则为寒，风则伤卫，寒则伤营，营卫俱病，故发热恶寒，寒热俱重，身体疼痛。本方是麻黄汤加重麻黄、甘草，减少杏仁，再加石膏、生姜、大枣所组成。方中重用麻黄，以增强发汗解表作用，故为君药；桂枝助麻黄发汗解表，为臣药；杏仁开泄肺气，佐麻、桂发汗解表，生姜、大枣调营卫而行津液，症见烦躁，故又于大队发汗解表药中配伍石膏辛甘大寒，清热除烦，又能制约大量麻、桂之辛温，使发汗解表而不助里热，以上均为佐药；使以甘草，调和诸药，且制麻、桂峻烈之性，防其汗出太过，又甘草得石膏，甘寒生津，更能除烦。诸药合而成方，俾汗出而邪热皆清，诸症自解。

[临床运用]

王旭高[7]说"发热恶寒，无汗烦躁八字，是大青龙着眼"，说明必须见有发热恶寒无汗的表寒证，并兼见烦躁的里热证，始可运用本方。若服后汗出表解烦除，即停后服。

小青龙汤《伤寒论》

[组成] 麻黄去节，三两（9克） 芍药三两（9克） 五味子半升（9克） 干姜三两（9克） 甘草三两，炙（9克） 桂枝三两，去皮（9克） 半夏半升，汤洗（9克） 细辛三两（9克）

[用法] 原方八味，以水一斗，先煮麻黄，减二升，去上沫，内诸药，煮取三升，去滓，温服一升。

现代用法：水煎服。

[功效] 解表散寒，温肺化饮。

[主治] 外感风寒，内停水饮，恶寒发热无汗，咳嗽喘息，痰多而稀，干呕不渴，苔白润滑，脉浮。或溢饮四肢浮肿，身体疼重者。

[方解]

风寒束表，毛窍闭塞，故恶寒发热无汗。方中麻黄发汗解表，宣肺平喘，为君药；桂枝助麻黄发汗解表，为臣药；半夏燥湿化痰，蠲饮降逆，干姜温脾肺之阳，散水寒之饮，细辛外可辛散风寒，内以温肺化饮，然干姜、细辛辛温大热，耗散肺气，故又用五味子收敛津气，以防肺气耗散太过，且五味子得干姜、细辛，有收有散，善于温肺止咳，芍药益阴养血，以上均为佐药；使以炙甘草调和诸药，得芍药酸甘化阴，以防麻、桂发汗太过，耗气伤阴。药共八味，配伍严谨，共奏解表散寒，温肺化饮之效。名小青龙者，谓其不若大青龙之兴云致雨也。

[临床运用]

本方为外寒内饮之证而设。若外寒已解而内饮未除，当改用温药和之之法，可投苓桂术甘汤之类以善其后。不宜久服小青龙汤，以免耗伤肺气，虚其虚也。

葱豉汤《肘后备急方》[8]

[组成]　葱白一虎口（5条）　豉一升（15克）

[用法]　原方以水三升，煮取一升，顿服取汗。不汗，复更作，加葛根二两、升麻三两，五升水，煎取二升，分再服，必得汗。若不汗，更加麻黄二两，又用葱汤研米二合，水一升煮之，少时下盐豉，后纳葱白四物，令火煎取三升，分服取汗也。

现代用法：水煎服。

[功效]　发汗散寒。

[主治]　外感风寒轻证，微恶风寒，或发微热，头痛无汗，鼻塞流涕，喷嚏，舌苔薄白，脉浮。

[方解]

此为外感风寒之轻证，故寒热不甚。方中葱白辛温，疏散表邪，通阳发汗，为君药；淡豆豉辛甘微温，发汗解表，为辅佐药。葱豉配伍，具有发汗散寒之效，乃轻可去实之剂也。

[临床运用]

本方药性平和，虽辛温而不燥，虽发散而不烈，无过汗伤津之弊，深为历代医家所重视。

香苏散《太平惠民和剂局方》[9]

[组成]　香附炒香，去毛　紫苏叶各四两（各120克）　陈皮二两，不去白（60克）甘草炙，一两（30克）

[用法]　原方为粗末，每服三钱，水一盏，煎七分，去滓，热服，不拘

时候，日三服。若作细末，只服二钱，入盐点服。

现代用法：为末，每次服 6 克，每日二三次。亦可水煎服，用量按原方比例酌减。

［功效］ 疏散风寒，理气和中。

［主治］ 外感风寒，内有气滞，形寒身热，头痛无汗，胸脘痞闷，不思饮食，舌苔薄白，脉浮。

［方解］

本方证乃因风寒客表，肝胃气滞所致。方中香附理气解郁，且能外达肌肤，解除表邪，苏叶疏散风寒，兼能理气和中，二味共为君药；陈皮理气和中，为辅佐药；炙甘草调和诸药，以为使。四药合用，外散肌表之风寒，内理肝胃之气滞，共奏疏散风寒、理气和中之效。

［临床运用］

本方适用于外感风寒，内有气滞之证，亦可用于素患肝气郁滞，脘胁胀痛而兼外感风寒者。临床多用于女性患者。

香薷散《太平惠民和剂局方》

［组成］ 香薷去土，一斤（500克） 白扁豆微炒 厚朴去粗皮，姜汁炙熟，各半斤（各250克）

［用法］ 原方为粗末，每三钱，水一盏，入酒一分，煎七分，去滓，水中沉冷，连吃二服，立有神效，随病不拘时。

现代用法：水煎待冷服，用量按原方比例酌减。

［功效］ 解表散寒，化湿和中。

［主治］ 夏月乘凉饮冷，外感于寒，内伤于湿，恶寒发热，头重头痛，无汗，胸闷，或四肢倦怠，腹痛吐泻，舌苔白腻者。

［方解］

暑月乘凉露卧，则外感于寒，邪在肌表。方中重用香薷辛温发散，解表散寒，化湿和脾，李时珍说"香薷乃夏月解表之药，犹冬月之用麻黄"，故为君药；厚朴苦辛温，化湿和中，为臣药；扁豆甘平，健脾化湿，为佐药；酒能温行血脉，以散寒湿，为使药。诸药配伍，对于外则表气不宣，内则脾胃不和者，实擅表里双解之功。

[临床运用]

本方即后世所称的三物香薷饮，既能散寒邪以解表，又能化湿滞而和胃，故常用于暑月乘凉饮冷，感受寒湿者。

第二节 辛凉解表

辛凉解表剂，适用于外感风热的表证。症见发热，微恶风寒，头痛，口渴，咽痛，舌尖红，苔薄白或薄黄，脉浮数等。盖辛以解表，凉以清热，故常用辛凉解表药如薄荷、牛蒡子、桑叶、菊花、连翘等为主组成方剂。根据病情的需要，亦有将辛温解表药与寒凉药配伍成为辛凉解表剂者，但方中辛温药决不能超过辛凉药的剂量。辛凉解表的代表方剂有银翘散、桑菊饮、麻黄杏仁石膏甘草汤等。

银翘散《温病条辨》[10]

[组成] 连翘一两（30克） 银花一两（30克） 苦桔梗六钱（18克） 薄荷六钱（18克） 竹叶四钱（12克） 生甘草五钱（15克） 荆芥穗四钱（12克） 淡豆豉五钱（15克） 牛蒡子六钱（18克）

[用法] 原方杵为散，每服六钱，鲜苇根汤煎，香气大出，即取服，勿过煎。肺药取轻清，过煎则味厚而入中焦矣。病重者，约二时一服，日三服，夜一服；轻者三时一服，日二服，夜一服；病不解者，作再服。

现代用法：加芦根适量，水煎服，用量按原方比例酌情增减。

[功效] 辛凉透表，清热解毒。

[主治] 温病初起，发热，微恶风寒，无汗或有汗不畅，头痛口渴，咳嗽咽痛，舌尖红，苔薄白或薄黄，脉浮数者。

[方解]

"温邪上受，首先犯肺""肺主气属卫"，外合皮毛，主一身之表。方中重用银花甘寒芳香，清热解毒，辟秽祛浊，连翘苦寒，清热解毒，轻宣透表，共为君药；薄荷辛凉，发汗解肌，除风热而清头目，荆芥、淡豆豉虽属辛温之品，但温而不燥，与薄荷相配，辛散表邪，共为臣药；牛蒡子、桔梗、甘草宣肺祛痰，解毒利咽，竹叶、芦根甘寒轻清，透热生津，均为佐药；甘草并能调和诸药，以为使。上药合而成方，共奏清热毒、散风热之效。

[临床运用]

1.《温病条辨》称本方为"辛凉平剂"，适用于温病初起，外感风热表证。

2.据编者临床体会，外感风热表证用本方治疗发热已退而余邪未尽，有咳嗽者，可用桑菊饮以善其后。

桑菊饮《温病条辨》

[组成] 杏仁二钱（6克） 连翘一钱五分（4.5克） 薄荷八分（2.4克） 桑叶二钱五分（7.5克） 菊花一钱（3克） 苦桔梗二钱（6克） 甘草八分（2.4克） 苇根二钱（6克）

[用法] 原方水二杯，煮取一杯，日二服。

现代用法：水煎服。

[功效] 疏散风热，宣肺止咳。

[主治] 太阴风温，但咳，身不甚热，微渴者。

[方解]

本方证乃风温之邪入侵手太阴肺经所致。方中桑叶、菊花甘苦微寒，疏散上焦风热，为君药；薄荷辛凉解表，助桑、菊疏风散热，从皮毛而解，杏仁、桔梗升降肺气，宣肺止咳，兼有解表作用，共为臣药；连翘苦寒，清热透表，芦根甘寒，清热生津，为佐药；甘草配桔梗，清利咽喉，且能调和诸药，以为使。诸药配伍，使上焦风热得以疏散，肺气得以宣畅，则邪去而咳止。

[临床运用]

1.《温病条辨》称本方为"辛凉轻剂"，适用于风温犯肺，以咳嗽为主要症状者。

2.据编者临床体会，若风温咳嗽，咳痰不爽者，可以本方加瓜蒌皮、浙贝母清化痰热。

麻黄杏仁石膏甘草汤《伤寒论》

[组成] 麻黄四两，去节（12克） 杏仁五十枚，去皮尖（9克） 甘草二两，炙（6克） 石膏半斤，碎，绵裹（24克）

[用法] 原方四味，以水七升，先煮麻黄，减二升，去上沫，内诸药，煮取二升，去滓，温服一升。

现代用法：水煎服。

[功效] 辛凉宣泄，清肺平喘。

[主治] 外感风邪，身热不解，有汗或无汗，咳逆气急，甚则鼻煽，口渴，舌质红，苔薄白或黄，脉浮滑而数者。

[方解]

本方证系表邪化热，壅遏于肺所致。方中麻黄辛苦温，宣肺平喘，李时珍说"麻黄乃肺经专药，虽为太阳发散之重剂，实发散肺经火郁之药也"；大量石膏辛甘大寒，清泄肺热，麻黄配石膏则为辛凉解热之剂，目的在于发泄郁热，故共为君药。杏仁苦温，得麻黄一升一降，宣畅肺气，止咳平喘，为辅佐药。甘草调和诸药以保胃气，使石膏大寒而不致伤胃，且甘草得石膏又能甘寒生津。因"汗出而喘"，肺热伤津故也，为使药。药仅四味，配伍严谨，共奏辛凉宣泄、清肺平喘之效。

[临床运用]

本方为宣肺泄热的主要方剂，以发热、喘急、苔黄、脉数为辨证要点，不论有汗无汗，均可运用。若汗出而喘，则为热壅于肺，皮毛开泄，原方石膏的用量为麻黄的一倍，但据临床实践证明，石膏的用量可五倍于麻黄，甚至十倍于麻黄。若无汗而喘，则为热闭于肺，皮毛亦闭，需加大麻黄用量，但麻黄用量仍当小于石膏。且此时用麻黄发表宣肺，是为郁热打开出路；用石膏清肺泄热，是为邪热杜绝来源。辛寒药量大于辛温药量，仍不失为辛凉之剂。

第三节 扶正解表

扶正解表剂，适用于体质素虚而又感受外邪，出现表证者。此时，扶正是为了解表，而不是单纯为了补虚。因为人体之所以能祛邪外出全凭正气，故正虚而有表证，必须扶正才能达到解表的目的。若单纯发汗，则势必伤阳气耗阴血，甚则有大汗亡阳之虞，可不慎乎！

正虚包括阳、气、阴、血之虚，故又有助阳（益气）解表与滋阴（养血）解表之不同。助阳（益气）解表法是为外感表证兼有阳气不足者而设，常用温阳益气药物如人参、附子等与解表药物如麻黄、细辛、羌活等同用，败毒散、麻黄附子细辛汤即其代表方。滋阴（养血）解表法是为外感表证兼有阴血不足者而设，常用滋阴养血药物如玉竹、麦冬等与解表药物如葱白、淡豆豉、薄荷等同用，加减葳蕤汤即其代表方。

败毒散（又名人参败毒散）《小儿药证直诀》[11]

[组成] 柴胡洗，去芦　前胡　川芎　枳壳　羌活　独活　茯苓　桔梗　人参各一两（3克）　甘草半两（1.5克）

[用法] 原方为粗末，每服二钱，水一盏，入生姜、薄荷各少许，同煎七分，去滓，不拘时候，寒多则热服，热多则温服。

现代用法：加生姜、薄荷各少许，水煎服。用量按原方比例酌减。

[功效] 益气解表，散风除湿。

[主治] 正气不足，外感风寒湿邪，恶寒壮热，头痛项强，肢体烦疼，无汗，鼻塞声重，咳嗽有痰，舌苔白腻，脉浮重按无力者。

[方解]

素体气虚，风寒湿邪客于肌表。方中羌活、独活辛苦而温，表散风寒，除湿止痛，共为君药；柴胡苦平，散热升清，川芎辛温，祛风止痛，以助二活发表止痛，为臣药；枳壳、桔梗一升一降，宽胸利气，前胡、茯苓宣肺化痰，生姜、薄荷辛散发表，尤妙在配伍人参扶正祛邪，俾气旺自能鼓邪外出，以上均为佐药；甘草和中健脾，调和诸药，是为使。本方有人参扶正祛邪，诸药配伍，疏导经络，表散邪滞，故方以"人参败毒"名之。

[临床运用]

1. 本方适用于气虚而外感风寒湿邪者。人参在本方中是为佐药，少用人参益气，可鼓邪外出，若用量过多，反而助湿，不利于祛邪。

2. 本方亦可治下痢初起而有风寒湿表证者。喻嘉言[12]认为痢疾初起之有表证，乃邪从表而陷里，以本方疏解表邪，表气疏通，里滞亦除，其痢自愈。邪从外入者，仍从外出，使其由里而出表，此即称为"逆流挽舟"之法。

麻黄附子细辛汤《伤寒论》

[组成] 麻黄二两，去节（6克） 细辛二两（6克） 附子一枚，炮，去皮，破八片（9克）

[用法] 原方三味，以水一斗，先煮麻黄，减二升，去上沫，内诸药，煮取三升，去滓，温服一升，日三服。

现代用法：水煎服。

[功效] 助阳解表。

[主治] 少阴证，始得之，反发热，脉沉者。

[方解]

少阴病本为阳气虚寒证，不应发热，其主症当为"脉微细，但欲寐"。今少阴病始得之而反发热，可知兼有太阳表证。太阳表证，当从汗解；少阴阳虚，又当温阳。方中麻黄散太阳之寒，发汗解表，附子温少阴之经，固护元阳，二味共为君药；细辛外解太阳之表，内散少阴之寒，既助麻黄发汗解表，又助附子温经散寒，为辅佐药。三药合用，俾太阳之风寒得以解散，少阴之元阳得以固护，真有制之师也。

[临床运用]

1. 本方主治，既有阳虚之本，又有感寒之标，是标本兼治之剂。临床以恶寒甚，发热轻，无汗，脉沉，舌苔白润为辨证要点。

2. 本方证虽属阳虚外感，但阳虚的程度并不太重，故可用助阳解表之法。若少阴阳气衰微，已见下利清谷，脉微欲绝等证，当急投四逆辈回阳救逆。若误发其汗，必致厥逆亡阳，应加留意。

加减葳蕤汤《重订通俗伤寒论》[13]

[组成] 生葳蕤二～三钱（6～9克） 生葱白二～三枚（2～3条） 桔梗一钱～一钱半（3～4.5克） 东白薇五分～一钱（1.5～3克） 淡豆豉三～四钱（9～12克） 苏薄荷一钱～钱半（3～4.5克） 炙甘草五分（1.5克） 红枣二枚（2枚）

[**用法**] 原书未著用法。

现代用法：水煎服。

[**功效**] 滋阴解表。

[**主治**] 素体阴虚，感受外邪，头痛身热，微恶风寒，无汗或有汗不多，咳嗽咽干，口渴心烦，舌红脉数。

[**方解**]

素体阴虚，感受外邪，易于化热。阴虚之体，汗源不充，感受外邪，不能作汗达邪。此时宜滋其液以充汗源，发其汗以解表邪。方中生葳蕤即生玉竹，滋阴润燥生津，为清补之品，《本草纲目》[14]谓其"主风温自汗灼热"，故为君药；臣以葱白、淡豆豉、薄荷疏散外邪；佐以白薇清热益阴，桔梗利咽止咳；使以炙甘草、红枣甘润增液，并能调和诸药。诸药配伍，可使发汗而不伤阴，滋阴而不留邪。

[**临床运用**]

本方由《小品方》[15]葳蕤汤（葳蕤、白薇、麻黄、独活、杏仁、川芎、甘草、青木香、石膏）加减而来，为素体阴虚，感受风邪者而设。大凡表证未解不宜使用滋阴之品，以免留邪。但阴虚之体复感外邪，若单纯发汗，不仅表邪不为汗解，反有劫液耗阴之弊，故唯有滋阴与解表同用，方是两全之法。

第二章

涌吐剂

根据《素问·阴阳应象大论》[16]"其高者，因而越之"的原则立法，凡以涌吐药物为主组成，具有涌吐作用，使停蓄在咽喉、胸膈、胃脘之间的痰涎、宿食、毒物等有形实邪上涌，从吐而出的方剂，统称涌吐剂，属于"八法"中的"吐法"。在"十剂"中属于"宣可去壅"的范畴。

本类方剂常以瓜蒂、白矾、食盐等涌吐药物为主组成，代表方有瓜蒂散、盐汤探吐方等。

瓜蒂散《伤寒论》

[组成] 瓜蒂一分，熬黄（1克） 赤小豆一分（1克）

[用法] 原方二味，各别捣筛，为散已，合治之，取一钱匕，以香豉一合，用热汤七合，煮作稀糜，去滓，取汁和散，温顿服之，不吐者，少少加，得快吐乃止。

现代用法：将瓜蒂、赤小豆分别研细末和匀，每服1～3克，用淡豆豉12克煎汤取汁，调药末送服。如急欲催吐，服药后可用洁净翎毛或压舌板探喉取吐。

[功效] 涌吐痰食。

[主治] 痰涎宿食，填塞胸脘，胸中痞硬，气上冲咽喉不得息，或手足厥冷，心下满而烦，欲吐不得出者。

[方解]

痰涎壅塞胸中，或宿食停于上脘。《素问·阴阳应象大论》说："其高者，因而越之。"病在胸脘，既非汗下所能及，又非消导所可行，唯当因势利导，使实邪从吐而解。方中瓜蒂苦寒有小毒，能涌吐痰涎宿食，为君药；赤小豆酸平，与瓜蒂相须为用，酸苦涌泄，善吐胸脘实邪，为臣药；香豉轻浮上行，以助瓜蒂宣越胸中陈腐浊邪，使其涌而出之，为佐使药。三药合用，涌吐痰涎宿食，宣越胸中陈腐之邪就近从上而解。如此则上焦得通，阳气得复，痞硬可消，胸中可和。若服之不吐，可"少少加，得快吐乃止"，唯恐伤气耗液也。

[临床运用]

本方乃涌吐剂之祖方。方中瓜蒂系生采之甜瓜蒂，入药以新而味苦者为佳，陈久者少效。若无甜瓜蒂，可以丝瓜蒂代之。

盐汤探吐方《金匮要略》[17]

[组成]　盐一升（适量）　水三升（适量）

[用法]　原方二味，煮令盐消，分三服，当吐出食，便差。

现代用法：将盐用沸水调成饱和盐汤，每服200毫升左右，服后用洁净翎毛或手指探喉助吐，以吐尽宿食为度。若服后不吐，可再进热盐汤探吐，务使得吐乃佳。

[功效]　涌吐宿食。

[主治]　宿食不消，心腹坚满疼痛。亦疗干霍乱，欲吐不得吐，欲泻不得泻，腹中绞痛，烦满不舒者。

[方解]

饮食不节，以致宿食停于胃脘，阻遏气机。《素问·至真要大论》说："咸味涌泄为阴。"本方以盐汤探吐，全在取其极咸之味，激起呕吐，《本经》即有"大盐令人吐"的记载。但盐汤涌吐之力较弱，故服后往往需用翎毛或手指、压舌板等探吐，以助药力，从而使不化之食从上涌而出之，则塞者可通，诸症可愈。

[临床运用]

本方药性平和，运用方便，收效迅速，为催吐常用方剂。

第三章

泻下剂

根据"其下者，引而竭之；中满者，泻之于内""其实者，散而泻之"（《素问·阴阳应象大论》）的原则立法，凡以泻利攻逐药物为主组成，具有通导大便，排除胃肠积滞，荡涤实热，攻逐水饮、寒积等作用，以治疗里实证的方剂，统称泻下剂，亦称攻里剂。属于"八法"中的"下法"。

第一节　寒　下

寒下剂，适用于里热积滞实证。症见大便秘结，腹部胀满疼痛，甚或潮热，苔黄、脉实等。本法以攻下积滞，荡涤邪热为目的，常用寒下药物如大黄、芒硝、芦荟等为主组成方剂。如燥屎宿食与实热结于胃肠，腑气不通，可与行气药如厚朴、枳实等配伍，以利于推荡宿食积热，代表方有大承气汤；如湿热瘀结肠间而为肠痈，可与利湿散瘀药如薏苡仁、冬瓜子、桃仁、牡丹皮等配伍，代表方有大黄牡丹汤；如肠胃燥热，心肝火旺，又可配合朱砂清心泻火，代表方有更衣丸。

大承气汤《伤寒论》

[组成]　大黄四两（12克）　厚朴半斤，去皮，炙（15克）　枳实五枚，炙（12克）　芒硝三合（9克）

[用法]　原方四味，以水一斗，先煮二物，取五升，去滓，内大黄，煮取二升，去滓，内芒硝，更上微火一二沸，分温再服。得下，余勿服。

现代用法：先用水煎厚朴、枳实，后入大黄，芒硝冲服。

[功效]　峻下热结。

[主治]

1.阳明腑实证，不恶寒，反恶热，日晡潮热，谵语神昏，矢气频转，大便不通，手足濈然汗出，腹满痛，按之硬，或目中不了了，睛不和，舌苔焦黄起刺，或焦黑燥裂，脉沉实。

2.热结旁流，下利清水，其气臭秽，脐腹疼痛，按之坚硬有块，口燥咽干，脉滑而数。

3.热厥、痉病、发狂之属于阳明腑实里热者。

[方解]

本方主治之症，前人归纳为"痞、满、燥、实"四字。"痞"作痞闷闭塞解，自觉脘腹胀满，此为肠胃气结，升降失常所致；"满"是脘腹胀满，按之有抵抗感，此为肠中宿食停滞，气机不得通畅所致；"燥"指热淫于内，消铄津液，肠中粪便既燥且坚，此时手按患者腹部有坚硬之块，即燥屎也；"实"乃指宿食积滞与热邪搏结于肠中，不得下行，而见便秘，腹满痛，或下利稀水臭秽而腹满不减。方中大黄苦寒，泻热通便，荡涤肠胃，为君药；臣以芒硝咸寒泻热，软坚润燥，与大黄相须为用，泻下热结之功颇大；积滞内阻，每致气滞不行，故又佐以枳实消痞，厚朴除满，下气推荡以助硝、黄攻下结热。四药合而成方，具有峻下热结之功。六腑以通为用，胃气以下降为顺。本方峻下热结，承顺胃气之下行，使塞者通，闭者畅，故方以"承气"名之。

[临床运用]

本方主治之症，必须具备痞、满、燥、实四症，才能运用本方。若误用本方损伤里气，恐有寒中、结胸、痞气等变端，应加注意。

大黄牡丹汤《金匮要略》

[组成]　大黄四两（12克）　牡丹皮一两（9克）　桃仁五十枚（9克）　冬瓜子半升（15克）　芒硝三合（9克）

[用法]　原方五味，以水六升，煮取一升，去滓，内芒硝，再煎沸，顿服之。

现代用法：水煎服前四味，芒硝冲服。

[功效] 泻热破瘀，散结消痈。

[主治] 肠痈初起，右少腹疼痛拒按，甚则局部肿痞，小便自调，时时发热，自汗出，复恶寒，或右足屈而不伸，舌苔薄腻而黄，其脉迟紧有力。

[方解]

肠痈是指肠内产生痈肿而出现右少腹部疼痛的一类疾患。方中大黄苦寒，泻热逐瘀，荡涤肠中热毒瘀滞，《本经》谓其"主下瘀血……荡涤肠胃，推陈致新"，牡丹皮辛苦微寒，清热凉血散瘀，《本经》谓其"除癥坚瘀血留舍肠胃"，二味共为君药；芒硝咸苦大寒，泻热导滞，软坚散结，助大黄荡涤肠胃，推陈致新，桃仁苦甘平，性善破血，助牡丹活血散瘀，且有润肠通便之功，二味共为臣药；冬瓜子甘寒，排脓散结，为治内痈要药，《本草纲目》记载"治肠痈"，故为佐药。诸药合用，使湿热瘀结荡涤消除，则热结通而痈自散，血行畅而痛自消，符合《素问·阴阳应象大论》"其下者引而竭之""其实者散而泻之"之旨。

[临床运用]

肠痈有湿热瘀滞与寒湿瘀滞之不同，本方只宜用于湿热瘀滞者。

更衣丸《先醒斋医学广笔记》[18]

[组成] 朱砂研如飞面，五钱（15克） 真芦荟研细，七钱（21克）

[用法] 原方滴好酒少许和丸，每服一钱二分，好酒吞，朝服暮通，暮服朝通，须天晴时修合为妙。

现代用法：黄酒和丸，每服4.5～6克，温开水送下。

[功效] 泻火通便。

[主治] 肠胃燥结，大便不通，或见心烦易怒，睡眠不安。

[方解]

大肠为传导之官，若肠胃燥热，耗伤津液，则大便干结不通。心烦易怒，睡眠不安，乃心肝火旺也。方中重用芦荟苦寒，入肝、胃、大肠经，泻火通便，清热凉肝，为君药；朱砂甘寒，泻心经邪热，重坠下达，为臣药；因芦荟气味秽恶，故用好酒少许辟秽和胃，为佐使药。诸药合用，以奏泻火通便之效。

[临床运用]

本方善治肠胃燥结，大便不通。对于心肝火旺所致的便秘，不宜用仁类润药者，本方颇为适合。

第二节 温 下

温下剂，适用于脏腑间有寒冷积滞之病，温以散寒，下以除积也。冷积的产生，多由素体阳虚内寒，复加饮食积滞而成。此证往往舌苔白滑，或舌根有厚腻苔。常用泻下药如大黄、巴豆配合温热药如附子、干姜、炙甘草等组成方剂。苦寒泻下药配入大队温热药中，则制其苦寒之性，而奏温下之功。代表方有温脾汤。至于暴病邪盛，寒滞食积，阻于肠胃，气机壅塞者，又当猛攻峻逐，如三物备急丸。

温脾汤《备急千金要方》

[组成] 大黄四两（12克） 附子大者一枚（9枚） 干姜 人参 甘草各二两（各6克）

[用法] 原方五味，㕮咀，以水八升，煮取二升半，分三服，临熟下大黄。

现代用法：水煎服，大黄后下。

[功效] 温补脾阳，攻下冷积。

[主治] 冷积便秘，或久利赤白，腹痛，手足不温，脉沉弦。

[方解]

脾阳不足，积滞内停。若单纯温补脾阳，则积滞不去；贸然予以攻下，又更伤中阳，故必须温补脾阳与攻下冷积并用。方中附子温补脾阳以散寒凝，大黄荡涤泻下而除积滞，共为君药；干姜、人参、甘草协助附子温补脾阳，为辅佐药；甘草并能调药和中，又为使药。诸药合用，共成温脾攻下之剂。

[临床运用]

本方为脾阳虚寒冷积不化所致的便秘或久利赤白而设。如腹痛较甚，可加肉桂、厚朴、木香以增强温中行气止痛之功；兼见呕吐，可加制半夏、砂仁以和胃降逆；如积滞较轻，可减少大黄剂量。

三物备急丸《金匮要略》

[组成] 大黄一两（3克） 干姜一两（3克） 巴豆一两，去皮、心，熬，外研如脂（3克）

[用法] 原方各须精新，先捣大黄、干姜为末，研巴豆内中，合治一千杵，用为散，蜜和丸亦佳，密器中贮之，莫令歇……以暖水若酒服大豆许三四丸，或不下，捧头起，灌令下咽，须臾当差；如未差，更与三丸，当腹中鸣，即吐下便差；若口噤，亦须折齿灌之。

现代用法：上药共为散，每服0.3～1.5克，温开水送下。若口噤不开，可用鼻饲法给药。

[功效] 攻逐寒积。

[主治] 寒凝食积，卒然心腹胀痛，痛如锥刺，气急口噤，暴厥者。

[方解]

寒凝食积阻于肠胃，气机痞塞。方中巴豆辛热，有大毒，入胃、大肠经，峻下去积，开通闭塞，为君药；干姜辛热，温中散结，助巴豆以祛寒，为臣药；大黄苦寒，荡涤肠胃，推陈致新，且能监制巴豆辛热之毒，为佐使药。三药配合，力猛效捷，以备暴急寒实之证而用，故方名三物备急丸。

[临床运用]

本方多用治饮食不调，食停肠胃，以致上焦不行，下脘不通，为卒起暴急寒实之病。当此之时，非急投本方，不能获效。

第三节 润　下

润下剂是滑润肠道，治疗便秘的方剂，适用于体虚便秘之症，其泻下之力较为和缓。如因于邪热伤津，或素体火盛，肠胃干燥，以致大便秘结者，其治疗方法，宜滋润与泻热通便相结合，润其燥而泻其热。常用滋润药物如麻子仁、杏仁、芍药等与泻下药物如大黄等组成方剂，代表方有麻子仁丸。如津伤肠燥而无火者，又当以五仁丸主之。

麻子仁丸（又名脾约麻仁丸）《伤寒论》

[组成] 麻子仁二升（500克） 芍药半斤（250克） 枳实半斤，炙（250克） 大黄一斤，去皮（500克） 厚朴一尺，炙，去皮（250克） 杏仁一升，去皮、尖，熬，别作脂（250克）

[用法] 原方六味，蜜和丸，如梧桐子大，饮服十丸，日三服。渐加，以知为度。

现代用法：上药为末，炼蜜为丸，每次服9克，每日1～2次，温开水送服。

[功效] 润肠通便，清热缓下。

[主治] 肠胃燥热，津液不足。大便干结，小便频数。

[方解]

本方证为肠胃燥热，脾约便秘。方中重用麻子仁甘平，润肠通便，《汤液本草》谓其"入足太阴、手阳明……《内经》谓'燥者润之'，故仲景以麻仁润足太阴之燥及通肠也"，故为君药；杏仁降气润肠，芍药养阴和里，为臣药；佐以枳实破结，厚朴除满，大黄清热通便；使以蜂蜜润燥滑肠，调和诸药。合而为丸，具有润肠通便，清热缓下之功。

[临床运用]

本方原治脾约之证，脾约证的辨证要点为小便数，大便难，舌苔黄。本方润肠药与泻下药同用，润而不腻，泻而不峻，而且原方只服桐子大十丸，渐加，以知为度，都说明本方意在缓下。

第四节 逐 水

逐水剂，适用于水饮停聚于胸腹及水肿而属体质强壮者，是用攻逐的方法使体内积水从大小便排出，以达到消除积水肿胀的目的。逐水法只能用治实证而正气未虚者，是急则治标之法。《素问·标本病传论》说："先病而后生中满者，治其标；小大不利，治其标。"故不能久用或过用逐水之剂，恐攻下伤正，逐水伤阴。本类方剂多有毒性，泻下作用峻烈，常用峻下逐水药如芫花、甘遂、大戟、牵牛子等为主组成方剂，代表方有十枣汤、舟车丸等。

十枣汤《伤寒论》

[组成] 芫花熬 甘遂 大戟各等分 大枣十枚

[用法] 原方三味等分，各别捣为散。以水一升半，先煮大枣肥者十枚，取八合，去滓，内药末。强人服一钱匕，羸人服半钱，温服之，平旦服。若下少，病不除者，明日更服，加半钱，得快下利后，糜粥自养。

现代用法：上三味等分为末，或以胶囊贮之，以大枣十枚煎汤，调服药末1.5～3克，每日一次，清晨空腹服。

[功效] 攻逐水饮。

[主治]

1. 悬饮，胁下有水气，以致咳唾胸胁引痛，心下痞硬，干呕短气，头痛目眩，或胸背掣痛不得息，舌苔滑，脉沉弦者。

2. 水肿腹胀，属于实证者，亦可用之。

[方解]

两胁为阴阳气机升降之道路，水停胸胁，络道被阻，升降失常，故咳嗽痰唾，胸胁牵引作痛，而成悬饮。本方为峻下逐水之剂。方中芫花辛温有毒，善消胸胁之水，《本草纲目》谓其"治水饮痰癖，胁下痛"，故为君药；甘遂苦寒有毒，善行经隧水湿，大戟苦寒有毒，善泻六腑之水，为辅佐药；《本草纲目》说："芫花、大戟、甘遂之性，逐水泄湿，能直达水饮窠囊隐僻之处，但可徐徐用之，取效甚捷，不可过剂，泄人真元也。"故又用大枣肥者十枚，取其益气扶正，培土制水，能缓和诸峻药之毒，使下不伤正，为使药。《医方论》[19]说："仲景以十枣命名，全赖大枣之甘缓以救脾胃，方成节制之师也。"故以十枣名汤，寓有深意。

[临床运用]

《丹溪心法》[20]将本方煮枣肉捣和为丸，名十枣丸。治水气，四肢浮肿，上气喘急，大小便不利者。改汤为丸，这在服用时较为方便，是"治之以峻，行之以缓"之法。

舟车丸《证治准绳》[21]引刘河间[22]方

[组成] 甘遂 芫花 大戟各一两，俱醋炒（各30克） 大黄二两（60克） 黑

牵牛研末，四两（120克） 青皮　陈皮　木香　槟榔各半两（各15克） 轻粉一钱
（3克）

[**用法**]　原方为末，水丸，空心服，初服五丸，日三服，加至快利后却
常服，以病去为度。

现代用法：研末，水泛为丸，每服3～6克，日服一次，清晨空腹温开水
送下。

[**功效**]　逐水行气。

[**主治**]　水肿水胀，形气俱实，口渴气粗，腹胀而坚，大小便秘，脉沉
数有力者。

[**方解**]

水湿之邪郁久化热，壅于脘腹经隧，肠胃气机受阻。方中重用黑丑，苦
寒有毒，通利二便，逐水退肿，为君药；大黄荡涤泻下，甘遂、大戟、芫花逐
水消肿，共为臣药；浊水停聚，每致气机升降失司，故以青皮破气散结，陈皮
理气燥湿，木香、槟榔疏利三焦之气，使气行则水行，又入少量轻粉，即水
银粉，辛寒大毒，取其走而不守，逐水通便。以上均为佐药。诸药合用，共
奏峻下逐水，行气破滞之功，使水热壅实之邪从二便排出，犹如顺流之舟，
下坡之车，顺势而下，故方以"舟车"名之。

[**临床运用**]

本方攻逐之力甚强，适用于阳水形气俱实者，故又名净腑丸。现多用治
肝硬化腹水，脉证俱实，正气尚可支持者。如肿势虽盛而体质虚弱，不可使
用。并忌与甘草同用。孕妇忌服本方。

第五节　攻补兼施

攻补兼施剂，适用于里实积结而正气内虚者。由于邪实正虚，若单纯攻
邪则正气不支，单纯补正又实邪愈壅，故宜泻下与补益并用，祛邪而又扶正，
方为两全之计。同时，正虚邪实之体，有时虽用峻剂攻逐，因正气大虚，无
力驱邪外出，燥屎终不能下，反更耗气伤阴，或实邪虽去，却造成正随邪脱
的危险。因此，将泻下药与补益药同用，是治疗里实积滞而正气内虚的妥善

方法。常用泻下药如大黄、芒硝与补益药如人参、当归、地黄、玄参等组成方剂，代表方有黄龙汤、增液承气汤。

黄龙汤《伤寒六书》[23]

[组成] 大黄（9克） 芒硝（9克） 枳实（6克） 厚朴（6克） 甘草（3克） 人参（6克） 当归（9克）[原书未著分量]

[用法] 原方以水二盏，姜三片，枣二枚，煎之后，再入桔梗一撮，热沸为度。

现代用法：上药加桔梗3克、生姜3片、大枣2枚，水煎服。

[功效] 扶正攻下。

[主治] 里热腑实而气血虚弱者。或因热病当下失下，心下硬痛，身热口渴，谵语，下利纯清水；或素体气血亏损，患阳明腑实之证；或因误治致虚，而腑实犹存，症见神倦少气，便秘，腹胀满硬痛，甚则循衣摸床，撮空理线，神昏肢厥，舌苔焦黄或焦黑，脉虚。

[方解]

本方原治热结旁流而兼气血两虚之证。若素体气血亏损，患阳明腑实之证，或因误治致虚，而腑实犹存，正虚甚则不能胜邪，犹当勉为图治。本方系大承气汤加人参、当归、甘草、桔梗、生姜、大枣而成。方中大黄、芒硝、枳实、厚朴泻热攻下，荡涤肠胃实热积滞，人参、当归双补气血，扶正以利于祛邪，使之下不伤正，为方中主要部分；佐以少量桔梗，开提肺气，疏通肠胃，欲降而先升；使以甘草、姜、枣扶其胃气，调和诸药，共成扶正攻下之剂。

[临床运用]

本方主治阳明腑实而气血两虚者。不攻则不能去其实，不补则无以救其虚，使用本方，较为合适。

增液承气汤《温病条辨》

[组成] 玄参一两（30克） 麦冬连心，八钱（24克） 细生地八钱（24克） 大黄三钱（9克） 芒硝一钱五分（4.5克）

[**用法**]　原方水八杯，煮取三杯，先服一杯，不知，再服。

现代用法：水煎，分三服，得下，余勿服。

[**功效**]　滋阴增液，通便泄热。

[**主治**]　阳明温病，热结阴亏，燥屎不行，下之不通者。

[**方解**]

温邪最易伤津耗液，阳明热结而津液枯燥，液愈亏而热愈炽，肠愈燥而液愈耗。方中重用玄参、生地、麦冬，甘凉濡润，滋阴增液，润肠通便；配合大黄、芒硝软坚润燥，泻热攻下，而成攻补兼施之剂。以图阴液来复，热结得下，则邪祛而正复。本方系增液汤合调胃承气汤去甘草，故名之曰"增液承气"。

[**临床运用**]

本方主要用于阳明温病，燥热内结而津液枯燥之证。若痔疮日久，大便燥结不通，属于阴虚热结者，亦可用之。

第四章

和解剂

凡是通过和解、调和的方法，以解除病邪的方剂称为和解剂。和解剂常用于治疗少阳病或肝脾不和、肠胃不和者，具有和解少阳、调和肝脾、调和肠胃等作用。属于"八法"中的"和法"。

第一节 和解少阳

和解少阳剂，适用于邪在少阳胆经。症见往来寒热，胸胁苦满，心烦喜呕，默默不欲饮食，口苦，咽干，目眩等。少阳位于半表半里，为阳经的枢机，病邪向外可从太阳透表而解，病邪向里亦可传入阳明或太阴，产生实热证或虚寒证。其病既不在表，亦不在里，故发汗、吐、下在所禁忌，当用和解一法。本法常用柴胡、黄芩、半夏、青蒿等为主组成方剂，代表方有小柴胡汤、大柴胡汤、蒿芩清胆汤等。

小柴胡汤《伤寒论》

[组成] 柴胡半斤（12克） 黄芩三两（9克） 人参三两（9克） 甘草三两，炙（6克） 半夏半升，洗（9克） 生姜三两，切（9克） 大枣十二枚，擘（4枚）

[用法] 原方七味，以水一斗二升，煮取六升，去滓，再煎，取三升，温服一升，日三服。

现代用法；水煎服。

[功效] 和解少阳。

[主治]

1.伤寒少阳病，往来寒热，胸胁苦满，默默不欲饮食，心烦喜呕，口苦，咽干，目眩，舌苔薄白，脉弦者。

2. 妇人中风，热入血室，经水适断，寒热发作有时。以及疟疾、黄疸等杂病见少阳证者。

[方解]

本方为和解少阳之主方。方中柴胡苦平，入肝胆经，能透泄少阳之邪从外而散，并能疏泄气机郁滞，故为君药；黄芩苦寒，助柴胡以清少阳邪热，柴胡升散，得黄芩降泄，则无升阳劫阴之弊，故为臣药；胆气犯胃、胃失和降，故佐以半夏、生姜降逆和胃，蠲饮止呕，人参、大枣扶助正气，俾正气旺盛，则邪无内向之机，可以直从外解；炙甘草助参、枣扶正，且能调和诸药，为使药。本方立法以和解少阳为主，柯琴[24]称其为"少阳枢机之剂，和解表里之总方"，故列于和解剂诸方之首。

[临床运用]

本方乃为少阳病而设，当以"往来寒热，胸胁苦满，默默不欲饮食，心烦喜呕，脉弦"为辨证要点。临床上只要抓住其中主症，便可用小柴胡汤，不必待其症候悉具。除治疗伤寒少阳病之外，对于妇人热入血室、产后郁冒以及疟疾、黄疸等杂病，凡见有上述主症者，均可运用本方治之。

大柴胡汤《伤寒论》

[组成] 柴胡半斤（12克） 黄芩三两（9克） 芍药三两（9克） 半夏半升，洗（9克） 生姜五两，切（15克） 枳实四枚，炙（9克） 大枣十二枚，擘（4枚） 大黄二两（6克）

[用法] 原方八味，以水一斗二升，煮取六升，去滓，再煎，温服一升，日三服。

现代用法；水煎服。

[功效] 和解少阳，内泻热结。

[主治] 少阳阳明并病，往来寒热，胸胁苦满，呕不止，郁郁微烦，心下痞硬，或心下满痛，大便不解或下利，舌苔黄，脉弦数有力者。

[方解]

此乃少阳病未解，传入阳明化热成实，故云少阳阳明并病。本方系由小柴胡汤去人参、甘草，加大黄、枳实、芍药而成。方中柴胡、黄芩和解少阳，以治往来寒热，胸胁苦满，为君药；大黄、枳实内泻热结，以治心下痞硬或满痛，郁郁微烦，大便不解或下利，为臣药；芍药和里，善治腹痛，且助柴、芩以清肝胆，半夏和胃降逆以治呕不止，共为佐药；重用生姜，既助半夏和胃止呕，又配大枣和营卫而行津液，共为使药。总之，本方为治少阳阳明并病，和解与泻下并用之方，较小柴胡汤专于和解少阳一经者力量为大，故名之曰"大柴胡汤"。

[临床运用]

本方为治少阳阳明并病的方剂。病在少阳，本当禁用下法，然而少阳阳明并病，若单用和解，则里实不去，单下热结，则少阳之证又不得解，故用本方外解少阳，内泻热结。汪昂 [25] 说："此加减小柴胡、小承气而为一方，少阳固不可下，然兼阳明腑证则当下。"如此既不悖于少阳禁下的原则，并可一药而解，实为一举两得之法。

蒿芩清胆汤《通俗伤寒论》[26]

[组成]　青蒿脑钱半至二钱（4.5～6克）　淡竹茹三钱（9克）　仙半夏钱半（4.5克）　赤茯苓三钱（9克）　青子芩钱半至三钱（4.5～9克）　生枳壳钱半（4.5克）　广陈皮钱半（4.5克）　碧玉散包，三钱（9克）

[用法]　原方未著用法。

现代用法：水煎服。

[功效]　清胆利湿，和胃化痰。

[主治]　湿遏热郁，寒热如疟，寒轻热重，口苦膈闷，吐酸苦水，或呕黄涎而粘，甚则干呕呃逆，胸胁胀疼，小便短少黄赤，舌红苔白腻，间现杂色，脉数而右滑左弦者。

[方解]

本方证乃湿遏热郁，阻于少阳胆与三焦所致。方中青蒿苦寒芳香，清透少阳邪热，黄芩苦寒，善清胆热，并能燥湿，二味共为君药；竹茹、枳壳、半夏、陈皮清热和胃，化痰降逆，为臣药；赤茯苓、碧玉散清热利湿，导邪从小便而去，且能和中，为佐使药。诸药合用，共奏清胆利湿、和胃化痰之效。

[临床运用]

本方具有清胆利湿，和胃化痰之效，主要适用于湿热郁阻少阳胆及三焦气分者。呕多，可加黄连、苏叶清热止呕；湿重，可加藿香、薏苡仁、白蔻仁、厚朴以化湿浊；小便不利，可加车前子、泽泻、通草治湿利小便。

第二节　调和肝脾

调和肝脾剂，适用于情志抑郁，肝脾失调的疾患。多见手足不温，脘腹胸胁胀痛，神疲食少，月经不调，腹痛泄泻等症。肝藏血，主疏泄，喜条达，内藏相火。若情志抑郁，疏泄失常，郁久化火，必耗阴血。反之，血虚无以濡养肝脏，肝气亦不得柔和调畅。可见肝郁足以导致血虚，血虚亦可导致肝郁。肝病可以传脾，此为木乘土；而脾为气血生化之源，脾虚化源不足，又可导致肝血虚，肝木失其柔和条达之性，亦致肝郁，此为土虚木郁。正因为肝脾关系密切，故调和肝脾为临床常用的治疗方法。常用疏肝健脾药如柴胡、芍药、白术、甘草等为主组成方剂，代表方有四逆散、逍遥散、痛泻要方等。

四逆散《伤寒论》

[组成]　甘草炙　枳实破、水渍，炙干　柴胡　芍药各等分（各6克）

[用法]　原方四味，各十分，捣筛，白饮和，服方寸匕，日三服。
现代用法；水煎服。

[功效]　透解郁热，疏肝理脾。

[主治]　阳气内郁，四肢厥逆，或脘腹疼痛，或泄利下重，脉弦者。

[方解]

四肢厥逆一证，有寒热之分。本方证属于热厥，乃由肝气郁结，气不宣通，阳气内郁，不能达于四肢而致。方中柴胡疏肝解郁，透达郁热，为君药；臣以芍药养血柔肝，和营止痛，柴胡得芍药，一散一收，则无升散太过耗劫肝阴之弊；枳实为佐，宽中下气；甘草为使，调和诸药。且柴胡与枳实同用，一升一降，加强疏肝理气之功；芍药与甘草同用，善能调和肝脾，缓急止痛。合而成方，共奏透解郁热、疏肝理脾之效。原方作散剂，主治"四逆"，故方名"四逆散"。

[临床运用]

本方乃疏肝理脾之平剂。临床上，凡肝郁而见四肢不温，肝脾不和所致的脘腹胁肋疼痛，泄利下重，均可用本方治之。

逍遥散《太平惠民和剂局方》

[组成] 柴胡去苗　当归去苗，锉，微炒　芍药白　白术　茯苓去皮，白者各一两（各30克）甘草微炙赤，半两（15克）

[用法] 原方为粗末，每服二钱，水一大盏，加烧生姜一块切破，薄荷少许，同煎至七分，去滓热服，不拘时候。

现代用法：共为散，每服6～9克，加煨姜、薄荷少许共煎汤温服，日三次。亦可作汤剂，水煎服，用量按原方比例酌情增减。亦有丸剂，每服6～9克，日服二次。

[功效] 疏肝解郁，养血健脾。

[主治] 肝郁血虚，两胁作痛，头痛目眩，口燥咽干，神疲食少，或见往来寒热，或月经不调，乳房作胀，脉弦而虚者。

[方解]

此为肝郁血虚之证。方中当归甘辛苦温，补血和血，且气香入脾，足以舒展脾气，白芍酸苦微寒，养血柔肝，敛阴益脾，归、芍同用，使血和则肝和，血充则肝柔，共为君药；木旺则土衰，肝病易传脾，故以白术、茯苓、甘草健脾益气，实土以御木侮，共为臣药；柴胡疏肝解郁，使肝木得以条达，薄荷少许，疏泄肝经郁热，发其郁遏之气，煨姜温胃和中，又能辛散解郁，共为佐使药。诸药合用，深合《素问·藏气法时论》"肝苦急，急食甘以缓之""脾欲缓，急食甘以缓之""肝欲散，急食辛以散之"之旨，务使血虚得养，脾虚得复，肝郁得疏，自然诸症自愈，气血调畅，故方以"逍遥"名之。

[临床运用]

1.本方为调和肝脾的要方，而肝藏血，脾统血，与月经有直接关系，故又为妇科调经的常用方剂之一。凡属肝郁血虚脾弱者，均可选用本方治疗。

2.肝郁多因情志不遂所致，治疗郁证，须嘱患者心情达观，方能获效。否则，药"逍遥"而人不逍遥，终无济也。

白术芍药散（又名痛泻要方）《景岳全书》[27] 引刘草窗 [28] 方

[组成] 炒白术三两（9克） 炒芍药二两（6克） 防风一两（3克） 炒陈皮一两半（4.5克）

[用法] 原方锉，分八帖，水煎或丸服。

现代用法：作汤剂，水煎服，用量按原方比例酌减。

[功效] 抑肝扶脾。

[主治] 肝木乘脾，肠鸣腹痛，大便泄泻，泻必腹痛，舌苔薄白，脉两关不调，左弦而右缓者。

[方解]

本方证系由肝木乘脾，肝脾不和，脾运失常所致。方中重用白术健脾，并能和中燥湿，白芍抑肝，并能缓急止痛，共为君药；配伍陈皮理气和中，防风具升散之性，辛能散肝郁，香能舒脾气，共为辅佐药。药仅四味，但补中寓疏，扶脾抑肝，调畅气机，痛泻自止。

[临床运用]

本方为治肝木乘脾，腹痛泄泻的常用方。痛泻之症，多见于肝郁性情急躁的患者，每因情绪影响而发作。除痛泻外，并见食欲不振，脘腹微胀，大便中夹有未完全消化的食物，很容易被误诊为伤食泻。但伤食腹痛，得泻便减；痛泻得泻后痛虽略缓，但须臾又腹痛而泻，症状不减，反复发作，以此为辨。

第三节　调和肠胃

调和肠胃剂适用于邪在肠胃，升降失常，寒热夹杂，出现心下痞、呕吐、肠鸣下利，腹中痛等症。纯属中气虚弱，寒热夹杂，故治宜辛开苦降，寒热并用，以调和肠胃。本法配伍特点是辛热药与苦寒药同用，滋补药与温清药共施，常以半夏、黄芩、干姜、黄连、人参、甘草等药物为主组成方剂。代表方有半夏泻心汤、黄连汤。

半夏泻心汤《伤寒论》

[组成] 半夏半升,洗（12克） 黄芩 干姜 人参各三两（各9克） 黄连一两（3克） 大枣十二枚,擘（4枚） 甘草三两,炙（9克）

[用法] 原方七味,以水一斗,煮取六升,去滓,再煮,取三升,温服一升,日三服。

现代用法；水煎服。

[功效] 和胃降逆,开结散痞。

[主治] 胃气不和,心下痞,但满而不痛,或呕吐,肠鸣下利,舌苔腻而微黄。

[方解]

痞者,寒热中阻,痞塞不通,上下不能交泰之谓,属于脾胃病变。方中重用半夏辛温,消痞散结,降逆止呕,以除痞满呕逆之症,故为君药；臣以干姜辛温散寒,黄芩、黄连苦寒泄热,夏、姜、芩、连苦辛并用,能通能降,足以开结散痞；佐以人参、大枣甘温益气,以补其虚；使以甘草补胃气而调诸药。本方寒热互用以和其阴阳,苦辛并进以调其升降,补泻兼施以调其虚实。务使中焦得和,升降复常,则心下痞满、呕吐、下利诸症自愈。本方以半夏为君药,有解除心下痞满之效,故方名半夏泻心汤。

[临床运用]

本方原为误下伤中,胃失和降,寒热互结,心下痞满者而设。后世运用范围很广,不仅伤寒误下成痞,即不由误下而寒热中阻致痞,以及脾胃虚弱,湿热留恋,升降失常致痞者,亦多用本方加减治之,疗效显著。

黄连汤《伤寒论》

[组成] 黄连 甘草炙 干姜 桂枝各三两（各9克） 人参二两（6克） 半夏半升,洗（9克） 大枣十二枚,擘（4枚）

[用法] 原方七味,以水一斗,煮取六升,去滓,温服一升,日三服,夜二服。

现代用法：水煎服。

[功效] 寒热并调,和胃降逆。

［主治］ 胸中有热，胃中有邪气，腹中痛，欲呕吐者。

［方解］

本方适用于胃肠升降失常，寒热夹杂的病证。胸中有热，故方中黄连苦寒清热，为君药；胃中有邪气，故以干姜、桂枝辛温散寒，为臣药，寒温并用，可使寒热调和；佐以半夏和胃降逆止呕，人参、大枣益气和中缓痛；炙甘草为使，善能缓急止痛，调和诸药。全方寒温互用，甘苦并施，能使寒散热消，上下调和，升降复常，诸症自愈。

［临床运用］

本方适用于胃肠升降失常，寒热夹杂的病证。以腹中痛，欲呕吐，舌苔水滑，上罩薄黄色为辨证要点。

第五章

温里剂

根据"寒者热之""清者温之""寒淫于内，治以甘热""寒淫所胜，平以辛热"（《素问·至真要大论》）的原则立法，凡以温热药物为主组成，具有温里祛寒，回阳救逆等作用，以治疗里寒证的方剂，统称温里剂。属于"八法"中的"温法"。

第一节　温中祛寒

温中祛寒剂，是治疗中焦脾胃虚寒证的方剂。脾胃属土，位居中州，胃主受纳，脾主运化，胃主降浊，脾主升清。若中焦脾胃阳气虚衰，则运化失职，升降失常，势必导致阴寒内生，出现肢体倦怠，四肢不温，脘腹胀满，腹中冷痛，不思饮食，口淡不渴，或呕吐下利，吞酸吐涎，舌淡苔白润，脉沉细或迟缓等症。常用温中祛寒药如干姜、吴茱萸、蜀椒、生姜等与健脾补气药如人参、饴糖、白术、炙甘草等配合组成方剂。代表方有理中丸、吴茱萸汤、小建中汤、大建中汤等。

理中丸《伤寒论》

[组成]　人参　干姜　甘草炙　白术各三两（各9克）

[用法]　原方四味，捣筛，蜜和为丸，如鸡子黄许大。以沸汤数合，和一丸，研碎，温服之，日三四服，夜二服；腹中未热，益至三四丸，然不及汤。汤法以四味依两数切，用水八升，煮取三升，去滓，温服一升，日三服。

现代用法：丸剂，每服6～9克，一日二三次，温开水送下；或作汤剂，水煎服，用量按原方比例酌定。

[功效] 温中祛寒，补气健脾。

[主治]

1.脾胃虚寒证，自利不渴，腹满呕吐，腹痛，食不下，舌苔白滑，脉缓弱或沉迟无力，以及霍乱属于脾胃虚寒者。

2.阳虚失血。

3.病后喜唾涎沫及小儿慢惊等症由中焦虚寒而致者。

[方解]

脾胃阳虚有寒，则运化失职，升降失常。中焦虚寒，非温则寒邪不去，非补则正气不复。方中干姜大辛大热，温中祛寒，《名医别录》[29]谓其"治寒冷腹痛，中恶霍乱，胀满"，《珍珠囊》[30]谓其"去脏腑沉寒痼冷"，故为君药；人参甘苦微温，补气健脾，且有温中之效，《别录》谓其"疗肠胃中冷"，故为臣药；脾虚寒湿不化，故以白术为佐，补脾气而燥脾湿，《珍珠囊》谓其"除湿益气，补中补阳"；炙甘草为使，补土温中，调和诸药。四药合用，有温有补有燥有和，而为温中祛寒，补气健脾之剂，为治理中焦虚寒的要方，故名曰"理中"。《素问·至真要大论》说："寒淫所胜，平以辛热，佐以甘苦。"此方是也。原方一方二法，可根据病情之缓急，而决定汤、丸之用。服药后可进热粥，以助药力温养中气。

[临床运用]

本方主要适用于中焦虚寒所致吐、泻、腹痛诸症。以蜜为丸，属于缓调之剂，宜于病情较轻者；若病情较急，宜改丸为汤，以收速效。服药后当以腹中热为度。

吴茱萸汤《伤寒论》

[组成] 吴茱萸一升，洗（9克） 人参三两（9克） 生姜六两，切（18克） 大枣十二枚，擘（4枚）

[用法] 原方四味，上以水七升，煮取二升，去滓，温服七合，日三服。现代用法：水煎服。

[功效] 温中补虚，降逆止呕。

[主治]

1. 胃中虚寒，食谷欲呕，或胃脘作痛，吞酸嘈杂，苔白滑，脉弦迟者。

2. 厥阴头痛，干呕，吐涎沫者。

3. 吐利，手足厥冷，烦躁欲死者。

[方解]

阴寒内盛，胃气不降，浊阴上逆。方中吴茱萸辛苦大热，温中散寒，降逆下气，《本经》谓其"主温中下气止痛"，故为君药；重用生姜为臣，取其辛温之性，助君药温中散寒，降逆止呕；佐以人参甘苦微温，补虚弱而益胃气；大枣甘温，甘能补中，温能益气，且能调和诸药，用以为使。合而成为温中补虚，降逆止呕之剂。

[临床运用]

本方辛苦甘温合用，具有温中补虚，降逆止呕之功。临床以呕吐涎沫，舌质不红，苔白滑，脉弦迟为辨证要点。

小建中汤《伤寒论》

[组成]　桂枝三两，去皮（9克）　芍药六两（18克）　甘草二两，炙（6克）　生姜三两，切（9克）　大枣十二枚，擘（4枚）　胶饴一升（30克）

[用法]　原方六味，以水七升，煮取三升，去滓，内胶饴，更上微火消解，温服一升，日三服。

现代用法：水煎去滓，加入饴糖溶化，温服。

[功效]　温中补虚，和里缓急。

[主治]　虚劳里急，腹中痛，喜得温按，按之则痛减，或心中悸动，虚烦不宁，面色无华，脉弦而涩，舌质淡嫩，苔薄白。

[方解]

虚劳腹痛，由于中气虚寒，不得温煦，故腹中拘急，时时作痛。本方即桂枝汤倍芍药加饴糖而成。方中饴糖甘温而润，温中补虚，缓急止痛，《千金要方》谓其"补虚冷，益气力"，故为君药；重用芍药敛阴，配以桂枝温阳，二味均为臣药；佐以炙甘草，得芍药则酸甘化阴，缓急止痛，得桂枝则辛甘化阳，温中补虚；使以生姜、大枣补脾胃，调营卫而和诸药。合而成方，共奏温中补虚，和里缓急，平补阴阳，调和气血之效。取"劳者温之"之义，俾中阳得运，化生气血，灌溉四旁，则虚劳何患其不愈。本方不用大温大补，而用平和醇厚之品，建立中焦脾胃之气，故方名"小建中汤"。

[临床运用]

本方虽从桂枝汤加味变化而来。但桂枝汤解肌发汗，调和营卫，治疗汗出恶风，营卫不和的中风表虚证；本方温中补虚，和里缓急，治疗中焦虚寒，里急腹痛的虚劳证。桂枝汤以桂枝为君药，本方以饴糖为君药，因为药物配伍和用量比例的不同，其功用和适应证亦就各不相同了。

大建中汤《金匮要略》

[组成]　蜀椒二合，去汗（6克）　干姜四两（12克）　人参二两（6克）

[用法]　原方三味，以水四升，煮取二升，去滓，内胶饴一升，微火煮取一升半，分温再服，如一炊顷，可饮粥二升，后更服，当一日食糜，温覆之。

现代用法：水煎去滓，加入饴糖15克，溶化，分二次温服。

[功效]　温中补虚，降逆止痛。

[主治]　中阳衰微，阴寒内盛，脘腹剧痛，手不可近，呕不能饮食，舌质淡，苔白滑，脉沉细迟。以及脏寒蛔动不安，上腹部剧痛者。

[方解]

中阳衰微，阴寒内盛。方中蜀椒大辛大热，温中散寒，下气止痛，并能驱蛔杀虫，为君药；干姜大辛大热，温中散寒，和胃止呕，为臣药；阴寒内盛由于中阳之虚，故用人参甘温，补益脾胃，扶持正气，为佐药；饴糖建中补虚，缓急止痛，且以缓和椒、姜辛烈之性，为佐使药。四药合用，而成温中补虚，降逆止痛之剂。本方大热大补，足以温健其中脏，使阴寒尽去，中阳建立，故方名"大建中汤"。

[临床运用]

本方以温中补虚，降逆止痛立法，临床常用于治疗腹痛、呕吐属中阳衰微，阴寒内盛者。本方证阴寒程度远较小建中汤证为甚，故本方散寒补虚之力也远较小建中汤为峻。

第二节　回阳救逆

回阳救逆剂，主治肾阳衰微所致的全身阴寒证。人体的真阳藏于肾中，若肾阳衰微，阴寒内盛，出现四肢逆冷，精神萎靡，恶寒蜷卧，下利清谷，脉微细等症时，非用大剂温热药物以回阳救逆不可。设不及时救治，必将亡阳虚脱，症见意识模糊，上气喘促，汗出如油如珠，四肢逆冷，脉微欲绝。急用回阳救逆，益气固脱之剂，庶可挽回生命。回阳救逆之剂主要由辛温燥热与甘温补气的药物配合组成，如附子、干姜、肉桂、人参、炙甘草之类。四逆汤、参附汤即其代表方。但阳气衰微见症不一，又有阳虚水泛者，肾不纳气者，故在具体运用回阳救逆法时，又需与化气利水、镇纳浮阳等法结合使用，如真武汤、黑锡丹等。阳虚阴盛，进而可出现阴盛格阳的证候。即在下利清谷、手足厥逆、脉微欲绝的同时，兼见身反发热或面赤戴阳的假热证。治疗真寒假热之证，切不能被假象所迷惑，应当抓住本质，迅予大剂回阳，才能挽救虚阳浮越的危象，如通脉四脉汤。

四逆汤《伤寒论》

[组成]　甘草二两，炙（6克）　干姜一两半（4.5克）　附子一枚，生用，去皮，破八片（9克）

[用法]　原方三味，以水三升，煮取一升二合，去滓，分温再服。强人可大附子一枚，干姜三两。

现代用法：以水久煎温服。

[功效]　回阳救逆。

[主治]　阴寒内盛，阳气衰微，四肢厥逆，恶寒蜷卧，神疲欲寐，呕吐腹痛，下利清谷，或大汗亡阳，脉沉或微细欲绝，舌质淡苔白滑或舌苔黑而滑润者。

[方解]

《素问·厥论》说："阳气衰于下，则为寒厥。"其主症为四逆，即指阳气衰微，四肢厥逆而言。《素问·至真要大论》说："寒淫所胜，平以辛热，佐以甘苦。"方中生附子大辛大热，入心、脾、肾经，为回阳救逆之要药，专补命门之火，通行十二经，无所不利，走而不守，为君药；干姜大辛大热，守而不走，善散里寒，助君药回阳救逆，为臣药；炙甘草甘温，益气温阳，并能缓和生附、干姜燥烈之性，为佐使药。三药合用，功专效宏，可迅达回阳救逆之功而四逆可愈，故方名"四逆汤"。

[临床运用]

本方为回阳救逆的代表方剂，《伤寒论》以此为治疗少阴病的主方。以四肢厥逆，神疲欲寐，脉微细为辨证要点。本方破阴寒回阳气，能挽回垂绝之阳于俄顷。

参附汤《济生续方》[31]

[组成] 人参半两（15克） 附子炮，去皮、脐，一两（30克）

[用法] 原方呋咀，分作三服，水二盏，生姜十片，煎至八分，去滓，食前温服。

现代用法：水煎服，用量按原方比例酌减。

[功效] 回阳益气固脱。

[主治] 阳气暴脱，手足逆冷，头晕气短，面色苍白，汗出脉微，舌淡苔薄白者。

[方解]

阳气暴脱，即为亡阳。方中重用人参甘温，大补元气，以固后天；附子大辛大热，温壮元阳，大补先天。二药相须，具有上助心阳，下温肾命，中补脾土之功。本方力专效宏，大温大补，最能振奋阳气，益气固脱，确为急救垂危之良方。

[临床运用]

1.本方为回阳益气固脱的代表方剂。临床不但用治阳气暴脱之证，对于妇女暴崩或产后血崩以致血脱亡阳者，亦可用本方救治，此为血脱益气之法也。

2.用本方回阳固脱，一般不能用党参代替人参。如人参无法办到，可用党参60～120克代替人参，量少则难以奏效。

真武汤《伤寒论》

[**组成**] 茯苓三两（9克） 芍药三两（9克） 生姜三两，切（9克） 白术二两（6克） 附子一枚，炮，去皮，破八片（9克）

[**用法**] 原方五味，以水八升，煮取三升，去滓，温服七合，日三服。

现代用法：水煎服。

[**功效**] 温阳利水。

[**主治**]

1.肾阳衰微，水气内停，小便不利，四肢沉重疼痛，腹痛，下利，或肢体浮肿，舌质淡苔白滑，脉沉迟者。

2.太阳病，发汗太过，其人发热，心下悸，头眩，身𥆧动，振振欲擗地者。

[**方解**]

肾为水脏，主化气而利小便，肾中真阳衰微，则气不化水，小便不利。肾主水液，故用附子大辛大热，温肾壮阳，为君药；制水在脾，故又臣以茯苓、白术健脾利水，生姜温散水寒之气；佐以白芍苦酸微寒，既能止腹痛利小便，《本经》谓其"主邪气腹痛……止痛，利小便"，又能缓和附子燥烈之性，使温阳利水而不伤阴。诸药合用，温肾阳以消阴翳，利水道以祛水邪。真武乃北方司水之神，本方有温阳利水之功，故名之曰"真武汤"。

[**临床运用**]

本方为治少阴阳衰，水气内停的方剂。据王绵之[32]教授经验，如有腹水，可加大茯苓剂量；如纳少腹胀，可酌加陈皮、木香，行气有助于利水。方中生姜一味，应按原方比例运用，不得轻视而作一般药引用。

黑锡丹《太平惠民和剂局方》

[**组成**] 金铃子蒸，去皮、核 葫芦巴酒浸，炒 木香 附子炮，去皮、脐 肉豆蔻面裹，煨 破故纸酒浸，炒 沉香镑 茴香舶上者，炒 阳起石研细，水飞，各一两（各30克） 肉桂去皮，半两（15克） 黑锡去滓称 硫黄透明者，结砂子，各二两（各60克）

[**用法**] 原方用黑盏或新铁铫内如常法结黑锡、硫黄砂子，地上出火毒，

研令极细，余药并杵，罗为细末，都一处和匀入研，自朝至暮，以黑光色为度，酒糊圆如梧桐子大，阴干入布袋内擦令光莹，每服三四十粒，空心盐姜汤或枣汤下，妇人艾醋汤下。

现代用法：酒糊丸，成人每服4.5克，小儿每服1.5～3克，空腹时用温开水或淡盐汤送下。如急救可用至9克。

[功效]　温补下元，镇纳浮阳。

[主治]

1.肾阳虚衰，肾不纳气，下虚上实，痰壅气喘，汗出肢厥，舌淡苔白，脉沉细或浮大无根者。

2.奔豚，气上冲胸，或肠鸣便溏，或男子阳痿，妇人血海虚寒，带下清稀者。

[方解]

肾阳虚衰，肾气摄纳无权，此为病之本，下虚是也；阳虚寒从内生，浊阴从而上泛，水泛为痰，胸中痰壅，此为病之标，上实是也。本方以黑锡、硫黄为君药。黑锡即铅，甘寒镇水，重坠以降逆气，坠痰涎，平其痰壅气喘之势；然肾为水火之脏，证属阳衰阴盛，故以硫黄酸温，补火助阳，温命门而消阴寒。二味合用，取阴阳互根，阴中求阳之意，善护真阴，温真阳，纳肾气，镇浮阳。臣以肉桂、附子温补命门，引火归原，葫芦巴、破故纸、茴香、阳起石均为温肾壮阳之品，使阳气充旺，则阴霾自散。寒则气滞，佐以木香调气，虚则气泄，又以肉豆蔻固下；又恐诸纯阳之品温燥太过，引动相火，故以金铃子苦寒以为反佐，且有清肝理气之功。使以沉香，质重性温，既降逆气，又纳肾气。合而成方，共奏温补下元，镇纳浮阳之效。

[临床运用]

本方为温肾纳气的代表方剂，历代医家经过临床实践，给本方以极高的评价。如喻昌说："凡遇阴火逆冲，真阳暴脱，气喘痰鸣之急证，舍此药再无他法可施。昌每用……藉手效灵，厥功历历可纪。"说明本方有急救垂危之功。如见足冷头汗，如油如珠，即将亡阳虚脱，须用独参汤或参附汤送服黑锡丹。

第三节　温经散寒

温经散寒剂，适用于经脉受寒，血行不畅所致的病证。此类疾患多由阴血虚弱，复受寒邪所伤；或阳气不足，阴寒之邪乘虚侵袭而成。故不宜纯用辛热之剂，而以温经散寒药如桂枝、细辛、肉桂、麻黄、姜炭等配合补益药如当归、白芍、熟地、杞子、鹿角胶等为主组成方剂，代表方有当归四逆汤、暖肝煎、阳和汤等。

当归四逆汤《伤寒论》

[组成]　当归三两(9克)　桂枝三两(9克)　芍药三两(9克)　细辛三两(4.5克)　甘草二两，炙(6克)　通草(按：即现在之木通)二两(6克)　大枣二十五枚，擘(8枚)

[用法]　原方七味，以水八升，煮取三升，去滓，温服一升，日三服。

现代用法：水煎服。

[功效]　温经散寒，养血通脉。

[主治]　血虚受寒，手足厥寒，脉细欲绝，舌淡苔白。并治寒伤血脉，腰、股、腿、足疼痛者。

[方解]

素体血虚，复受寒邪所伤，血脉凝滞，运行不畅，四肢失于温养，故手足厥寒。本方即桂枝汤去生姜，倍大枣，加当归、细辛、木通而成。血虚寒凝，故用当归补血和血，温通血脉，为君药；臣以桂枝温通经脉，芍药养血和营；佐以细辛温经散寒，木通通利血脉；使以炙草、大枣补脾气而调诸药。且《别录》载甘草能"通经脉，利血气"。合而成为温经散寒，养血通脉之剂。因方中以当归为君药，用以治疗血虚寒凝所致的手足厥寒证，故方名"当归四逆汤"。

[临床运用]

1.本方温经散寒，养血通脉，主治血虚有寒的手足厥寒，肢体疼痛等症。若妇女血虚寒凝而致月经不调，经行后期，经来腹痛、量少色黯者，亦可用本方治疗。

2.冻疮初起或未溃，可使用本方熏洗或煎服以温经散寒。

暖肝煎《景岳全书》

[组成]　当归二、三钱（6～9克）　枸杞三钱（9克）　小茴香二钱（6克）　肉桂一、二钱（3～6克）　乌药二钱（6克）　沉香一钱（3克，或木香亦可）　茯苓二钱（6克）

[用法]　原方水一盅半，加生姜三五片，煎七分，食远温服。

现代用法：加生姜三五片，水煎服。

[功效]　温补肝肾，散寒行气。

[主治]　肝肾阴寒，小腹疼痛，疝气等症。

[方解]

素体肝肾不足，复因阴寒内盛，下焦受寒，厥阴经气失于疏泄。方中当归、枸杞温补肝肾，为君药；小茴香、肉桂温经散寒，为臣药；佐以乌药、沉香温通理气，茯苓淡渗利湿；使以生姜温散水寒之气。本方温补肝肾以治其本，散寒行气以治其标，标本兼顾，以奏暖肝之效，故方名"暖肝煎"。

[临床运用]

本方适用于肝肾阴寒所致的小腹疼痛、疝气等症。方中沉香如缺，据张景岳[33]自注："或木香亦可。"

阳和汤《外科证治全生集》[34]

[组成]　熟地一两（30克）　白芥子炒，研，二钱（6克）　鹿角胶三钱（9克）　肉桂去皮，研粉，一钱（3克）　姜炭五分（1.5克）　麻黄五分（1.5克）　生甘草一钱（3克）

[用法]　原方煎服。

现代用法：水煎服。

[功效]　温阳补血，散寒通滞。

[主治]　一切阴疽、贴骨疽、流注、鹤膝风等，属于阴寒之证。患处漫肿无头，色白或黯，不红不热，口不渴，舌淡苔白，脉沉细或迟细者。

[方解]

阴疽多由气血虚寒，寒凝痰滞，阻于肌肉、筋骨、血脉之中而成。方中重用熟地滋养精血，《纲目》载其"填骨髓，长肌肉，生精血，补五脏内伤不足，通血脉"，故为君药；鹿角胶助阳补髓，强壮筋骨，《纲目》谓其又治"疮疡肿毒"，为臣药；佐以肉桂补命门之火，消散阴寒，温通血脉，姜炭破阴回阳，以解寒凝，更有少量麻黄发越阳气，开其腠理，使寒凝之毒从外而解，白芥子祛痰散结，治皮里膜外之痰，非此不达。使以生甘草甘以缓之，协和诸药，不使诸辛热之性一发而过，且能解毒。本方虽有熟地、鹿角胶之滋腻，但得姜、桂、麻黄之宣通，则补而不滞；虽有姜、桂、麻黄之辛散，但得大量熟地、鹿角胶之滋补，则宣发而不伤正，相辅相成，其效益彰。全方配伍奇妙，具有温阳补血，宣通血脉，散寒祛痰之功，使阴疽得以消散，犹如阳和一转，寒凝悉解，故方名"阳和汤"。

[临床运用]

本方为治疗外科阴证疮疡的名方，主治一切阴疽。

第六章

清热剂

根据"热者寒之，温者清之"（《素问·至真要大论》）的原则立法，凡以清热药为主组成，具有清热泻火、凉血解毒等作用，以治疗里热证的方剂，统称清热剂。属于"八法"中的"清法"。

第一节　清气分热

清气剂，适用于热在气分，见有壮热、烦渴、汗出、脉洪大滑数、苔黄而干，或热扰胸膈，心烦懊憹等症。常用清热泻火药如石膏、知母、竹叶、黄芩、栀子等为主组成方剂。由于热邪易于耗气伤阴，故又每配益气养阴之品，如人参、麦冬、甘草等。代表方有白虎汤、竹叶石膏汤、栀子豉汤、凉膈散等。

白虎汤《伤寒论》

［组成］　石膏一斤，碎（30克）　知母六两（9克）　甘草二两，炙（6克）　粳米六合（15克）

［用法］　原方四味，以水一斗，煮米熟汤成，去滓，温服一升，日三服。
现代用法：水煎至米熟汤成，去滓温服。

［功效］　清热生津。

［主治］　阳明经热证，不恶寒但恶热，面赤气粗，口干舌燥，烦渴引饮，大汗出，脉洪大有力或浮滑而数，舌质深红，苔黄而干。

［方解］

本方证乃外感寒邪，化热入里，或温邪传入气分的实热证。方中石膏辛甘大寒，辛能解肌热，寒能清胃火，功擅清热泻火，除烦止渴，有达热出表之能，故为君药；臣以知母苦寒质润，清泄肺胃之热，且能滋阴润燥，石膏、知母相配，则清热止渴除烦之力尤强。炙甘草、粳米益胃生津，和中泻火，使大寒之品而无损伤脾胃之虑，石膏、知母得甘草、粳米则清热生津之功尤胜。全方药仅四味，但配伍精当，专清阳明气分之热，犹如金风送爽，炎暑自解。白虎为西方金神，故名之曰"白虎汤"。

[临床运用]

《伤寒论》以本方为治疗阳明热证的主方，《温病条辨》以本方为治疗肺胃气分热证的主方。使用本方应以身大热、口大渴、汗大出、脉洪大等四大症为辨证要点。

竹叶石膏汤《伤寒论》

[组成] 竹叶二把（9克） 石膏一斤（30克） 半夏半升，洗（9克） 人参三两（9克） 甘草二两，炙（6克） 麦门冬一升，去心（18克） 粳米半升（15克）

[用法] 原方七味，以水一斗，煮取六升，去滓，内粳米，煮米熟汤成，去米，温服一升，日三服。

现代用法：水煎服。

[功效] 清热生津，益气和胃。

[主治] 热病，邪热未清，气阴已伤，身热汗出，口干唇燥，烦渴欲饮，虚羸少气，气逆欲吐，脉虚数，舌红少苔者。

[方解]

邪热未清，热淫于内。本方由白虎汤合麦门冬汤加减而成。方中竹叶、石膏清热除烦，据《本草求真》[35]记载：竹叶"合以石膏同治，则能解除胃热，而不致烦渴不止"，故为君药；臣以人参、麦冬益气养阴，《本经》谓麦冬主"胃络脉绝，羸瘦短气"；佐以半夏和胃降逆止呕，配合大量麦冬，尤有妙用，盖半夏得麦冬则不燥，麦冬得半夏则不腻，于清热养阴，和胃降逆方中用此最宜；使以甘草、粳米益胃和中，且防竹叶、石膏寒凉伤胃。合而用之，清热而兼和胃，补虚而不恋邪，确为清补并行的良方。

[临床运用]

本方不仅用于热病后期，余热未清，气阴两伤之证，凡温热病邪在气分，见到气阴已伤之证者，均可使用。尤其对于暑温、伏暑发热，气阴受伤者，使用本方最为合适。

栀子豉汤《伤寒论》

[组成]　栀子十四个，擘（9克）　香豉四合，绵裹（9克）

[用法]　原方二味，以水四升，先煮栀子，得二升半，内豉，煮取一升半，去滓，分为二服，温进一服。得吐者，止后服。

现代用法：水煎服。

[功效]　清热除烦。

[主治]　身热懊憹，虚烦不眠，胸闷胸痛，但按之软而不硬，舌苔微黄者。

[方解]

外感热病，邪气入里，热扰胸膈。方中栀子苦寒，清热除烦，《别录》谓其"疗心中烦闷"；豆豉苦寒，其性轻浮，宣散郁热，《别录》谓其治"伤寒头痛寒热……烦躁满闷"。二药相配，为清宣胸中郁热，治疗虚烦懊憹之良方。

[临床运用]

《伤寒论》以本方治伤寒"发汗、吐、下后，虚烦不得眠，若剧者，必反复颠倒，心中懊憹"之症。后世对本方的运用有所发展，凡温热病邪初入气分，热扰胸膈，症见发热，心烦懊憹，卧起不安，舌苔微黄者，均可用之。

凉膈散《太平惠民和剂局方》

[组成]　川大黄　朴硝　甘草燿，各二十两（各600克）　山栀子仁　薄荷叶去梗　黄芩各十两（各300克）　连翘二斤半（1250克）

[用法]　原方为粗末，每二钱，水一盏，入竹叶七片，蜜少许，煎至七分，去滓，食后温服；小儿可服半钱，更随岁数加减服之。得利下，住服。

现代用法：上药共为粗末，每服9～12克，加竹叶3克，蜜少许，水煎服。亦可作汤剂，水煎服，用量按原方比例酌减。

[功效] 清热泻火，通便。

[主治] 上中二焦热邪炽盛，烦躁口渴，面赤唇焦，口舌生疮，胸膈烦热，咽痛吐衄，便秘溲赤，谵语狂妄，及小儿急惊，舌红苔黄，脉滑数者。

[方解]

上中二焦热邪炽盛，上焦心火上炎，肺热熏蒸，中焦胃腑燥热上冲。本方重用连翘清热解毒，配合黄芩、山栀清热泻火，薄荷、竹叶发散火郁，共泻热于上；而以大黄、朴硝咸寒攻下，以荡涤于中，配甘草、白蜜既能缓和硝、黄之急下，有利于中焦燥热之荡涤，又能解热毒、润燥结、存胃津，使缓下而不伤正气。全方清热、泻下并用，使火热之邪借阳明为出路，体现了"以下为清"的治疗方法。《素问·至真要大论》说："热淫于内，治以咸寒，佐以甘苦。"本方咸寒甘苦并用，深合经旨，能使上中二焦邪热上清下泄，则胸膈自清，诸证可解。方名"凉膈"，即是此意。

[临床运用]

据编者临床体验，咽喉红肿疼痛，甚则腐烂，壮热不退，烦渴欲饮，大便秘结，舌红苔黄燥者，投本方收效甚捷。如咽喉腐烂较甚，可加用锡类散吹喉。

第二节 清营凉血

清营凉血剂，适用于邪热入营或热入血分之证。邪热入营，症见身热夜甚，口渴或反不渴，心烦不寐，神昏谵语，舌绛而干，脉虚数。热入血分较邪热入营病势更为深重，除出现上述种种症状外，其主要表现为血热动血，迫血妄行，而见吐血、衄血、便血、溺血，或热甚发斑，舌质深绛，脉数等症。本类方剂多以性味咸寒（如水牛角、玄参）和甘寒（如生地、麦冬）的药物组成。叶天士[36]《外感温热篇》说："入营犹可透热转气……入血就恐耗血动血，直须凉血散血。"故病入营分，应该在清营的基础上配伍银花、连翘、竹叶心等清气透热之品，使营分之热转出气分而解。热入血分，耗血动血，则应配伍赤芍、丹皮等凉血散血之品，使血宁火熄，瘀祛新生。代表方有清营汤、犀角地黄汤等。

清营汤《温病条辨》

[组成] 犀角三钱（现水牛角代，30克） 生地五钱（15克） 玄参三钱（9克）竹叶心一钱（3克） 麦冬三钱（9克） 丹参二钱（6克） 黄连一钱五分（4.5克） 银花三钱（9克） 连翘连心用，二钱（6克）

[用法] 原方水八杯，煮取三杯，日三服。

现代用法：水煎服。

[功效] 清营解毒，透热养阴。

[主治] 温邪初传营分，身热夜甚，烦渴或反不渴，夜寐不安，时有谵语，舌绛而干，脉虚数，或见斑点隐隐者。

[方解]

温邪在气分不解，深入发展可导致热入营分。《素问·至真要大论》说："热淫于内，治以咸寒，佐以甘苦。"方中犀角（现水牛角代）咸寒，能入心经，清营解毒，散血中之热，故为君药；热甚必伤阴液，臣以生地、玄参、麦冬甘寒与咸寒并用，养阴增液而清营热；佐以黄连苦寒，清心泻火解毒，丹参苦微寒，清热凉血除烦，银花、连翘并能清热解毒；使以少量竹叶心，辛淡甘寒，善清心热。又银花、连翘、竹叶心性寒质轻，轻清透泄，使入于营分之邪热有外达之机，仍转气分而解。合而用之，共奏清营解毒，透热养阴之效，为治疗热伤营阴之主方。

[临床运用]

本方用于温热病邪热入营之证。邪初入营而气分之邪尚未尽解者，亦可用之，有气营两清之效。若兼见痉厥、手足瘛疭，为营热动风，可加入钩藤、丹皮、羚羊角，或少许紫雪丹以清热熄风。

犀角地黄汤《备急千金要方》[37]

[组成] 犀角一两（水牛角代，30克） 生地黄八两（24克） 芍药三两（9克）牡丹皮二两（6克）

[用法] 原方四味㕮咀，以水九升，煮取三升，分三服。

现代用法：水煎服。

[功效] 清热养阴，凉血散血。

[主治]

1. 温热之邪深入血分，热甚动血，吐血、衄血、便血、尿血，斑色紫黑，或神昏谵语，舌绛起刺，脉数者。

2. 蓄血留瘀，喜忘如狂，漱水不欲咽，腹不满但自言腹满，大便黑而易解者。

[方解]

温热之邪深入血分，迫血妄行。方中犀角咸寒，清热凉血解毒，《本草纲目》谓其"治吐血、衄血、下血及伤寒蓄血，发狂谵语，发黄发斑……泻肝凉心，清胃解毒"，生地甘寒，养阴清热，凉血止血，共为君药；赤芍苦微寒，和营泄热，凉血散血，丹皮辛苦微寒，泻血中伏火，凉血散瘀，共为辅佐药，既能增强犀角、生地凉血之功，又可防止瘀血停滞，使止血而不留瘀。热入血分，耗血动血，不清其热则血不宁，不滋其阴则火不熄，不化其瘀则新血不生。本方清热之中兼以养阴，使热清血宁而无耗血之虑；凉血之中兼以散瘀，使血止而无留瘀之弊。药仅四味，但配伍精当，功专效宏。

[临床运用]

本方专为温热之邪燔于血分而设，是治疗热入血分而致各种失血证的重要方剂。方中生地以用鲜生地为好，取其清热凉血止血作用，较干生地尤佳。方中芍药，一般多用赤芍，其凉血散瘀作用较白芍为优。若阴血损伤较甚者，亦可用白芍。

第三节 清热解毒

清热解毒剂，适用于瘟疫、温毒或疮疡疔毒等症。瘟疫、温毒系感受外邪所致，有强烈的传染性，常见烦躁狂乱，热甚发斑或头面红肿，口渴咽痛等症。疮疡疔毒由于发生的部位不同，症状也各有不同。总之，热毒有在全身者，有在局部者，有在气分者，有入血分者，当根据患者临床表现具体分析。本节方剂常用清热解毒药如黄连、黄芩、黄柏、栀子、银花、连翘、板蓝根、玄参、蒲公英、紫花地丁等为主组成，又根据具体症状的不同，分别配伍凉血、活血、行气、疏风之品，代表方有黄连解毒汤、清瘟败毒饮、普济消毒饮、仙方活命饮、五味消毒饮等。

黄连解毒汤《外台秘要》[38] 引崔氏方

[组成] 黄连三两（9克） 黄芩 黄柏各二两（6克） 栀子十四枚，擘（9克）

[用法] 原方四味，切，以水六升，煮取二升，分二服。

现代用法：水煎服。

[功效] 泻火解毒。

[主治] 一切火热实证，狂躁烦心，口燥咽干，大热干呕，错语不眠，吐血衄血，甚至发斑，以及外科痈肿疔毒，舌苔黄腻，脉数有力者。

[方解]

火热毒邪，充斥三焦。火热炽盛，蕴积而成毒，是以解毒必须泻火，泻火即所以解毒也。方中重用黄连为君药，大泻心火且泻中焦之火；黄芩泻上焦之火，黄柏泻下焦之火，栀子通泻三焦之火，导热下行，从膀胱而出，共为辅佐药。四药合用，苦寒直折，使火邪去而热毒解，故方名"黄连解毒汤"。

[临床运用]

1. 本方为治火热毒邪壅盛三焦的代表方，故集三黄、栀子大苦大寒之品为一炉，以热毒虽盛而津液未伤，舌苔黄腻，脉数有力者为宜。若热伤阴液，舌质红绛，脉虚数者，不可用之，恐苦寒之品易于化燥伤阴。

2. 本方在临床运用时，多与银花、连翘相配伍，其清热解毒作用更强。治疗痈肿疔毒，更可加入蒲公英、紫花地丁、绿豆衣、甘中黄等。若大便不畅或秘结，方中可加大黄以通大便，使热毒从二便而出。本方若为末水丸，则名栀子金花丸（《景岳全书》）。急攻则用汤，缓祛则用丸，略有区别。

清瘟败毒饮《疫疹一得》[39]

[组成] 生石膏大剂六～八两，中剂二～四两，小剂八钱～一两二钱（24～250克）小生地大剂六钱～一两，中剂三～五钱，小剂二～四钱（12～30克） 乌犀角大剂六～八钱，中剂三～五钱，小剂二～四钱（水牛角代，30～60克） 真川连大剂四～六钱，中剂二～四钱，小剂一～一钱半（3～18克） 栀子（9克） 桔梗（6克） 黄芩（9克） 知母（9克） 赤芍（9克） 玄参（15克） 连翘（9克） 甘草（6克） 丹皮（9克）

鲜竹叶（15克）[以上十味，原书未著剂量]

[用法] 原方先煮石膏数十沸，后下诸药，犀角磨汁和服。

现代用法：水煎服。

[功效] 清气凉血，泻火解毒。

[主治] 瘟疫热毒，气血两燔，头痛如劈，狂躁烦心，口干咽痛，大热干呕，错语不眠，吐血衄血，热甚发斑，舌刺唇焦，脉沉伏或沉细而数，或沉而数，或浮大而数者。

[方解]

瘟疫系感受疫疠邪气所致的具有强烈传染性的温病。本方系由白虎汤、犀角地黄汤、黄连解毒汤三方加减而成。气血两燔，热毒充斥，非大剂清凉莫救。方中重用石膏为君药，直清胃热。盖胃为水谷之海，气血生化之源，十二经脉之气皆来源于胃，阳明又为多气多血之经，阳明胃热得清，则十二经之火自消，淫热自退；配合犀角、黄连、黄芩清上焦心肺之火，丹皮、栀子、赤芍清肝经之火，生地、知母清热救阴，共为臣药；更加连翘清热解毒，玄参养阴解毒，竹叶清心除烦，桔梗载药上行，共为佐药；甘草解热毒，调诸药而和胃气，为使药。诸药合用，共奏清气凉血、泻火解毒之功。因本方专治瘟疫热毒，故名曰"清瘟败毒饮"。

[临床运用]

本方用治瘟疫热毒充斥周身表里上下，气血两燔者。临床应根据病势轻重，掌握各药剂量。若热毒猖獗，病势沉重者，宜投大剂，方可救治。但本方寒凉过甚，若病势较轻者，剂量宜轻，不可过重，徒伤胃气。

普济消毒饮子《东垣试效方》[40]

[组成] 黄芩 黄连各五两（15克） 橘红 玄参 生甘草各二钱（各6克）连翘 鼠粘子 板蓝根 马勃 薄荷各一钱（各3克） 白僵蚕炒 升麻各七分（各2克） 柴胡 桔梗各二钱（各6克）[一方无薄荷，有人参三钱]

[用法] 原方共为细末，半用汤调，时时服之；半蜜为丸，噙化之。

现代用法：水煎服，用量按原方比例酌情增减。

[功效] 清热解毒，疏风散邪。

[主治] 大头瘟，初起恶寒发热，肢体沉重，继则头面红肿，目不能开，咽喉不利，口渴舌燥，苔黄，脉浮数有力。

[方解]

大头瘟，又名大头天行，乃感受风热疫毒之邪，壅于上焦，攻冲头面所致。方中重用黄芩、黄连清泄上焦热毒，为君药；玄参养阴生津，泻火解毒，软坚散结，橘红理气化痰，生甘草泻火解毒，共为臣药；连翘、板蓝根、马勃清热解毒，其中连翘并能散结消肿，马勃且能清利咽喉，鼠粘子、薄荷、僵蚕疏散风热，其中鼠粘子、僵蚕又可清利咽喉，散结消肿，以上均为佐药；升麻、柴胡升举清阳，疏散风热，桔梗清利咽喉，载药上行，共为使药。全方有清有散，有降有升，共奏清热解毒，疏风散邪之效。大头瘟流行之时，用本方时时服之，能够普遍救济，消散温毒，故名之曰"普济消毒饮子"。

[临床运用]

本方为治疗大头瘟的常用方。原方后注："如大便硬，加酒煨大黄一钱至二钱以利之。"则其效尤佳。正虚者，可酌加党参以扶正祛邪。

仙方活命饮《校注妇人良方》[41]

[组成] 白芷　贝母　防风　赤芍药　当归尾　甘草节　皂角刺炒　穿山甲炙　天花粉　乳香　没药各一钱（各3克）　金银花　陈皮各三钱（各9克）

[用法] 原方用酒一大碗，煎五七沸服。

现代用法：水煎服，或水、酒各半煎服。

[功效] 清热解毒，消肿溃坚，活血止痛。

[主治] 疮疡肿毒初起，红肿焮痛，身热恶寒，苔薄白或微黄，脉数有力，属阳证者。

[方解]

疮疡肿毒，多由热毒壅结，气血壅滞而成。方中重用金银花清热解毒，消散疮痈，乃痈疽圣药，《本草纲目》谓其"治诸肿毒，痈疽……散热解毒"，故为君药；防风、白芷祛风消肿，归尾、赤芍活血通络，乳香、没药散瘀止痛，陈皮理气化滞，共为臣药；贝母、花粉清热化痰，散结消肿，甘草节泻火解毒，散痈消肿，共为佐药；穿山甲、皂角刺消肿溃坚，性专行散，直达病所，酒能活血通络以行药势，共为使药。合而用之，共奏清热解毒，消肿溃坚，活血止痛之效。

[临床运用]

1.本方乃疮疡肿毒初起之首方。凡疮疡肿毒初起，红肿焮痛，属于阳证体实者，均可使用。脓未成者，服之可使消散；脓已成者，服之可使外溃，故《医宗金鉴》谓本方"乃疮痈之圣药，诚外科之首方也"。

2.若疮疡痛不甚者，可减乳香、没药；红肿痛甚者，可加紫花地丁、蒲公英、连翘；便秘者，可加大黄；大热大渴伤津者，宜去白芷、防风、陈皮。

五味消毒饮《医宗金鉴》

[组成] 金银花三钱（20克） 野菊花 蒲公英 紫花地丁 紫背天葵子各一钱二分（各9克）

[用法] 原方水二盅，煎八分，加无灰酒半盅，再滚二三沸时热服，渣如法再煎服，被盖出汗为度。

现代用法：水煎，加酒一二匙和服。

[功效] 清热解毒消肿。

[主治] 各种疔毒，局部红肿热痛，初起如粟，坚硬根深如钉状，舌红苔黄，脉数有力者。

[方解]

《素问·生气通天论》说："膏粱之变，足生大丁。"疔毒多由感受温热火毒以及恣食膏粱厚味，内生积热，气血壅滞而成。方中重用金银花清热解毒，凉血消肿，为君药；野菊花、紫背天葵善消疔毒，蒲公英、紫花地丁清热解毒消肿，共为辅佐药；少量黄酒助药势，行血脉，为使药。本方五味药皆以清热解毒见长，故方名"五味消毒饮"。

[临床运用]

本方为治疗疔疮肿毒的有效方剂。据岳美中[42]教授经验，本方加金线重楼（蚤休）、半枝莲、粉甘草，疗效尤佳。

第四节　清脏腑热

清脏腑热的方剂，适用于热邪偏盛于某一脏腑所产生的火热之证。其临床表现根据邪热偏盛于某一脏腑而有所不同。清脏腑热的方剂，是根据各个脏腑的特点而由不同的清热药物组成的。如清心火多用黄芩、黄连、竹叶，清肝火多用龙胆草、黄芩、黄连、黑山栀，清脾胃火多用石膏，清肺热则多用芦根、桑白皮，清大肠热多用黄芩、白头翁。代表方有泻心汤、导赤散之清心火，龙胆泻肝汤、左金丸之清肝火，清胃散之清胃热，苇茎汤、泻白散之清肺热，芍药汤、葛根黄芩黄连汤、白头翁汤之清大肠，均属"热者寒之""有余折之"（《素问·至真要大论》）的治疗方法。

泻心汤《金匮要略》

[组成]　大黄二两（6克）　黄连一两（3克）　黄芩一两（9克）

[用法]　原方三味，以水三升，煮取一升，顿服之。

现代用法：水煎服。

[功效]　泻火泄热。

[主治]　心胃火热内炽，迫血妄行，吐血衄血，便秘溲赤，舌苔黄腻，脉数有力。亦治三焦积热，目赤肿痛，口唇生疮及外科痈肿等症。

[方解]

心胃积热，邪火内炽，热伤阳络，迫血妄行。方中重用大黄为君药，取其泻火泄热，苦降行瘀，唐容川谓："大黄一味，能推陈致新……既速下降之势，又无遗留之邪。"辅佐黄连、黄芩泻火清热，配合大黄，使火降热清则血自宁，不止血而血自止。本方止血而无留瘀之弊，故为治疗血热吐衄之良方。

[临床运用]

《金匮要略》以本方治"心气不足，吐血、衄血"。心气不足是由于火热有余，本方泻火泄热，可收止血之效。盖泻心即是泻火，泻火即可以止血。本方亦可用治妇人倒经、产后恶露不净属心火炽盛，迫血妄行者。据已故日本名医大塚敬节[43]之经验，"出血时冷服为佳"。

导赤散《小儿药证直诀》

[组成] 生地黄 木通 生甘草梢各等分

[用法] 原方为末，每服三钱，水一盏，入竹叶同煎至五分，食后温服。

现代用法：加入竹叶适量，水煎服，用量按原方比例酌情增减。

[功效] 清心利水。

[主治] 心经有热，面赤烦躁，口渴意欲饮冷，口糜舌疮，或心热移于小肠，小便赤涩刺痛，舌尖红，脉数者。

[方解]

心经有热，火炎于上；心与小肠相为表里，心热移于小肠。方中生地甘苦寒，清热凉血养阴，既能清心热、凉心血，又能养心阴、滋肾水，使肾水上济心火，则心热自清，故为君药；臣以木通苦寒，降火利水，引心经之热从小肠而出，配伍生地，则利水而不伤阴；佐以竹叶辛淡甘寒，清心利水，且能除烦；生甘草梢清热泻火并能缓急止痛，为使药。四药相合，清心而兼养阴，利水而能导热。赤色属心，本方能引导心与小肠之热从小便而去，故方名"导赤散"。

[临床运用]

1.本方上清心火，下清小肠，为清心利水的代表方剂。原方后云："一方不用甘草，用黄芩；一方用灯芯。"据编者临床体会，如心火炽盛，加黄芩疗效更好；如小便短赤涩痛，加灯芯其效尤著。

2.治血淋涩痛，可用本方加旱莲草、白茅根、血余炭、车前子、阿胶珠等凉血止血、利水通淋之品。

龙胆泻肝汤《医方集解》[44]

[组成] 龙胆草酒炒（6克） 黄芩炒（6克） 栀子酒炒（9克） 泽泻（9克） 木通（6克） 车前子（9克） 当归酒洗（9克） 生地黄酒炒（12克） 柴胡（4.5克） 甘草生用（3克）[原书未著剂量]

[用法] 原方未著用法。

现代用法：水煎服。或作丸剂，日服两次，每服6克，温开水送下。

[功效] 泻肝火，清湿热。

[主治]

1.肝胆实火，胁痛头痛，口苦目赤，耳聋耳肿。

2.肝经湿热下注，小便淋浊，阴痒阴肿，筋痿阴湿，赤白带下，舌边红苔黄腻，脉弦数有力。

[方解]

方中龙胆草大苦大寒，专泻肝胆实火，除下焦湿热，为君药；黄芩、山栀苦寒泻火，清热燥湿，助龙胆草泻肝火清湿热，共为臣药；佐以泽泻、木通、车前子清利湿热，使实火湿热俱从小便而去，肝为藏血之脏，肝火炽盛易伤阴血，加之苦燥清利，泻之过甚，亦耗阴血，故用当归、生地滋养肝血，使邪去而正不伤；使以柴胡条达肝气，且为肝胆引经之药，甘草调和诸药，使诸苦寒之品不致伤胃。本方配伍之妙在于寓补于泻，既能泻肝火清湿热，又使泻火利湿之品不致耗伤阴血，诚良方也。

[临床运用]

1.本方清肝胆利湿热，凡肝胆实火或肝经湿热，津液未伤者，均可以本方苦寒直折。

2.本方药多苦寒，易伤脾胃，应中病即止，毋使过剂。原方龙胆草、栀子皆用酒炒，黄芩亦炒用，均恐苦寒易伤胃气。方中龙胆草用量不宜过大，当在3～6克。

左金丸（又名回令丸）《丹溪心法》

[组成]　黄连六两（180克）　吴茱萸一两（30克）

[用法]　原方为末，水丸或蒸饼为丸，白汤下五十丸。

现代用法：为末，水泛为丸，每服2～3克，温开水送服。亦可作汤剂，水煎服，用量按原方比例酌定。

[功效]　清肝泻火，降逆止呕。

[主治]　肝火犯胃，胁肋作痛，脘痞嗳气，吞酸吐酸，口苦，舌边红苔黄，脉弦数者。

[方解]

本方为清肝泻火之正剂。方中重用黄连大苦大寒，入心泻火，心为肝之子，心火清则肝火自平，乃"实则泻子"之法，故为君药；少佐吴茱萸大辛大热，疏肝开郁，降逆止呕，且制黄连苦寒之性，以免损伤胃气，又防黄连苦寒直折而产生火盛格拒的反应。吴茱萸仅用黄连的六分之一，故对清肝泻火并无妨害，且成反佐之功。二药合用，一寒一热，相反相成，共奏清肝泻火，降逆止呕之效。本方重用黄连以清火，使火不克金，金能制木，则肝木平矣。佐金以制木，此"左金"所以得名也。

[临床运用]

本方多用于肝经火旺所致的胁痛实证，若肝血不足所致的胁痛虚证，则当用养血柔肝之法，不适用本方。吞酸、吐酸属胃气虚寒者，亦忌用本方。

清胃散《兰室秘藏》[45]

[组成] 当归身（6克） 黄连如连不好，更加二分，夏月倍之（4.5克） 生地黄酒制，以上三分（12克） 牡丹皮五分（9克） 升麻一钱（6克）

[用法] 原方为细末，都作一服，水一盏半，煎至一盏，去滓，待冷服之。

现代用法：水煎服。

[功效] 清胃泻火凉血。

[主治] 胃中积热上冲，上下牙痛，牵引头脑，满面发热，其齿喜冷恶热，或牙龈溃烂，或牙宣出血，或唇口颊腮肿痛，口气热臭，口干舌燥，舌红苔黄，脉滑大而数者。

[方解]

《灵枢·经脉》[16]说："胃足阳明之脉……下循鼻外，入上齿中，还出挟口，环唇，下交承浆，却循颐后下廉，出大迎，循颊车，上耳前，过客主人，循发际，至额颅。""大肠手阳明之脉……贯颊，入下齿中。"方中黄连苦寒，泻火清热，为君药；生地、丹皮凉血清热，为臣药；阳明为多气多血之经，故佐以当归身滋养阴血而退阳热；使以升麻，既为阳明引经药，又善解阳明热毒，升胃家清阳，清升则热降，热降则肿消而痛止。诸药合用，共奏清胃泻火凉血之功。

[临床运用]

1. 本方原为胃火牙痛而设，其实凡胃热之证，血热而火郁者，均可使用。据《医方集解》"一方加石膏"，则清胃泻火之力尤强，临证当酌情加入。

2. 若热盛伤津，本方可加麦冬、花粉；大便秘结者，加入大黄导热下行，收效尤捷。

玉女煎《景岳全书》

[组成] 石膏三五钱（9～15克） 熟地三五钱或一两（9～30克） 麦冬二钱（6克） 知母 牛膝各钱半（各4.5克）

[用法] 原方水一盅半，煎七分，温服或冷服。

现代用法：水煎服。

[功效] 清胃热、滋肾阴。

[主治] 少阴不足，阳明有余，烦热口渴，头痛，牙疼，吐衄失血，脉浮洪滑大，重按则现虚象，舌质红绛，苔黄而干。

[方解]

阳明胃热伤津，少阴阴虚液耗。方中石膏辛甘大寒，清阳明胃火之有余，熟地甘温，滋少阴肾水之不足，共为君药；知母苦寒质润，既助石膏清胃泻火，无苦燥伤津之虑，且能滋肾养阴，麦冬甘寒，养肺胃之阴，与熟地同用，取金水相生之意，使水足则火自平，均为辅佐药；牛膝苦酸而平，补益肾阴，且能引血下行，以降炎上之火，使血不上溢，为使药。诸药合用，共奏清热壮水之效。

[临床运用]

1. 本方常用于水亏火盛所致的烦热口渴，头痛、牙疼，吐衄失血等症。原书加减法："如火之盛极者，加栀子、地骨皮之属亦可；如多汗多渴者，加北五味子十四粒；如小水不利，或火不能降者，加泽泻一钱五分或茯苓亦可；如金水俱亏，因精损气者，加人参二三钱尤妙。"

2. 根据编者临床体验，本方以生地易熟地，则清热作用更强。如热甚失血，可用大量鲜生地，并加赤芍、丹皮、白茅根之类。

苇茎汤《备急千金要方》

[组成] 苇茎切，二升，以水二斗，煮取五升，去滓（30～60克） 薏苡仁半升（15～30克） 瓜瓣半升（15～30克） 桃仁三十枚（9克）

[用法] 原方四味㕮咀，内苇汁中，煮取二升，服一升。当有所见，吐脓血。

现代用法：水煎服。

[功效] 清肺化痰，逐瘀排脓。

[主治] 肺痈，咳有微热，甚则咳吐臭痰脓血，胸中隐隐作痛，口干咽燥而不渴饮，烦满，胸中甲错，脉滑数，苔黄腻。

[方解]

风热外袭（或风寒郁而化热），痰热内结，内外合邪，熏蒸于肺，以致痰热瘀血互结肺中，蕴酿而成肺痈。方中苇茎即芦苇的嫩茎，性味甘寒，清肺泄热，除烦止渴，为治肺痈君药，用量宜大。臣以薏苡仁甘淡微寒，清热利湿，化痰排脓；瓜瓣即冬瓜子，甘寒清热，滑痰排脓，亦为内痈要药。佐以桃仁苦甘而平，润肺止咳，逐瘀行滞。药仅四味，方虽平淡，但其清热化痰、逐瘀排脓之效甚伟。具有"重不伤峻，缓不伤懈"的特点。

[临床运用]

1. 本方为治肺痈（肺脓疡）的常用方，不论肺痈之将成、已成，均可服用。将成者服之可使消散，已成者服之可使肺中痰浊脓瘀排出体外，则肺脏治节得以恢复而病亦自愈。

2. 肺痈成痈期如热毒瘀结，痰味腥臭者，可以本方合犀黄丸以解毒化瘀。溃脓期如咳吐脓血，状如米粥，可以本方合桔梗、甘草、象贝母、鱼腥草以增强清热解毒，化痰排脓之效。

泻白散《小儿药证直诀》

[组成] 地骨皮 桑白皮炒，各一两（各30克） 甘草炙，一钱（3克）[周学海复刻本曰："聚珍本甘草作半两。"]

[用法] 原方锉散，入粳米一撮，水二小盏，煎七分，食前服。

现代用法：入粳米一撮，水煎服，用量按原方比例酌情增减。

[功效]　泻肺清热，止咳平喘。

[主治]　肺热咳嗽，甚则气喘，皮肤蒸热，日晡尤甚，舌红苔黄，脉细数。

[方解]

肺主气，宜清肃下降。方中桑白皮甘寒，泻肺清热，止咳平喘，为君药；地骨皮甘淡寒，助君药泻肺中伏火，善于退热，为臣药；甘草润肺止咳，养胃和中，粳米补益脾肺之气，且防桑白皮、地骨皮寒凉伤胃之弊，共为佐使药。四药合用，泻肺清热，止咳平喘而不伤正，故对肺有伏火，正气不太伤者，用之较为适合。方名"泻白"，乃取肺色白，本方能泻肺中伏热之意。

[临床运用]

本方用治肺有伏热，气逆不降所致的咳喘。若肺经热甚，本方清热之力嫌弱，宜加黄芩、知母以增强清肺泄热之效；咳甚者，可加杏仁、川贝、瓜蒌皮以润肺止咳；口渴者，可加天花粉以生津止渴。

芍药汤《素问病机气宜保命集》[46]

[组成]　芍药一两（15克）　当归　黄连各半两（各9克）　槟榔　木香　甘草炒，各二钱（各6克）　大黄三钱（6克）　黄芩半两（9克）　官桂二钱半（1.5克）

[用法]　原方叹咀，每服半两，水二盏，煎至一盏，食后温服。清如血痢，则渐加大黄；如汗后脏毒，加黄柏半两，依前服。

现代用法：水煎服。

[功效]　行血调气，清热解毒。

[主治]　湿热痢，腹痛便脓血，赤白相兼，里急后重，肛门灼热，脉滑数，苔黄腻。

[方解]

本方证乃由湿热疫毒之邪蕴蓄肠中所致。方中重用芍药和血而止腹痛，《神农本草经》谓其"主邪气腹痛"，《本草纲目》谓其"主下痢腹痛后重"，故为君药；臣以当归行血，合芍药以和营，能治下痢腹痛，黄芩、黄连清热燥湿，并能解毒；佐以木香、槟榔调气导滞，大黄清湿热，破积而行血；反佐肉桂少许取其辛温行血，且防大量苦寒伤胃之弊；使以甘草缓急止痛，调和诸药。又芍药得甘草，善止腹痛；大黄与木香、槟榔同用，增强破积导滞之功，乃"通因通用"之法；且大黄得肉桂，行血之力更著，肉桂得大黄，则无辛热助火之虑。河间云："行血则便脓自愈，调气则后重自除。"此方是也。

[临床运用]

本方为治湿热痢之常用方。若热甚者，可去肉桂之温热；痢下赤多白少，甚或纯下鲜紫脓血者，除去肉桂外，当归可改用当归炭，并加丹皮炭、炒银花等以凉血止血。

葛根黄芩黄连汤《伤寒论》

[组成] 葛根半斤（15克） 甘草二两，炙（6克） 黄芩三两（9克） 黄连三两（9克）

[用法] 原方四味，以水八升，先煮葛根，减二升，内诸药，煮取二升，去滓，分温再服。

现代用法：水煎服。

[功效] 清里解表。

[主治] 外感表证未解，热邪入里，身热下利，胸脘烦热，口中作渴，喘而汗出，舌红苔黄，脉数或促者。

[方解]

外感表证初起，邪在太阳，理应解表。方中重用葛根为君药，既能外解肌表之邪，又能升发脾胃清阳之气而止泻利；辅佐黄芩、黄连清泄里热，厚肠止利；使以甘草甘缓和中，协调诸药，共成清里解表之剂。原方先煮葛根，后纳诸药，则解肌之力缓而清里之力强，乃三表七里之治也。

[临床运用]

本方为治身热下利的代表方剂，虽能外解肌表之邪，内清肠胃之热，但以清里热为主，对于热泻、热痢，不论有无表证，皆可用之。若兼呕吐，可加半夏、竹茹以降逆止呕；挟有食滞，加山楂、神曲以消食；腹胀而痛，加煨木香、炒白芍行气缓急止痛。

白头翁汤《伤寒论》

[组成]　白头翁二两（12克）　黄柏　黄连　秦皮各三两（各9克）

[用法]　原方四味，以水七升，煮取二升，去滓，温服一升，不愈，再服一升。

现代用法：水煎服。

[功效]　清热解毒，凉血止痢。

[主治]　热利下重，渴欲饮水，腹痛便脓血，肛门灼热，舌红苔黄，脉弦数。

[方解]

《伤寒论·厥厥阴篇》说："热利下重者，白头翁汤主之。"又说："下利欲饮水者，以有热故也，白头翁汤主之。"方中白头翁苦寒，清热解毒，凉血止痢，《别录》谓其"止毒利"，为治疗热毒赤痢之君药；黄连、黄柏苦寒，清热燥湿治痢，秦皮苦寒而涩，清热燥湿，断下止痢，均为辅佐药。四药合用，具有清热解毒，凉血止痢之效。

[临床运用]

本方为治疗热毒赤痢的常用方剂。若发病急骤，痢下鲜紫脓血，壮热口渴，腹痛剧烈，舌质红绛，脉大而数，属疫毒痢者，可用本方加赤芍、丹皮、炒银花以治之。

第五节　清热祛暑

清热祛暑剂，适用于夏月感暑之证。以身热烦渴，汗出体倦，脉虚为主症。《素问·热论》说："先夏至日者为病温，后夏至日者为病暑。"但夏月天暑下迫，地湿上蒸，暑湿之邪易于相因为患，故有"暑多挟湿"之说。暑为阳邪、热邪，大热伤气耗津，每多出现气虚津伤等证。大抵纯系感受暑热，症见热势鸱张，烦渴自汗，面垢齿燥，宜清暑为主，佐以益气生津，如白虎加人参汤（见清热剂）；兼表寒者，往往天气炎热，纳凉露卧所致，症见高热头痛，无汗恶寒，宜祛暑解表，如香薷饮（见解表剂）；感暑挟湿，法当清暑利湿，《明医杂著》[47]认为："治暑之法，清心利小便最好。"代表方有六一散；暑能伤气耗津，津气耗伤较甚者，宜用清暑益气法，代表方有清暑益气汤。

使用祛暑剂，需掌握兼证的有无及主次轻重。如暑病兼湿而暑重湿轻者，则湿易化燥，用药不宜过于温燥，以免燥伤津液；如湿重暑轻者，则暑蕴湿中，凉润甘寒之剂又当慎用，以免湿邪缠绵不解。

六一散（原名益元散）《伤寒直格》[48]

[组成] 滑石六两，白腻好者（180克）　甘草一两（30克）

[用法] 原方为细末，每服三钱，蜜少许，温水调下，或无蜜亦可，每日三服，或饮冷饮者，新井泉调下亦得。

现代用法：为细末，每服9～15克，温开水调服，或布包入汤剂煎服。

[功效] 清暑利湿。

[主治] 感受暑湿，身热心烦口渴，小便不利或呕吐泄泻，苔黄腻。亦治膀胱湿热，小便赤涩，癃闭淋痛，以及砂淋等。

[方解]

暑为阳热之邪，暑气通于心。方中重用滑石甘淡而寒，质重体滑，其淡能利湿，寒能清热，重能下降，滑能利窍，功擅清暑利湿通淋，《神农本草经》谓其"主身热泄澼，女子乳难，癃闭，利小便"，故为君药；少量甘草和其中气，且以缓和滑石寒滑之性，使邪去而正不伤，为佐使药。二药配合，清暑利湿，使内蕴之暑湿从小便排泄，则热可退、渴可解、利可止。《明医杂著》所谓："治暑之法，清心利小便最好。"正合本方立方之意，亦为暑病挟湿的治疗大法。本方以滑石六两、甘草一两，作散剂服，故名"六一散"。亦寓"天一生水，地六成之"之义。

[临床运用]

1.本方为治暑湿证之要方，临床每多配伍清暑利湿之品，如藿香、佩兰、青蒿、通草、西瓜翠衣、竹叶等。

2.膀胱湿热下注，小便赤涩，癃闭淋痛，可以本方酌加车前子、泽泻、萹蓄、瞿麦之类；砂石淋者，更可酌加金钱草、海金沙、石韦、冬葵子等化石通淋；血淋者，可以本方加生侧柏叶、生车前草、生藕节治之，名三生益元散（《医方集解》）。

清暑益气汤《温热经纬》[49]

[组成] 西洋参（4.5克） 石斛（12克） 麦冬（9克） 黄连（3克） 竹叶（6克） 荷梗（12克） 知母（6克） 甘草（3克） 粳米（15克） 西瓜翠衣（30克）
[原方未著分量]

[用法] 原方未著用法。

现代用法：水煎服。

[功效] 清暑益气，养阴生津。

[主治] 感受暑热，气津两伤，身热汗多，心烦口渴，四肢困倦，精神不振，脉虚数。

[方解]

暑为阳邪，最易耗气伤津。方中西洋参苦甘凉，益气生津，为君药；石斛、麦冬甘寒生津，养阴清热，为臣药；黄连苦寒，竹叶辛淡甘寒，均能清心除烦；荷梗苦平，清热解暑，通气宽胸，知母苦寒质润，滋阴清热，西瓜翠衣甘寒，清热涤暑，以上均为佐药；甘草、粳米益胃和中，为使药。诸药合用，共奏清暑益气、养阴生津之效，故方名"清暑益气汤"。

[临床运用]

1.本方用治感受暑热，耗气伤津者。以身热汗多，心烦口渴，体倦少气，脉虚数，舌苔薄白而干，舌质红，病发于暑天为辨证要点。

2.方中黄连用量宜小，防其苦寒化燥，反伤津液。

第六节　清虚热

清虚热剂适用于热病后期，邪热未尽，阴液已伤，热留阴分，出现暮热早凉，热退无汗，舌红少苔，或因肝肾阴亏，虚火内扰而致的骨蒸劳热，唇红颧赤，形瘦盗汗等症，常用养阴药如鳖甲、生地、知母与清热药如青蒿、地骨皮、银柴胡等为主组成方剂。代表方有青蒿鳖甲汤、清骨散。

青蒿鳖甲汤《温病条辨》

[组成] 青蒿二钱（6克） 鳖甲五钱（15克） 细生地四钱（12克） 知母二钱（6克） 丹皮三钱（9克）

[**用法**] 原方水五杯，煮取二杯，日再服。

现代用法：水煎服。

[**功效**] 养阴透热。

[**主治**] 温病后期，阴液已伤，邪热未尽，深伏阴分，症见夜热早凉，热退无汗，能食形瘦，舌红少苔，脉细数者。

[**方解**]

人体卫阳之气，日行于表而夜入于里。温病后期，阴液已伤，邪热未尽，深伏阴分，阳气入阴，助长邪热。方中鳖甲咸寒，直入阴分，养阴清热，青蒿芳香苦寒，清热凉血，透邪外出，共为君药；细生地、知母助鳖甲养阴清热，丹皮助青蒿透泄阴分伏热，共为辅佐药。吴鞠通[50]认为："此方有先入后出之妙，青蒿不能直入阴分，有鳖甲领之入也；鳖甲不能独出阳分，有青蒿领之出也。"故青蒿、鳖甲兼有引经使药的作用。诸药相合，滋中有清，清中能透，养阴而不留邪，祛邪而不伤正，为邪少虚多者设，是养阴透热，清除阴分余邪的良方。

[**临床运用**]

本方常用于温病后期，阴液已伤，邪热未尽，深伏阴分之证。以夜热早凉，热退无汗，至夜复热为辨证要点。对于杂病阴虚，夜热不退者，可以本方酌加石斛、地骨皮、天花粉等养阴清热。

清骨散《证治准绳》

[**组成**] 银柴胡一钱五分（4.5克） 胡黄连 秦艽 鳖甲醋炙 地骨皮 青蒿 知母各一钱（各3克） 甘草五分（1.5克）

[**用法**] 原方水二盅，煎八分，食远服。

现代用法：水煎服。

[**功效**] 清虚热，退骨蒸。

[**主治**] 阴虚骨蒸劳热，唇红颧赤，形瘦盗汗，舌红少苔，脉细数。

[**方解**]

本方证乃肝肾阴亏，虚火内扰所致。方中重用银柴胡清虚热退骨蒸，而无苦泄升散之弊，《本草经疏》[51]谓其"专用治劳热骨蒸"，故为君药；地骨皮、胡黄连、知母能除阴分之热，从内而清，青蒿、秦艽能除肝胆之热，从外而散，鳖甲滋阴清热，又能引药入里，以退骨蒸，共为辅佐药；少量甘草调和诸药，以免苦寒之品损伤胃气，为使药。本方集清热退蒸之品而用之，侧重于清，故方以"清骨"名之。

[临床运用]

本方为治疗骨蒸劳热的常用方剂，对于阴虚火旺，骨蒸潮热者，甚为有效。若阴虚较甚，潮热又不太严重，可去胡黄连、银柴胡、秦艽，加入生地、丹皮滋阴清热。

第七章

开窍剂

凡以芳香开窍药物为主组成，具有开窍启闭的作用，以治疗窍闭神昏之症的方剂，统称开窍剂。

第一节 凉 开

凉开剂适用于温邪热毒内陷心包，痰热蒙蔽心窍的热闭证。症见高热、神昏、谵语，甚则痉厥。其他如感触秽恶之气，卒然昏倒，不省人事，或中风窍闭，见有热象者，亦可选用。

本类方剂常用清热解毒泻火的牛黄、犀角、黄连、石膏等配伍芳香开窍的麝香、冰片、安息香等组成。若热盛动风，出现抽搐痉厥者，多配伍羚羊角、玳瑁等凉肝熄风之品。清热解毒的目的在于消除温邪热毒，以去内陷心包之病因；芳香开窍的目的在于治疗窍闭神昏的主症。代表方有安宫牛黄丸、紫雪丹、至宝丹等。

安宫牛黄丸《温病条辨》

[组成] 牛黄 郁金 犀角 黄连 朱砂 山栀 雄黄 黄芩各一两（各30克） 梅片 麝香各二钱五分（各7.5克） 珍珠五钱（15克） 金箔衣

[用法] 原方为极细末，炼老蜜为丸，每丸一钱，金箔为衣，蜡护。脉虚者人参汤下，脉实者银花、薄荷汤下，每服一丸。兼治飞尸卒厥，五痫中恶，大人小儿痉厥之因于热者。大人病重体实者，每再服，甚至日三服；小儿服半丸，不知，再服半丸。

现代用法：共为极细末，炼蜜为丸，每丸 3 克，金箔为衣（或有不用者），每服一丸，日服一至二次，水调服。小儿根据年龄酌减。

[功效]　清热解毒，豁痰开窍。

[主治]　温热病，热邪内陷心包，痰热蒙蔽心窍而致高热烦躁，神昏谵语，舌蹇肢厥，舌赤中黄浊，口气重。亦治中风窍闭、小儿惊厥属痰热内闭者。

[方解]

叶天士《外感温热篇》说："温邪上受，首先犯肺，逆传心包。"热毒内陷，必以清解心包热毒为主，但痰热相搏，痰浊不祛，热邪难清，故欲清心包之热邪，必当开泄痰浊之闭阻。方中牛黄清心解毒，熄风定惊，豁痰开窍，一药而三用，犀角（现水角牛代）清热凉血，解毒定惊，二味共为君药；珍珠、朱砂助犀角善清心热，镇心定惊，郁金清热凉血，冰片芳香开窍，雄黄劫痰解毒，麝香开窍辟秽，且后四味药均具芳香之性，使包络邪热温毒一齐由内透达于外，并能豁痰开窍，则秽浊自消，神明可复，黄连、黄芩、山栀清热解毒，使邪热一齐俱散，以上均为辅佐药；金箔入心经，镇心坠痰，蜂蜜调和诸药，共为使药。诸药合用，共奏清热解毒、豁痰开窍之效。心包乃心之宫城，《灵枢·邪客》说："心者，五脏六腑之大主也，精神之所舍也，其脏坚固，邪弗能容也。客之则心伤，心伤则神去，神去则死矣。故诸邪之在于心者，皆在于心之包络。"本方能清心包之热，又以牛黄为君药，制成丸剂，故名"安宫牛黄丸"。

[临床运用]

本方为清热解毒、豁痰开窍的重要方剂，凡属痰热蒙蔽心包，神昏谵语者，均可使用。中风、小儿惊厥属痰热内闭者，亦可配合清热涤痰药同用。

紫雪丹（原名紫雪、紫雪散）《外台秘要》引苏恭 [52] 方

[组成]　石膏　寒水石　磁石　滑石各三斤（各1500克）犀角屑　羚羊角屑　青木香　沉香各五两（各150克）玄参　升麻各一斤（各500克）甘草炙，八两（250克）丁香一两（30克）黄金百两（3000克）朴硝精者，十斤（5000克）硝石四升（1500克）朱砂研，三两（90克）麝香研，五分（1.5克）

[用法] 原方以水一斛，先煮五种金石药，得四斗，去滓后内八物，煮取一斗五升，去滓，取硝石四升，芒硝亦可，用朴硝精者十斤，投汁中，微炭上煮，柳木篦搅勿住手，有七升，投在木盆中，半日欲凝，内成研朱砂三两，细研麝香当门子五分，内中搅调，寒之二日成霜雪紫色。病人强壮者，一服二分，当利热毒，老弱人或热毒微者，一服一分，以意节之。

现代用法：制成散剂，每服1.5～3克，日服1～2次，冷开水调下，小儿用量酌减。

[功效] 清热解毒，镇痉开窍。

[主治] 温热病，热邪内陷心包，壮热烦躁，昏狂谵语，口渴唇焦，尿赤便闭，甚至痉厥，舌赤无苔，以及小儿热盛痉厥。

[方解]

本方证乃因热邪炽盛，内陷心包，营热动风所致。方中石膏、寒水石清热泻火，除烦止渴，滑石寒能清热，滑能利窍，引邪热从小便而去，三石合用，以退壮热而除烦渴；犀角清心凉血解毒，且其气清香，寒而不遏，善透包络邪热，羚羊角凉肝熄风，清热解毒，犀、羚并用，为治心营热盛，营热动风之良剂；麝香辛温走窜，芳香开窍，以上诸药，为方中主要部分。玄参、升麻、甘草泻火解毒，其中玄参并能养阴生津，甘草兼以和胃安中；黄金、磁石、朱砂重镇安神；木香、沉香、丁香行气化浊，以助麝香芳香开窍；朴硝、硝石泻热润燥，泻火通便，导邪热从大便而出，以上诸药，均为方中辅助部分。诸药合用，共奏清热解毒，熄风镇痉，开窍安神之效。药成霜雪紫色，其性大寒，故名之曰"紫雪"。

[临床运用]

本方为清热解毒，镇痉开窍的重要方剂。主要用治温热病热毒炽盛，热邪内陷心包，心营热盛，引动肝风而致的壮热烦躁，昏狂谵语，痉厥等症，亦可用治小儿热盛惊厥属营热动风者。并治小儿麻疹，热毒内盛，疹色紫红，或透发不畅，高热、喘促、昏迷，指纹紫红者。

至宝丹《太平惠民和剂局方》

[组成] 生乌犀屑研 朱砂研飞 雄黄研飞 生玳瑁屑研 琥珀研，各一两

（各30克） 麝香研 龙脑研，各一分（各0.3克） 金箔半入药，半为衣 银箔研，各五十片（各50片） 牛黄研，半两（15克） 安息香一两半，为末，以无灰酒搅，澄，飞过，滤去沙土，约得净数一两，慢火熬成膏（45克）

[用法] 原方将犀角、玳瑁为细末，入余药研匀。将安息香膏重汤煮凝成后，入诸药中和搜成剂，盛不津器中，并旋丸如桐子大，用人参汤化下三丸至五丸。又疗小儿诸痫急惊心热，卒中客忤，不得眠睡，烦躁风涎搐搦，每二岁儿服二丸，人参汤化下。

现代用法：每服一丸（重3克），研碎，温开水和服，小儿半丸。

[功效] 化浊开窍，清热解毒。

[主治] 中暑、中风、中恶（感触秽浊之气，卒然昏不知人，气闷欲绝）及温病痰热内闭，神昏不语，痰盛气粗，身热烦躁，舌质红绛苔黄垢腻，脉滑数，以及小儿惊厥属于痰热内闭者。

[方解]

本方所治诸症，皆是热邪内扰，痰浊蒙蔽心包所致。方中犀角清营凉血解毒，善透包络邪热，牛黄清热解毒，开窍豁痰，两味共为君药；玳瑁助犀角清热解毒，龙脑芳香，走窜开窍，麝香芳香走窜，开窍辟秽，安息香香而不燥，窜而不烈，芳香开窍，辟秽化浊，三香合用，助牛黄化浊豁痰开窍，以上四味共为臣药；又有雄黄劫痰解毒，琥珀、朱砂镇心安神，为佐药。金银箔入心经，重镇安神，为使药。诸药合用，共奏化浊开窍，清热解毒之功。因本方药物贵重，疗效卓著，故名之曰"至宝丹"。

[临床运用]

本方以化浊开窍为主，清热解毒为辅，是治疗痰热蒙蔽心包，神昏内闭的重要方剂。原书服法用人参汤化下本方，确有深意。在病情复杂，正气危殆之际，借助人参益气养心之力，与辛香开窍药同用，对启复神明，扶正祛邪，极著功效。但应以兼见脉虚，汗出肢冷，属内闭外脱者为宜。原书另有用童子小便合生姜自然汁化下本方一法，以加强清热开窍之效，适用于脉滑数实者，在临床上亦有参考价值。

第二节 温 开

温开剂适用于中风、痰厥、中恶突然昏倒，牙关紧闭，不省人事，苔白脉迟，属于寒邪痰湿气闭之证。常用芳香开窍药如苏合香、冰片、麝香等，配伍辛温行气化浊的药物为主组成方剂。代表方有苏合香丸。温开剂除了温通开窍，以治疗寒闭证外，并能理气止痛，辟秽解毒，用治胸腹疼痛，霍乱吐泻等症。

苏合香丸《外台秘要》引《广济方》[53]

[组成] 吃力伽（即白术） 青木香 乌犀屑 香附 朱砂 诃黎勒 檀香 安息香 沉香 麝香 丁香 荜茇各二两（各60克） 龙脑 苏合香 薰陆香（即乳香）各半两（各15克）

[用法] 原方十五味捣筛，白蜜和为丸，每朝取井华水服如梧子四丸，于净器中研破服之。老小一丸。

现代用法：加炼蜜为丸，每丸重3克，每服一丸，温开水送下，小儿用量酌减。

[功效] 温通开窍，行气化浊。

[主治]

1. 中风、中气，猝然昏倒，双手紧握，牙关紧闭，面白唇青，呼吸粗促有力，不省人事，脉沉滑，苔白滑腻。或感触秽恶之气，胸腹满痛，甚则昏不知人。

2. 感触寒湿秽浊之气，霍乱吐利，时气瘴疟，苔白滑腻。

[方解]

本方为"温开"法的代表方剂。方中苏合香开窍逐秽，《本经逢原》[54]谓其"聚诸香之气而成，能透诸窍脏，辟一切不正之气。凡痰积气厥，必先以此开导，治痰以理气为本也"；安息香开窍逐秽，香而不燥，窜而不烈；龙脑、麝香辟秽开窍，走窜经络。以上四药，为本方主要部分。沉香、檀香、丁香、木香、乳香、香附子诸香行气解郁，散寒化浊，以解除脏腑气血之郁滞；荜茇助上述十种香药，以增强温中散寒之功；并取犀角咸寒，清心解毒，其气清香，清灵透发，寒而不遏，朱砂镇心安神，以心为火脏，不受辛热散气之品，故反佐之；更有白术甘温健脾以固中气，并助诸药运化输布于周身，诃子温涩敛气，与诸香配伍，以防辛散太过，耗伤正气；以上诸药，为本方辅助部分。全方集辛香之品于一炉，但又有升有降，有散有收，共奏温通开窍，行气化浊之功。

[临床运用]

本方为"温开"法的代表方剂，凡中风、中气、感触秽恶之气（中恶），而见猝然昏倒，牙关紧闭，不省人事，苔白滑腻，属阴闭者，均可用之。

第八章

补益剂

凡以补益药为主组成，能补益人体气血阴阳的不足，用以治疗各种虚证的方剂，统称补益剂。属于"八法"中的"补法"。

补益的方剂较多，在临床运用时，主要针对气、血、阴、阳之虚，而分为补气、补血、气血双补、补阴、补阳等五类。

第一节　补　气

补气剂，适用于脾肺气虚的病证。症见倦怠乏力，少气懒言，语言轻微，面色萎白或萎黄，动则气促，食少便溏，形体瘦弱，脉虚弱或虚大，舌质淡苔薄白，舌边或有齿痕。常用补气药如人参、党参、黄芪、白术、山药、炙甘草等为主组成方剂。气贵流通，故补气方中每配少量理气的陈皮、木香、砂仁之类，以防甘药壅气之弊。代表方有四君子汤、参苓白术散、补中益气汤、生脉散等。

四君子汤《鸡峰普济方》[55]

[组成]　人参　白术　茯苓　甘草各一两（各30克）

[用法]　原方为细末，每服二钱，水一盏，入生姜三片、枣一枚，同煎至六分，去滓温服，不以时。

现代用法：水煎服，用量按原方比例酌减，或作丸剂，温开水送服6～12克，日服二次。

[功效]　益气补中，健脾养胃。

[主治] 脾胃气虚，面色萎黄或萎白，言语轻微，四肢无力，食少便溏，舌质淡苔薄白，脉来虚弱。

[方解]

脾主运化，胃司受纳，为气血生化之源。方中人参甘苦温，大补元气，健脾养胃，为君药；脾喜燥恶湿，脾虚不运，每易生湿，故以白术苦甘温，健脾益气，燥湿和中，为臣药；茯苓甘淡平，健脾补中渗湿，黄宫绣[56]说："茯苓入四君，则佐参、术以渗脾家之湿。"张秉成[57]亦说："渗肺脾之湿浊下行，然后参、术之功益彰其效。"故为佐药；炙甘草甘温益气，补中和胃，为使药。诸药合用，共奏益气补中，健脾养胃之功。本方四味，皆平和之品，具冲和之德，故名之曰"四君子"。

[临床运用]

本方为治疗脾胃气虚的基本方剂。很多补气健脾的方剂，是从本方衍化而来的。对于各种原因引起的脾胃气虚，均可以本方加减运用。

参苓白术散《太平惠民和剂局方》

[组成] 莲子肉　薏苡仁　缩砂仁　桔梗炒令深黄色，各一斤（各500克）白扁豆姜汁浸，微炒，一斤半（750克）　白茯苓　人参去芦　甘草炒　白术　山药各二斤（各1000克）

[用法] 原方为细末，每服二钱，枣汤调下，小儿量岁数加减。

现代用法：为细末，每服6克，枣汤调下，日服二次。或作丸剂吞服。也可作汤剂，水煎服，用量按原方比例酌减。

[功效] 健脾益气，和胃渗湿。

[主治] 脾胃虚弱，湿自内生，饮食不消，或吐或泻，面色萎黄，四肢无力，胸脘胀满，苔白腻，脉虚缓。

[方解]

脾胃强者，自能胜湿。若脾胃虚弱，则运化失职，湿自内生。本方由四君子汤加山药、扁豆、莲肉、薏苡仁、砂仁、桔梗等组成。方中参、苓、白术益气健脾，为君药；臣以山药、扁豆、莲肉、薏苡仁以增强君药益气健脾之效，且茯苓、白术、扁豆、薏苡仁健脾而兼渗湿；佐以炙甘草益气和中，砂仁芳香化湿，和胃理气；桔梗为使，载药上行，升清即所以降浊，湿祛则有助于健脾。诸药合用，补其虚，除其湿，行其滞，调其气，俟脾健湿去，诸症自愈。

[临床运用]

本方药性平和，温而不燥，是健脾益气，和胃渗湿的常用方剂。本方尚能补肺气之虚，理气化痰，增进食欲，故亦能用治肺虚劳损，乃培土生金之法。

补中益气汤《脾胃论》[58]

[组成] 黄芪病甚劳役热甚者一钱（18克） 甘草炙，以上各五分（9克） 人参去芦，三分（9克） 当归酒焙干或晒干，二分（6克） 橘皮不去白，二分或三分（6克）升麻二分或三分（6克） 柴胡二分或三分（6克） 白术三分（9克）

[用法] 原方㕮咀，都作一服，水二盏，煎至一盏……去渣，食远稍热服。

现代用法：水煎服。或作丸剂，每服6～9克，每日2～3次，温开水送服。

[功效] 补中益气，升阳举陷。

[主治]

1.气虚发热，身热有汗，渴喜热饮，头痛恶寒，懒言恶食，脉虽洪大，按之虚软；或脾胃气虚，四肢倦怠，不耐作劳，动则气喘，舌质淡苔薄白。

2.气虚下陷，脱肛，子宫脱垂，久疟，久痢，便血，崩漏，大便泄泻，小便淋漓不禁，及一切清阳下陷诸症。

[方解]

《脾胃论》说："真气又名元气，乃先身生之精气也，非胃气不能滋之。""脾胃之气既伤，而元气亦不能充，而诸病之所由生也。"又说："饮食不节则胃病……形体劳役则脾病。"本方系李东垣[59]根据《素问·至真要大论》"劳者温之""损者益之"之旨而制。方中重用黄芪，味甘微温，入脾肺经，补肺气而固表，益中气而升阳，故为君药；臣以人参、炙甘草甘温，补脾益气，助黄芪益气补中。东垣说："参、芪、甘草，泻火之圣药。"盖烦劳则虚而生热，得甘温以补元气，虚热自退；佐以白术健脾，当归补血，陈皮理气；使以升麻、柴胡，升举清阳，配合君药升提下陷之阳气。正如《本草纲目》所说："升麻引阳明清气上行，柴胡引少阳清气上行，此乃禀赋素弱，元气虚馁，及劳役饥饱，生冷内伤，脾胃引经最要药也。"诸药合用，共奏补中益气，升阳举陷之效。

[临床运用]

1. 本方为补气升阳的代表方剂，临床用治中气不足，气虚下陷之证，确有疗效。

2. 升提药与补气药同用是本方配伍特点。若不用升提药，则升阳举陷之功不显；若不用补气药，升提无济于事。气虚而后清阳下陷，故必以补气药为主，气足则陷自升。升提药只用少量即可，不必过多。

生脉散《内外伤辨惑论》[60]

[组成]　人参（10克）　麦冬（15克）　五味子（6克）[原方未著分量]

[用法]　原方未著用法。

现代用法：水煎服。

[功效]　益气生津，敛阴止汗。

[主治]

1. 热伤元气，气阴两虚，气短倦怠，口渴多汗，脉虚细或虚数，甚则大汗不止，喘喝欲脱，脉散大无根，舌干红无苔。

2. 久咳肺虚，咳呛少痰，短气自汗，口干舌燥，脉虚者。

[方解]

热伤元气，气阴两虚。方中人参甘温，大补元气，止渴生津，为君药；臣以麦冬甘寒，养阴清热，润肺生津；佐以五味子酸温，敛肺止汗而生津。其中麦冬并能清心育阴，五味子又可固肾气，敛心气。三药合用，一补、一清、一敛，共成益气养阴，敛汗生津之功。汪昂说："人有将死脉绝者，服此能复生之，其功甚大。"本方能使气充而脉复，故以"生脉"名之。

[临床运用]

本方为治疗热伤元气，气阴两虚的常用方剂，可用于温热病伤津耗气所致的津气欲脱之证，有补气生津，敛阴固脱之效。夏季暑热耗伤气阴，汗出过多，神疲口渴者，亦可运用本方治疗。

第二节 补 血

补血剂，适用于血虚的病证。症见头晕眼花，面色苍白或萎黄，爪甲无华，心悸怔忡，失眠多梦，筋脉挛急，皮肤干燥，头发干枯，脉细弱或细涩，舌质淡苔薄白。妇女则月事不调，多见经行后期，量少色淡，甚至闭经。常用补血药物如熟地、当归、白芍、龙眼肉等为主组成方剂。然而有形之血不能自生，生于无形之气；气为血之帅，血为气之母，气血相互依存，若失血过多，往往气亦随之而衰。故补血剂中常配伍人参、黄芪之类益气生血。代表方有四物汤、当归补血汤、归脾汤等。

四物汤《太平惠民和剂局方》

[组成] 当归去芦，酒浸微炒　川芎　白芍药　熟地黄酒蒸，各等分

[用法] 原方为粗末，每服三钱，水一盏半，煎至八分，去渣热服，空心食前。若妊娠胎动不安，下血不止者，加艾十叶，阿胶一片，同煎如前法。或血脏虚冷，崩中去血过多，亦加胶艾煎。

现代用法：水煎服，用量按原方比例酌情增减。

[功效] 补血和血调经。

[主治] 营血虚滞，症见惊惕，头晕，目眩，爪甲无华，妇人经水不调，或月经量少，或经闭不行，脐腹作痛，舌质淡苔白，脉弦细或细涩。

[方解]

心主血，肝藏血。方中熟地甘微温，滋阴补血，为君药；臣以当归甘辛苦温，补血养肝，和血调经；佐以白芍苦酸微寒，养血柔肝，和营止痛；使以川芎辛温，活血理气。其中地、芍为血中之阴药，归、芎为血中之阳药，四药相合，可使补而不滞，营血调和。因此，不仅血虚之证可用本方补血，即血滞之证亦可用本方和血，补中有散，散中有收，而为治理血分疾病的基本方剂。

[临床运用]

1. 本方为补血和血的基本方,亦为调经的常用方。凡血虚、血滞、月经不调及胎前产后诸症,常可用本方加减治之。

2. 临床若以补血为主,本方可加重熟地、白芍用量,当归改用当归身,少用或不用川芎;若以和血为主,本方可加重当归、川芎用量,白芍改为赤芍;若血虚有热,可将熟地改为生地。

当归补血汤《内外伤辨惑论》

[组成] 黄芪一两(30克) 当归酒洗,二钱(6克)

[用法] 原方㕮咀,都作一服,水二盏,煎至一盏,去渣温服,空心食前。

现代用法:水煎服。

[功效] 补气生血。

[主治] 劳倦内伤,血虚气弱,阳浮外越,肌热面赤,烦渴引饮,脉洪大而虚,重按则微,以及妇女月经过多、崩漏,产后血虚发热,或疮疡溃后,久不愈合。

[方解]

劳倦内伤,元气不足,阴血亦亏。有形之血生于无形之气,故方中重用黄芪甘温补气,以资生血之源,《本草备要》[61]且谓其"泻阴火,解肌热";配以当归甘辛苦温,为养血之要品,补营之圣药。黄芪剂量五倍于当归,取阳生阴长,气旺血自生之义。

[临床运用]

本方为补气生血的代表方剂,多用于血虚发热之证。以脉洪大而虚,重按则微为辨证要点。

归脾汤《济生方》[62]

[组成] 白术(9克) 茯神去木(12克) 黄芪去芦(12克) 龙眼肉(12克)酸枣仁炒去壳,各一两(12克) 人参(9克) 木香不见火,各半两(6克) 甘草炙,二钱半(4.5克) 当归(9克) 远志各一钱(3克)[后二味从《校注妇人良方》补入]

［**用法**］ 原方㕮咀，每服四钱，水一盏半，生姜五片，枣子一枚，煎至七分，去渣，温服，不拘时候。

现代用法：加生姜3片，大枣5枚，水煎服。或作丸剂，每服6～9克，每日2～3次，温开水送下。

［**功效**］ 益气补血，健脾养心。

［**主治**］ 思虑过度，损伤心脾，怔忡健忘，惊悸盗汗，四肢倦怠，食少不眠；或脾虚不能摄血，而见吐血、衄血、便血；以及妇女月经不调，崩中漏下。舌质淡苔薄白，脉细弱。

［**方解**］

心藏神而主血，脾主思而统血，思虑过度则损伤心脾。方中黄芪、人参甘微温，补脾益气，龙眼肉甘平，补心安神，益脾养血，共为君药；白术苦甘温，助参、芪补脾益气，茯神、酸枣仁甘平，助龙眼养心安神，当归甘辛苦温，滋养营血，与参、芪配伍，补血之力更强，以上并为臣药；远志苦辛温，交通心肾，宁心安神，木香辛苦温，理气醒脾，使诸益气养血之品补而不壅，共为佐药；炙甘草甘温益气，调和诸药，生姜、大枣调和营卫，共为使药。合而成方，养心与健脾同用，养心不离补血，健脾不离补气，气血充足则心神安而脾运健。本方多用益气健脾药，因为心血是由脾转输的精微所化，《灵枢·决气》说："中焦受气取汁，变化而赤，是谓血。"补脾气即所以养心血也。脾统血，脾气健旺则能统血摄血，血自归脾，故名之曰"归脾汤"。

［**临床运用**］

本方为治疗心脾两虚，气血不足的常用方剂，以惊悸怔忡，健忘失眠，倦怠食少，舌质淡苔薄白，脉细弱为辨证要点。

第三节　气血双补

气血双补剂，适用于气血俱虚的病证。症见面色无华，头晕目眩，心悸气短，食少倦怠，舌质淡苔薄白，脉细弱无力。常用补气药如人参、黄芪、甘草、大枣与补血药如地黄、当归、白芍、阿胶等为主组成方剂。代表方有八珍汤、薯蓣丸、炙甘草汤等。

八珍汤《正体类要》[63]

[组成]　人参　白术　白茯苓　当归　川芎　白芍药　熟地黄各一钱（各9克）甘草炙，五分（4.5克）

[用法]　原方姜、枣煎服。

现代用法：加生姜3片、大枣5枚，水煎服。

[功效]　气血双补。

[主治]　气血两虚，面色苍白或萎黄，头晕目眩，四肢倦怠，气短懒言，心悸怔忡，纳食不馨，舌质淡苔薄白，脉细弱或虚大无力。亦治失血过多，恶寒发热，烦躁作渴，或疮疡久溃，不能愈合。

[方解]

本方统治气血两虚的病症。本方由四君子汤合四物汤组成。方中参、术、苓、草以益气，地、芍、归、芎以养血，姜、枣调和营卫，合成气血双补之剂，共奏阳生阴长之功。

[临床运用]

本方常用于久病虚弱，妇人月经不调、崩漏、胎萎不长、产后虚损、疮疡久不收口等证属气血两虚者。

薯蓣丸《金匮要略》

[组成]　薯蓣三十分（22.5克）当归　桂枝　神曲　干地黄　豆黄卷各十分（各7.5克）甘草二十八分（21克）人参七分（5.3克）芎䓖　芍药　白术　麦门冬　杏仁各六分（各4.5克）柴胡　桔梗　茯苓各五分（3.8克）阿胶七分（5.3克）干姜三分（2.3克）白蔹二分（1.5克）防风六分（4.5克）大枣百枚为膏（30枚）

[用法]　原方二十一味，末之，炼蜜和丸如弹子大，空腹酒服一丸，一百丸为剂。

现代用法：研末，炼蜜为丸，每服6～9克，每日2次，温开水或黄酒送下。

[功效]　补虚祛风。

[主治]　虚劳，头目眩晕，纳减羸瘦，身重少气，肢痛麻木。

[方解]

虚劳怯弱，外风容易侵袭人体。方中重用薯蓣（即山药），味甘性平，补脾胃，疗虚损，《神农本草经》谓其"主伤中，补虚赢，除寒热邪气，补中，益气力，长肌肉，强阴"，兼擅补虚祛风之长，故为本方君药；参、术、苓、草、干姜、大枣益气温阳，地、芍、归、芎、麦冬、阿胶养血滋阴，以助薯蓣补虚益损，共为臣药；桂枝、柴胡、防风、白蔹升散走表，祛风清热，杏仁、桔梗升降气机，大豆黄卷专泄水湿，神曲消食和胃，使诸补益之品补而不滞，共为佐药；甘草、大枣又能调和诸药，为使药。全方补中寓散，用小量丸剂缓缓调治，则虚损渐复，风气渐去。

[临床运用]

1.《千金方》将本方载入风眩门，添了黄芩，改阿胶为鹿角胶，用治虚劳风眩。

2. 根据岳美中教授经验，本方适用于老年人气血虚损，常有周身不适，头眩、肢痛麻木诸证，所谓"风眩""风痹"或"五劳七伤"者。而且，本方对平素睡眠欠佳，精神不支，阴阳气血不足者，俱可运用，有滋补强壮作用。

炙甘草汤（又名复脉汤）《伤寒论》

[组成] 甘草四两，炙（12克） 生姜三两，切（9克） 桂枝三两，去皮（9克）人参二两（6克） 生地黄一斤（30克） 阿胶二两（6克） 麦门冬半升，去心（12克）麻仁半升（12克） 大枣三十枚，擘（10枚）

[用法] 原方九味，以清酒七升，水八升，先煮八味，取三升，去滓，内胶烊消尽，温服一升，日三服。

现代用法：水中加白酒60克煎药取汁，再入阿胶烊消后服用。

[功效] 滋阴养血，益气通阳。

[主治]

1.心脏阴阳气血俱虚，脉结代，心动悸，虚赢少气，舌淡红少苔或淡嫩而干。

2.肺痿，咳嗽，涎唾多，短气赢瘦，心悸，自汗，咽干舌燥，大便干结，脉虚数或迟者。

[方解]

《素问·脉要精微论》说"代则气衰"。成无己说："结代之脉，动而中止能自还者，名曰结；不能自还者，名曰代。由血气虚衰，不能相续也。心中悸动，知真气内虚也。"说明脉结代、心动悸，为心之阴阳气血俱虚所致，阴血不足则心失所养，阳气不振则鼓动无力。仲景此方，命名为炙甘草汤，显系以炙甘草为君药，取其甘温益气，《别录》谓其"通经脉，利血气"，故能用治"脉结代，心动悸"；臣以生地、麦冬、阿胶、麻仁滋阴养血，人参、大枣益气生津；佐以桂枝、生姜辛温通阳，调和血脉，且大队补益药中配伍桂枝、生姜，则滋阴养血而不腻，益气生津而不壅，使补益药更好地发挥作用；使以清酒，活血以通经脉，血脉流通，脉始复常。且方中地黄用量独重，以酒煎煮，则不至于滋腻损伤脾胃，而养血滋阴之功益著。合而用之，滋心阴，养心血，益心气，温心阳，使气血充足，阴阳调和，则能定悸复脉，故又名之曰"复脉汤"。

[临床运用]

本方为治疗心脏阴阳气血俱虚，脉结代、心动悸的效方。《千金翼方》[64]以本方"治虚劳不足，汗出而闷，脉结心悸，行动如常，不出百日，危急者二十一日死"。《外台秘要》以本方"治肺痿涎唾多，心中温温液液者"。《医方集解》引喻嘉言曰："《外台》所取在于益肺气之虚，润肺金之燥，至于桂枝辛热，似有不宜，不知桂枝能通营卫，致津液，则肺气自能转输，涎沫以渐而下，尤为要紧，所以云治心中温温液液也。"

第四节 补 阴

补阴剂，适用于阴虚的病证。症见形体消瘦，口燥咽干，虚烦不眠，肠燥便秘，头晕耳鸣，腰酸腿软，甚则骨蒸盗汗，喘咳咯血，颧红，消渴，遗精梦泄，舌红少苔，脉细数。阴虚则生内热，往往可见虚火上炎的症状，此时若单用苦寒清热，不能收效。《素问·至真要大论》说："诸寒之而热者，取之阴。"王冰说："壮水之主，以制阳光。"都是指补阴方法而言，补阴则虚火自降。本类方剂，常用补阴药如地黄、龟板、沙参、麦冬、枸杞子、知母、山药、山茱萸等为主组成，代表方有六味地黄丸、左归饮、大补阴丸、一贯煎等。

六味地黄丸（原名地黄丸）《小儿药证直诀》

[组成]　熟地黄八钱（24克）　山茱肉　干山药各四钱（各12克）　泽泻　牡丹皮　白茯苓去皮，各三钱（各9克）

[用法]　原方为末，炼蜜丸如梧子大，空心温水化下三丸。

现代用法：研细末，炼蜜为丸，每服6～9克，每日2～3次，空腹用温开水或淡盐汤送下，亦可作汤剂，水煎服。

[功效]　滋阴补肾。

[主治]　肾阴不足，腰膝酸软，头晕目眩，耳鸣耳聋，盗汗，遗精，消渴，骨蒸潮热，手足心热，小便淋沥，牙齿动摇，舌干咽痛，足跟作痛，以及小儿囟开不合，舌红少苔，脉细数或尺脉虚大。

[方解]

肾藏精，为先天之本，肾阴不足，则变生诸症。方中重用熟地甘微温，入肝肾经，滋阴补血，填精益髓，大补真阴，为壮水之要药，故为君药。山茱肉酸涩微温，入肝肾经，补肝肾，秘精气，肾气受益则封藏得度，肝阴得养则疏泄无虞；山药甘平，入肺脾肾三经，健脾补肺，固肾益精，取土旺生金，金盛生水之义，均为臣药。以上三药以补肾为主，或兼补肝，或兼补脾，是为三补。泽泻甘寒，入肾、膀胱经，利水渗湿泄热，祛肾中之邪水；丹皮辛苦微寒，入心肝肾经，清热凉血，和血消瘀，泻阴中之伏火，以治虚火上炎；茯苓甘淡平，入心脾肺经，补益心脾，淡渗利湿，助山药以益脾，配泽泻以利水，共为佐使药。以上三药，是为三泻。合而成方，"非但治肝肾不足，实三阴并治之剂。有熟地之腻补肾水，即有泽泻之宣泄肾浊以济之；有茱肉之温涩肝经，即有丹皮之清泻肝火以佐之；有山药之收摄脾经，即有茯苓之淡渗脾湿以和之。药止六味，而大开大合，三阴并治，洵补方之正鹄也"（《医方论》）。总之，本方滋补而不留邪，降泄而不伤正，以补为主，补中有泻，寓泻于补，则补而不滞，为通补开合之剂，非专事蛮补者可比。

[临床运用]

本方系钱乙[65]从《金匮要略》肾气丸去桂、附而成，原为主治小儿肾虚诸病。肾主藏精，又主水液，故以"三补"填其精，苓、泽利其水，阴虚则火旺，故用丹皮泻相火。方中"三补"补其正，"三泻"泻其邪，祛邪是为了更好地补正。"三补"为主，故用量较重，而"三泻"的用量则较轻。临床上凡见上述肾阴不足的证候，均可运用本方加减治之。

左归饮《景岳全书》

[组成]　熟地二三钱或加至一二两（6～60克）　山药二钱（6克）　枸杞二钱（6克）　茯苓一钱五分（4.5克）　山茱萸一二钱，畏酸者少用之（3～6克）　炙甘草一钱（3克）

[用法]　原方水二盅，煎七分，食远服。

现代用法：水煎服。

[功效]　补肾养阴。

[主治]　真阴不足，腰酸，遗泄，盗汗，口渴欲饮，舌光红，脉细略数。

[方解]

真阴，又名元阴、真精，藏于肾。《素问·上古天真论》说："肾者主水，受五脏六腑之精而藏之。"本方为纯甘壮水之剂。方中重用熟地滋肾水，填真阴，以为君药；臣以枸杞子、山茱萸补益肝肾，助君药补肾养阴；佐以山药滋肾阴，养胃阴，茯苓健脾气，养胃阴；使以炙甘草调和诸药，且能滋养脾胃气阴，盖土润可以滋肾，先天之精须赖后天水谷之精，方能不断资生。诸药合用，滋肾水并养肝阴，补先天不忘后天，共奏补益肾水，滋养真阴之功。因其能补左肾真水，使阴精得归其原，故方以"左归"名之。

[临床运用]

本方导源于六味地黄丸，也由六味药组成，但两者略有不同。六味地黄丸寓泻于补，适用于阴虚火炎之证；本方为纯甘壮水之剂，以证属纯虚，故无取泽泻之泄，丹皮之凉。

大补阴丸（原名大补丸）《丹溪心法》

[组成] 黄柏炒褐色 知母酒浸，炒，各四两（各120克） 熟地黄酒蒸 龟板酥炙，各六两（各180克）

[用法] 原方为末，猪脊髓、蜜丸，服七十丸，空心盐白汤下。

现代用法：为细末，猪脊髓适量蒸熟，捣如泥状，再加炼蜜和丸，如梧桐子大，每服6～9克，早晚各服一次，盐开水送下；或作汤剂，水煎服，用量按原方比例酌减。

[功效] 降火滋阴。

[主治] 阴虚火旺，骨蒸潮热，盗汗遗精，咳嗽咯血，心烦易怒，足膝疼热，舌红少苔，尺脉数而有力。

[方解]

真阴不足，相火必旺。方中黄柏苦寒，坚真阴而制相火，知母苦寒，滋阴降火，润肺清金，《本草纲目》谓其"下则润肾燥而滋阴，上则清肺金而泻火"。黄柏、知母相须为用，能平相火而保真阴，有金水相生之妙，此属清源之举。熟地甘微温，滋肾养阴，填精补髓；龟板咸甘平，滋阴潜阳，壮水制火，为肾经要药；猪脊髓乃血肉有情之品，以髓补髓，均能益肾水以退虚火，此属培本之图。合而成为降火滋阴之剂，使相火得清，真阴得补，诸症自愈，故方名"大补阴丸"。

[临床运用]

本方为降火滋阴的代表方。朱丹溪[66]说："阴常不足，阳常有余，宜常养其阴，阴与阳齐，则水能制火，斯无病矣。"本方即依据这一理论而制定。尤其对于以阴虚火旺为临床特征的劳瘵病，丹溪认为："火旺致此病者，十居八九；火衰成此疾者，百无二三。"因此，滋阴必先降火，火降方能保存真阴，并使滋阴之品益显其功。

一贯煎《续名医类案》[67]

[组成] 北沙参（9克） 麦冬（9克） 生地黄（15克） 当归（9克） 枸杞（9克） 川楝子（4.5克）[原方未著剂量]

[用法] 原方未著用法。

现代用法：水煎服。

[功效] 滋阴疏肝。

[主治] 肝肾阴虚，肝气不舒，脘胁胀痛，吞酸吐苦，咽干口燥，脉细弱或虚弦，舌红少津。亦治疝气瘕聚。

[方解]

肝体阴而用阳，喜条达而恶抑郁。方中生地黄滋阴养血，补益肝肾，为君药；枸杞、当归养血柔肝，沙参、麦冬滋阴增液，善养肺胃之阴，知木能乘土，必先培土，又清金之所以制木，以上均为臣药；佐以川楝子疏肝理气泄热，遂肝木条达之性，虽属苦寒之品，但配入大队甘凉养阴药中，则使肝体得养，肝气条畅，诸症自除，诚为治疗阴虚脘胁疼痛的良方。

[临床运用]

1.魏玉璜[68]运用本方，尚多加减方法。如口苦燥者，加酒川连三至五分；大便秘结，加瓜蒌仁；有虚热或汗多，加地骨皮；痰多，加贝母；舌红而干，阴亏过甚，加石斛；胁胀痛，按之硬，加鳖甲；烦热而渴，加知母、石膏；腹痛，加芍药、甘草；脚弱，加牛膝、薏苡仁；不寐，加酸枣仁等等。

2.治疗脘胁胀痛一般多以理气药为主，但理气药大多性味香燥，用于肝肾阴虚之体，每致伤津耗液，反使病情增剧。故对肝肾阴虚血不养肝，肝气郁结所致的脘胁胀痛，编者多以本方为基本方。若加白芍、甘草，则柔肝止痛作用更强；加佛手、生大麦芽、绿萼梅，则疏肝理气之效尤佳，且药性平和，理气而不伤阴。

第五节 补 阳

补阳剂，是治疗阳虚证的方剂。但阳虚之中，又有心阳虚、脾阳虚、肾阳虚等不同。有关治疗心脾阳虚的方剂，已于温里剂中介绍，本节主要讨论治疗肾阳虚的方剂。凡神疲乏力，腰膝酸痛，腰以下有冷感，下肢软弱，小便清白频数，溺后余沥，阳痿早泄，脉沉细，尺部尤甚，舌质淡苔白，均属肾阳虚衰，下元失于温养之症。《素问·至真要大论》说："诸热之而寒者，取之阳。"王冰说："益火之源，以消阴翳。"都是指温补肾阳法而言。常用肉桂、附子、鹿角胶、杜仲、菟丝子、熟地、萸肉、仙茅、仙灵脾等为主组成方剂。若阳虚不能温化，气化不行，邪水停留，则应在补阳的基础上适当配伍利水药以消除邪水，恢复肾脏主水之权。代表方有肾气丸、右归饮等。

肾气丸《金匮要略》

[组成] 干地黄八两（250克） 山茱萸 薯蓣各四两（各125克） 泽泻 茯苓 牡丹皮各三两（各90克） 桂枝 附子炮,各一两（各30克）

[用法] 原方八味，末之，炼蜜和丸，梧子大，酒下十五丸，日再服。

现代用法：研末，炼蜜为丸，每服6～9克，日服二次，温开水或淡盐汤送下。也可作汤剂，水煎服，用量按原方比例酌减。

[功效] 温肾化气。

[主治] 肾阳不足，腰痛脚弱，身半以下常有冷感，少腹拘急，小便不利，或小便反多，入夜尤甚，舌淡而胖，尺脉沉细。以及痰饮、消渴、脚气、转胞等症。

[方解]

肾为先天之本，中寓命门之火，肾阳不足，不能温养下焦。方中重用干地黄滋阴补肾，为君药；臣以薯蓣固肾益精，山茱萸补肝肾，涩精气，桂枝、附子温肾扶阳；佐以牡丹皮凉肝，茯苓、泽泻利水泄浊。桂、附、山萸得丹皮则温而不燥，地黄、薯蓣、山萸配苓、泻，则补而不滞。本方在大队滋阴药中配入少量桂、附，意在微微生火，以鼓舞肾气，取"少火生气"之义，故方剂名"肾气"。阴阳互为其根，无阳则阴无以化，无阴则阳无以生。本方水火并补，滋阴助阳，使邪去正复，肾气自充。正如张景岳所说："善补阳者，必于阴中求阳，以阳得阴助，则生化无穷。"而奏"益火之源以消阴翳"之效，乃治肾之祖方。

[临床运用]

本方为治疗肾阳不足的常用方。后世运用本方时，常以熟地黄易干地黄，以肉桂易桂枝，可供参考。

右归饮《景岳全书》

[组成] 熟地二三钱或加至一二两（6～60克） 山药炒，二钱（6克） 山茱萸一钱（3克） 枸杞二钱（6克） 甘草炙，一二钱（3～6克） 肉桂一二钱（3～6克） 杜仲姜制，二钱（6克） 制附子一二三钱（3～9克）

[用法] 原方水二盅，煎七分，食远温服。

现代用法：水煎服。

[功效] 温肾填精。

[主治] 肾阳虚衰，气怯神疲，腹痛腰酸，肢冷脉细，舌淡苔白，或阴盛格阳，真寒假热之症。

[方解]

《素问·灵兰秘典论》说："肾者，作强之官，伎巧出焉。"本方从肾气丸变化而来，也由八味药组成。方中重用熟地甘微温，滋肾填精，为君药；山药甘平，健脾固肾益精，山茱萸酸微温，补肝肾，涩精气，肉桂辛甘大热，补命门不足，益火消阴，附子大辛大热，峻补元阳，益火之源，以上均为臣药；枸杞甘平，滋补肝肾，补虚益精，杜仲甘温，补肝肾，益精气，壮筋骨，共为佐药；炙甘草温中健脾，调和诸药，以为使。诸药合用，妙在阴中求阳，温肾填精，能补右肾命门之火，使元阳得归其原，故以"右归"名之。

[临床运用]

本方亦属于"益火之源"的方剂。原书说："如治阴盛格阳，真寒假热等证，宜加泽泻二钱，煎成，用凉水浸冷服之尤妙。"此即《素问·五常政大论》"治寒以热，凉而行之"的服药方法。

第九章

固涩剂

根据《素问·至真要大论》"散者收之"的原则立法，凡以收敛固涩药物为主组成，具有收敛耗散、固涩滑脱的作用，用以治疗气、血、精、津液耗散滑脱之证的方剂，统称固涩剂。属于"十剂"中"涩可固脱"的范畴。

第一节　固表止汗

固表止汗剂，适用于体虚卫外不固，阴液不能内守而致的自汗、盗汗。常以固表止汗的药物如黄芪、牡蛎、麻黄根、浮小麦等为主组成方剂，代表方有牡蛎散。本节某些方剂则于固表的同时并能消除汗出之因，如玉屏风散的以补为固，用治表虚自汗；当归六黄汤的滋阴泻火，固表止汗，用治阴虚火扰而致的盗汗，均体现了这一配伍精神。

牡蛎散《太平惠民和剂局方》

[组成]　黄芪去苗，土　麻黄根洗　牡蛎米泔浸，刷去土，火烧通赤，各一两（各30克）

[用法]　原方三味为粗散，每服三钱，水一盏半，小麦百余粒，同煎至八分，去渣热服，日二服，不拘时候。

现代用法：为粗散，每服9克，加浮小麦30克，水煎服。或加浮小麦作汤剂，用量按原方比例酌减。

[功效]　益气固表，敛阴止汗。

[主治]　体虚卫外不固，阴液外泄，常自汗出，夜卧更甚，心悸惊惕，短气烦倦，舌质淡红，脉细弱。

[方解]

《素问·阴阳应象大论》："阴在内，阳之守也；阳在外，阴之使也。"方中煅牡蛎咸涩微寒，敛阴潜阳，固涩止汗，为君药；生黄芪味甘微温，益气实卫，固表止汗，为臣药；麻黄根甘平，功专止汗，为佐药；浮小麦甘凉，专入心经，养心气，退虚热，止自汗，为使药。合而成方，益气固表，敛阴止汗，使气阴得复，自汗可止。

[临床运用]

本方为卫气不固，阴液外泄的自汗证而设，但亦可用治盗汗。如属阳虚，可加白术、附子以助阳固表；如属气虚，可加人参、白术以健脾益气；如属阴虚，可加生地、白芍以养阴止汗。自汗应重用黄芪，盗汗可再加稽豆衣、糯稻根等，则疗效尤佳。

玉屏风散《医方类聚》[69] 引《究原方》[70] 方

[组成]　防风一两（30克）　黄芪蜜炙　白术各二两（各60克）

[用法]　原方㕮咀，每三钱重，水盏半，枣一枚，煎七分，去滓，食后热服。

现代用法：研为粗末，每服6～9克，每日二次，水煎服。

[功效]　益气固表止汗。

[主治]　表虚自汗，以及虚人易感风邪者。症见自汗恶风，面色萎白，舌淡苔白，脉浮虚软。

[方解]

气虚不能卫外，卫气不固，营阴易泄。方中黄芪甘温益气，固表止汗，为君药；白术健脾益气，固表止汗，为臣药；芪、术合用，大补脾肺之气，俾脾胃健旺，肌表充实，则汗不易泄，邪不易侵。佐以防风，走表以祛风邪，且升脾中清阳，助黄芪益气御风。《本草纲目》引李杲曰："防风能制黄芪，黄芪得防风其功愈大，乃相畏而相使者也。"且黄芪得防风，固表而不恋邪；防风得黄芪，祛邪而不伤正。三药配伍，使卫强则腠理固密而邪不复侵，脾健则正气自复而内有所据，邪去则外无所扰而诸恙易愈。实为补中兼疏的安内攘外之剂。其效犹如御风的屏障，而又珍贵如玉，故名之曰"玉屏风散"。

[临床运用]

本方为益气固表止汗之良剂，主治气虚自汗及虚人易感风邪者。又可用治气虚感受风邪，自汗不解，不任表药发散者。

当归六黄汤《兰室秘藏》

[组成] 当归 生地黄 熟地黄 黄柏 黄芩 黄连以上各等分（各6克）黄芪加倍（12克）

[用法] 原方为粗末，每服五钱，水二盏，煎至一盏，食前服。小儿减半服之。

现代用法：水煎服，用量按原方比例酌情增减。

[功效] 滋阴泻火，固表止汗。

[主治] 阴虚火扰，盗汗发热，面赤心烦，口干唇燥，便难溲赤，舌红，脉数。

[方解]

素体阴虚内热。方中当归、生地黄、熟地黄滋阴养血，阴血充则火自降，共为君药；辅以黄柏、黄芩、黄连清热泻火，火热去则阴自坚，共为臣药；汗出过多，不仅耗损阴血，亦且伤及阳气，导致卫外不固，腠理不密，故倍用黄芪益气固表，以为佐药。诸药合用，使阴复热退，卫强汗止。

[临床运用]

1. 本方用治阴虚火扰之盗汗，甚为合拍。若纯属阴虚而无火者，则不宜用黄芩、黄连、黄柏等苦寒沉降之品，而当用生脉散、六味地黄丸等养阴增液为主。

2. 本方固涩之力不足，故盗汗严重者可酌加麻黄根或浮小麦、牡蛎等，其效更佳。

第二节　涩精止遗

涩精止遗剂，适用于肾虚封藏失职，精关不固所致的遗精滑泄，或肾气不足，膀胱失约所致的尿频遗尿等证。常用涩精止遗的药物如桑螵蛸、龙骨、牡蛎、芡实、莲须、金樱子等为主组成方剂。代表方有桑螵蛸散、金锁固精丸等。

桑螵蛸散《本草衍义》[71]

[组成] 桑螵蛸 远志 菖蒲 龙骨 人参 茯神 当归 龟板醋炙，以上各一两（各30克）

[用法] 原方为末，夜卧人参汤调下二钱。

现代用法：研末，每日临卧时服6克，以人参汤调服。亦可作汤剂，水煎服，用量按原方比例酌减。

[功效] 调补心肾，涩精止遗。

[主治] 心肾两虚，小便频数，或遗尿滑精，心神恍惚，健忘，舌淡苔白，脉细弱。

[方解]

本方证乃由心气不足，肾虚不摄所致。方中桑螵蛸补肾固精止遗，《别录》谓其"疗男子虚损，五脏气微，梦寐失精，遗溺"，故为君药；臣以龙骨收敛固涩且安心神，《别录》谓其"缩小便……养精神，安魂魄"，桑螵蛸得龙骨则固涩作用大为增强，小便频数，遗尿滑精可止；佐以人参大补元气，茯神益气安神，且降心气下交于肾，菖蒲善开心窍，远志安神定志，且通肾气上达于心，如此则心肾相交，更以当归补心血，龟甲滋肾阴，且人参、当归合用，能双补气血。诸药合而成方，确有交通心肾，补益气血，涩精止遗之效。

[临床运用]

本方用治心肾两虚而致小便频数或遗尿滑精者，尤宜于小儿睡中遗尿或时欲小便而不能控制者。

金锁固精丸《医方集解》

[组成] 沙苑蒺藜炒 芡实蒸 莲须各二两（各60克） 龙骨酥炙 牡蛎盐水煮一日一夜，煅粉，各一两（各30克）

[用法] 原方莲子粉糊为丸，盐汤下。

现代用法：为细末，以莲子粉糊为丸，每服6～9克，日服二次，空腹淡盐汤送下。

［功效］ 补肾固精。

［主治］ 肾虚精关不固，遗精滑泄，神疲乏力，腰痛耳鸣，舌淡苔白，脉细弱。

［方解］

《素问·六节藏象论》说："肾者主蛰，封藏之本，精之处也。"方中沙苑蒺藜甘温，补肾固精，《本草纲目》谓其"补肾，治腰痛泄精，虚损劳气"，《本经逢原》亦谓其"为泄精虚劳要药，最能固精"，故为君药；臣以芡实、莲子甘涩而平，俱能益肾固精，且补脾气，莲子并能交通心肾；佐以龙骨甘涩平，牡蛎咸平微寒，俱能固涩止遗，莲须甘平，尤为收敛固精之妙品。合而用之，既能补肾，又能固精，实为标本兼顾之良方。以其能秘肾气，固精关，专为肾虚精滑者设，故美其名曰"金锁固精丸"。

［临床运用］

本方以补肾固精为主，兼能交通心肾，用治肾虚精关不固之症。若女子带下属肾虚滑脱者，亦可运用本方。

第三节 涩肠固脱

涩肠固脱剂，适用于泻痢日久，邪气已衰，脾肾虚寒，以致大便滑脱不禁的病证。常用涩肠固脱的药物如肉豆蔻、诃子、赤石脂、禹余粮等为主组成方剂。代表方有桃花汤、四神丸等。

桃花汤《伤寒论》

［组成］ 赤石脂一斤，一半全用，一半筛末（24克，一半全用，一半筛末） 干姜一两（6克） 粳米一斤（24克）

［用法］ 原方三味，以水七升，煮米令熟，去滓，温服七合，内赤石脂末方寸匕，日三服。若一服愈，余勿服。

现代用法：水煎，米熟汤成，去渣，加入赤石脂末6克，日服二次。

［功效］ 温涩止利。

［主治］ 下利不止，便脓血，色黯不鲜，日久不愈，腹痛喜温喜按，舌淡苔白，脉迟弱或微细。

［方解］

少阴阳衰，阴寒之邪在里，寒湿阻滞下焦，肠络受伤，变为脓血，滑利下脱，故下痢不止，便下脓血。方中重用赤石脂温涩固下以止泄痢，《神农本草经》谓其"主泄痢，肠澼脓血"，《别录》谓其"疗腹痛肠澼，下痢赤白"，为久痢不止，肠道滑脱者设，尤妙在以赤石脂一半筛末冲服，令其留着于肠中，则收涩之力更强，故为君药；干姜大辛大热，温中散寒，止血止痢，《神农本草经》谓其"温中止血"，主"肠澼下利"，故为臣药；粳米甘平，养胃和中，助石脂、干姜以固肠胃，为佐使药。诸药合用，共奏涩肠止痢之效。方名桃花汤者，据张志聪说："赤石脂色如桃花，故名桃花汤。"而柯韵伯则谓："名桃花者，取春和之义，非徒以色言耳。"王晋三[72]也说："桃花汤非名其色也，肾脏阳虚用之，一若寒谷有阳和之致，故名。"二说均有至理，并存可也。

［临床运用］

本方偏于温涩固下而止泄痢，故对少阴阳衰，下痢便脓血，滑脱不禁者，最为适合。若兼见手足厥冷，脉沉微者，是少阴阳衰重证，还可加用附子等药，可参考《肘后方》"疗伤寒若下脓血者赤石脂汤方"（赤石脂二两碎，干姜二两切，附子一两炮破，以水五升，煮取三升，去滓，温分三服。脐下痛者，加当归一两、芍药二两，用水六升）。

四神丸《内科摘要》[73]

［组成］ 肉豆蔻二两（60克） 补骨脂四两（120克） 五味子 吴茱萸各二两（各60克）

［用法］ 原方为末，生姜四两，红枣五十枚，用水一碗，煮姜、枣，水干，取枣肉，丸桐子大，每服五七十丸，空心食前服。

现代用法：以上四味为细末，用水适量，加生姜125克、红枣50枚同煮，待红枣熟烂，去姜取枣，去皮核，用肉和药末为丸，每服6～9克，日服二次，饭前及临睡用温开水送下。亦可作汤剂，水煎服，用量按原方比例酌减。

［功效］ 温肾暖脾，固涩止泻。

［主治］ 脾肾虚寒，五更泄泻，不思饮食，食不消化，或腹痛肢冷，舌质淡苔薄白，脉沉迟无力。

[方解]

五更泄泻，又称鸡鸣泄、肾泄。《素问·金匮真言论》说："鸡鸣至平旦，天之阴，阴中之阳也，故人亦应之。"方中重用补骨脂辛苦大温，补命门之火，以温养脾土，《本草纲目》谓其"治肾泄"，故为君药；肉豆蔻辛温，温脾暖胃，涩肠止泻，配合补骨脂，则温肾暖脾，固涩止泻之功相得益彰，故为臣药；五味子酸温，固肾益气，涩精止泻，吴茱萸辛苦大热，温暖脾胃，以散阴寒，共为佐药；生姜温胃散寒，大枣补脾养胃，共为使药。诸药合用，俾火旺土强，肾泄自愈。方名"四神"者，正如王晋三所说："四种之药，治肾泄有神功也。"

[临床运用]

本方用治五更泄泻属脾肾虚寒者。若腰酸肢冷较甚，可配合右归丸，以增强补肾温阳之功。

第四节　固崩止带

固崩止带剂，适用于妇人血崩不止及带下日久不止等症，兼见心悸气短，面色少华，舌淡苔白，脉来微弱。常以固崩止带的药物如龙骨、牡蛎、海螵蛸、五倍子等为主组成方剂。代表方有固冲汤、完带汤等。

固冲汤《医学衷中参西录》[74]

[组成]　白术一两，炒（30克）　生黄芪六钱（18克）　龙骨八钱，煅，捣细（24克）　牡蛎八钱，煅，捣细（24克）　萸肉八钱，取净核（24克）　生杭芍四钱（12克）　海螵蛸四钱，捣细（12克）　茜草三钱（9克）　棕边炭二钱（6克）　五倍子五分，轧细，药汁送服（1.5克）

[用法]　原方未著用法。

现代用法：水煎服，其中五倍子轧细末，以药汤送服。

[功效]　益气健脾，固冲摄血。

[主治]　脾气虚弱，冲脉不固，妇人血崩或月经过多，色淡质稀，心悸气短，舌质淡，脉微弱者。

[方解]

冲为血海，而脾为气血生化之源，主统血摄血。方中重用白术、黄芪补气健脾，俟脾气健旺则统摄有权，冲脉得固，故为君药；妇人血崩，最易耗伤阴血，故以山萸肉、生白芍补益肝肾，养血敛阴，共为臣药；煅龙骨、煅牡蛎、棕边炭、五倍子收涩止血，而止血须防留瘀，故又有海螵蛸、茜草化瘀止血，使血止而无留瘀之弊，以上共为佐药。冲为血海，血崩则冲脉空虚，而本方有益气健脾，固冲摄血之效，故方名"固冲汤"。

[临床运用]

本方为治脾气虚弱，冲脉不固，而致崩漏或月经过多的常用方。若兼见肢冷汗出，脉微欲绝者，为阳脱之象，需加重黄芪用量，并配合参附汤以益气回阳。

完带汤《傅青主女科》[75]

[组成]　白术一两，土炒（30克）　山药一两，炒（30克）　人参二钱（6克）白芍五钱，酒炒（15克）　车前子三钱，酒炒（9克）　苍术三钱，制（9克）　甘草一钱（3克）　陈皮五分（1.5克）　黑芥穗五分（1.5克）　柴胡六分（1.8克）

[用法]　原方水煎服。

现代用法：与原方相同。

[功效]　补脾舒肝，化湿止带。

[主治]　脾虚肝郁，湿浊下注，白带绵绵，日久不止，甚则臭秽，面色少华，倦怠乏力，舌苔白，脉缓者。

[方解]

带下者，因带脉不能约束而有此病，故以带名之。方中大量土炒白术补气健脾燥湿，炒山药补气健脾涩精，使脾土水谷精气不致下流，故为君药；臣以中等量的人参、苍术补脾气且燥脾湿，君臣相配，则脾气健旺，湿无由生；佐以白芍，能于土中泻木，配合君药白术，善于补脾疏肝，车前子因势利导，渗利既成之湿，尤妙在小量柴胡、陈皮、黑芥穗，用柴胡升提肝本之气，配白芍补肝体而助肝用，陈皮理气健脾，配白术、山药，则补气而不致壅气，黑芥穗能入血分，收湿止带，且能疏肝散风；使以甘草，补气健脾，调和诸药。合而成方，肝脾同治，量大者补养，量小者消散，寓补于散之中，寄消于升之内，共奏补脾疏肝，化湿止带之效，故方以"完带"名之。

[临床运用]

本方为治脾虚肝郁，湿浊下注，带下不止的常用方剂。

第十章

安神剂

凡用重镇安神或滋养安神的药物为主组成，具有安神作用，以治疗神志不安疾患的方剂，统称安神剂。

第一节　重镇安神

根据《素问·至真要大论》"惊者平之"的原则立法，凡用重镇的金石药或介类药为主组成，具有镇惊安神作用的方剂，统称重镇安神剂。在"十剂"中属于"重可镇怯"的范畴。

本节方剂多用治惊狂、癫痫、怔忡、失眠、躁扰不宁等症，常用重镇安神药物如朱砂、磁石、龙骨等为主组成。代表方有朱砂安神丸、磁朱丸等。

朱砂安神丸《内外伤辨惑论》

[组成]　朱砂五钱，另研，水飞为衣（15克）　甘草五钱五分（17克）　黄连去须净，酒洗，六钱（18克）　当归去芦，二钱五分（7.5克）　生地黄二钱五分（7.5克）

[用法]　原方除朱砂外，四味共为细末，汤浸蒸饼为丸，如黍米大，以朱砂为衣，每服十五丸或二十丸，津唾咽下，食后。或温水、凉水少许送下亦得。

现代用法：研细末为丸，朱砂为衣，每服4.5～9克，临睡前温开水送下。亦可作汤剂，水煎服，用量按原方比例酌减，其中朱砂研细末水飞，以药汤送服。

[功效]　镇心安神，清热养血。

［主治］ 心火上炎，灼伤阴血，心神烦乱，怔忡惊悸，胸中气乱而热，有似心中懊侬之状，失眠多梦，舌尖红，脉细数。

［方解］

《素问·灵兰秘典论》说："心者，君主之官也，神明出焉。"《素问·六节藏象论》说："心者，生之本，神之处也。"心火上炎，当清其火；心阴不足，当补其阴。若补而不清，邪热依然伤阴；若清而不补，阴血难以恢复。方中朱砂甘而微寒，入心经，重可镇怯，寒能清热，长于镇心安神，且清心火，《神农本草经》谓其"养精神，安魂魄"，《本草从新》[76]谓其"泻心经邪热，镇心定惊"，故为君药；黄连苦寒，清心除烦，助君药以泻心火，故为臣药；生地黄甘苦大寒，清热泻火，滋阴养血，当归甘辛苦温，补养心血，配伍生地，则不致于助热，均为佐药；甘草泻火补气，且制黄连苦寒之性，使苦寒清热而不致于化燥伤阴，有调和诸药之效，故为使药。合而用之，泻心火而宁心神，养心阴且补心血，为治疗火旺伤阴，心神烦乱，怔忡失眠的良方。

［临床运用］

本方为治疗心火上炎，灼伤阴血，而致怔忡失眠的常用方剂。以怔忡失眠，舌尖红，脉细数为辨证要点。

磁朱丸（原名神曲丸）《备急千金要方》

［组成］ 磁石二两（60克） 朱砂一两（30克） 神曲四两（120克）

［用法］ 原方三味末之，炼蜜为丸，如梧子大，饮服三丸，日三。

现代用法：上药研细末，曲糊，酌加炼蜜为小丸，每服6克，日服二次，用米汤或温开水送下。

［功效］ 益阴潜阳，镇心明目。

［主治］ 心肾不交，两目昏花，视物模糊，耳鸣耳聋，心悸失眠。亦治癫痫。

［方解］

本方证乃由肾阴（精）不足，心火偏亢，心肾不交，水火不济所致。方中磁石辛寒入肾，益阴潜阳，重镇安神，为君药；朱砂甘寒入心，泻心经邪热，镇心安神，为臣药。二药相合，能镇摄浮阳，交融水火，使心肾相交，则精气得以上输，心火不致上炎。神曲甘辛温，和胃以助消化，使金石药物不碍胃气，且精生于谷，神曲能消化五谷，则谷可化精，故为佐药。蜂蜜补中和胃，为使药。总之，本方合用摄纳浮阳，镇心明目，以及助运中宫之品，使水火交融，诸症悉平。

[临床运用]

本方用治心肾不交而致两目昏花，视物模糊，耳鸣耳聋，心悸失眠等症。若能配合六味地黄汤同用，疗效更佳。

第二节　滋养安神

滋养安神剂，适用于心肝血虚所致的虚烦不眠，心悸怔忡等症。常用具有滋养安神作用的药物，如酸枣仁、柏子仁、五味子、茯苓、小麦等为主组成方剂。代表方有酸枣仁汤、天王补心丹、甘草小麦大枣汤等。

酸枣仁汤《金匮要略》

[组成]　酸枣仁二升（12克）　甘草一两（3克）　知母二两（6克）　茯苓二两（6克）　芎䓖二两（6克）

[用法]　原方五味，以水八升，煮酸枣仁，得六升，纳诸药，煮取三升，分温三服。

现代用法：水煎服。

[功效]　养血安神，清热除烦。

[主治]　虚劳虚烦不得眠，脉弦细者。

[方解]

肝藏血、藏魂，人卧则血归于肝。虚劳之人，肝气不荣，肝血不足，不能藏魂。《素问·六节藏象论》说："肝者，罢极之本，魂之居也。"《素问·五脏生成》说"肝欲酸"，方中重用酸枣仁，甘酸而平，入心、肝经，养血安神，《别录》谓其"治烦心不得眠"，故为君药；《素问·藏气法时论》说："肝欲散，急食辛以散之，以辛补之。"川芎辛温，疏肝气，调营血，与酸枣仁配伍，酸收辛散并用，相反相成，更好地发挥养血调肝之效，为臣药；茯苓甘平，助君药宁心安神，且能培土以荣木，知母苦寒，清热除烦，又能缓和川芎温燥之性，共为佐药；《素问·藏气法时论》说："肝苦急，急食甘以缓之。"甘草培土缓肝，调和诸药，既可助茯苓培土荣木，亦可助知母清热除烦，为使药。诸药合用，共奏养血安神，清热除烦之效。如此则肝血足，虚烦除，睡眠自宁。

[临床运用]

本方主要用治肝血不足，血虚内热所致的虚烦不眠证。据编者临床体验，血虚甚者可配合四物汤，疗效更佳。

天王补心丹《校注妇人良方》

[组成] 人参去芦 茯苓 玄参 丹参 桔梗 远志各五钱（各15克） 当归酒浸 五味 麦门冬去心 天门冬 柏子仁 酸枣仁炒，各一两（各30克） 生地黄四两（120克）

[用法] 原方为末，炼蜜为丸，如梧桐子大，朱砂为衣，每服二三十丸，临卧，竹叶煎汤送下。

现代用法：为末，炼蜜为丸，如梧桐子大，朱砂为衣，每服6～9克，日服二次，温开水送下；亦可作汤剂，水煎服，用量按原方比例酌减。

[功效] 滋阴清热，补心安神。

[主治] 阴亏血少，心悸怔忡，睡眠不安，神疲健忘，大便干燥，口舌生疮，舌红少苔，脉细而数。

[方解]

《素问·灵兰秘典论》说："心者，君主之官也，神明出焉。"方中大量生地入心肾经，滋阴清热，水盛则足以伏火，故为君药。玄参、天冬、麦冬助君药滋阴清热，其中玄参、天冬入肾经，壮水制火，使肾水上升则心火不亢；麦冬入心经，甘寒清润，长于滋心阴，清心热，共为臣药。当归补血润燥，丹参养血清热，使心血充足，心神自安；血生于气，人参、茯苓，所以益心气，气旺则血自生，并均具有宁心安神之效；酸枣仁、远志、柏子仁养心安神，其中远志且通肾气上达于心，有交通心肾之妙；五味子酸温，以敛心气之耗散，以上共为佐药。桔梗载药上行，使药力作用于胸膈之上，不使速下；朱砂为衣，取其色赤入心，寒以清热，重可宁神，均为使药。诸药合用，共奏滋阴清热，补心安神之效。据《成方切用》[77]记载："终南宣律师课诵劳心，梦天王授以此方。"故名之曰"天王补心丹"。

[临床运用]

本方滋阴清热，补心安神，适用于心经阴亏血少所致的心悸怔忡，睡眠不安，神疲健忘，大便干燥，口舌生疮等症。

甘草小麦大枣汤（又名甘麦大枣汤）《金匮要略》

[组成] 甘草三两（9克） 小麦一升（30克） 大枣十枚（10枚）

[用法] 原方三味，以水六升，煮取三升，温分三服。亦补脾气。

现代用法：水煎服。

[功效] 养心安神，缓急和中。

[主治] 脏躁，喜悲伤欲哭，不能自主，呵欠频作，舌红少苔，脉细而数。

[方解]

脏，心脏也。心虚血少，则发为脏躁，而致虚火内扰，心神不宁。本病虽有虚火，不宜苦降；又非大虚，无需大补。根据《素问·藏气法时论》"肝苦急，急食甘以缓之"，《灵枢·五味》"心病者，宜食麦"的治则，只宜以甘平之品缓肝之急，养心之气。方中重用小麦甘平，补养心气以安心神，肝心为子母之脏，小麦又能补养肝气，《别录》有小麦"养肝气"的记载，故为君药；甘草甘平，补养心气，和中缓急，为臣药；大枣甘温质润，益气和中，润燥缓急，为佐使药。药仅三味，而甘润滋养，具有养心安神，缓急和中之效。原方后注："亦补脾气。"因三药均有补脾益气之功，且火为土母，心得所养，则火能生土，乃虚则补母之法；又见肝之病，知肝传脾，当先实脾，为肝虚治法，亦即《难经·第十四难》[78]"损其肝者缓其中"之意也。

[临床运用]

本方用治思虑过度，脏阴不足而致的脏躁。此病不拘于妇人，男子亦有患此者，然以妇人为多见。始则知觉过敏，睡眠不安，发作时自觉烦闷急躁，或悲伤哭泣，或作痉挛，或口出妄言，状似癫狂，不能自主，出现种种神志失常之症。此时使用本方，疗效卓著。

第十一章

治风剂

凡用辛散疏风或滋阴潜阳、平肝熄风的药物为主组成，具有疏散外风或平熄内风的作用，以治疗风病的方剂，统称治风剂。

第一节　疏散外风

疏散外风剂，适用于外风所致诸病。《灵枢·五变》说："肉不坚，腠理疏，则善病风。"说明人体正气不足，腠理疏松，极易感受外界风邪，导致风病。外风从外而入，必须用驱风之品使之从外而出，所谓外风宜散，治疗多以疏散为主。由于风邪伤人经络，津液不得流通，凝聚成痰，故在疏散外风的同时常配合化痰药。本节方剂常用川芎、羌活、防风、白芷、荆芥、僵蚕等疏风之品为主组成，并常与白附子、南星等化痰药同用。

"治风先治血，血行风自灭"，风邪伤人经络，气血凝滞不通，常须配合活血化瘀药如乳香、没药、地龙、当归等，使血脉流通，滞留的风邪也可随之消除。风为阳邪，郁而化热，伤血耗血，故有时还当配合养血凉血之品，如生地、赤芍、丹皮等。

疏散外风的代表方剂有川芎茶调散、牵正散、玉真散、活络丹等。本类方剂所用药物性多温燥，对于素体津液不足，阴虚阳亢者应当慎用。

川芎茶调散《太平惠民和剂局方》

［组成］　白芷　甘草㷧　羌活各二两（各60克）　荆芥去梗　川芎各四两（各120克）　细辛去芦，一两（30克）　防风一两半（45克）　薄荷叶不见火，八两（250克）

［用法］　原方为细末，每服二钱，食后茶清调下。

现代用法：共为细末，每服 6 克，日服二次，饭后用茶叶水调下，亦可作汤剂，水煎服，用量按原方比例酌减。

[**功效**] 疏风止痛。

[**主治**] 外感风邪，偏正头痛，或恶寒发热，目眩鼻塞，舌苔薄白，脉浮者。

[**方解**]

《素问·太阴阳明论》说："伤于风者，上先受之。"方中川芎辛温升散，善于祛风止痛，为治头痛要药，尤善治少阳、厥阴经头痛（两侧、巅顶痛），《本经》谓其"主中风入脑头痛"，为君药；羌活辛苦温，表散风寒，善治太阳经头痛（后头痛牵连项部），白芷辛温，发表祛风，善治阳明经头痛（前额痛），《本草纲目》引李杲"头痛必用川芎，如不愈，加各引经药，太阳羌活，阳明白芷"均为臣药；风为阳邪，善行数变，日久可郁而化热，故用大量薄荷辛凉散风，荆芥辛温，祛风而清头目，更有防风辛甘微温，善祛风邪，细辛辛温，祛风止痛，以上均为佐药；甘草和中益气，使升散不致耗气，且能调和诸药，茶清苦寒降火，上清头目，可制风药之辛燥升散，使升中有降，均为使药。服于食后，是使药性留恋于上，不致速趋于下。本方集大队辛散之品，疏风而止头痛，正如《医方集解》所说："头痛必用风药者，以巅顶之上，惟风可到也。"因本方君药为川芎，剂型为散剂，用茶清调服，故方名"川芎茶调散"。

[**临床运用**]

本方乃疏风散邪，以治头风头痛的良方。对于外感头痛、头风头痛而偏于风寒者，较为适用。

牵正散《杨氏家藏方》[79]

[**组成**] 白附子　白僵蚕　全蝎去毒，各等分，并生用

[**用法**] 上为细末。每服一钱，热酒调下，不拘时候。

现代用法：共为细末，每服 3 克，热酒或温开水送下；亦可作汤剂，水煎服，用量按原方比例酌情增减。

[**功效**] 祛风化痰。

［主治］ 风痰阻络，口眼㖞斜，面部肌肉抽动。

［方解］

本方证系风痰阻于头面经络所致。方中白附子辛甘温，散而能升，善祛风痰，治头面之风，为君药；僵蚕咸辛平，祛风化痰，全蝎辛平，熄风镇痉，共为辅佐药；并用热酒调服，取酒性善走，宣通血脉，以助药势直达头面受病之所，为使药。诸药合用，力专效宏，可使风去痰消，经络通畅，则㖞斜之口眼自可牵正，故方以"牵正"名之。

［临床运用］

本方为治疗风痰阻络，口眼㖞斜的常用方剂。但方中白附子、全蝎均为有毒之品，用量不宜过大。

活络丹（又名小活络丹）《太平惠民和剂局方》

［组成］ 川乌炮，去皮、脐　草乌炮，去皮、脐　地龙去土　天南星炮，各六两（各180克）　乳香研　没药研，各二两二钱（各66克）

［用法］ 原方为细末，入研药令匀，酒面糊为丸，如梧桐子大，每服二十丸，空心日午冷酒送下，荆芥茶下亦得。

现代用法：共为细末，酒面糊为丸，每丸重3克，每次服一丸，每日一至二次，空腹用陈酒或温开水送服。

［功效］ 温经通络，搜风除湿，祛痰逐瘀。

［主治］ 风寒湿邪留滞经络，流注手脚，筋脉挛急，屈伸不利，或疼痛游走不定。亦治中风后手足不仁，日久不愈，经络中有湿痰死血，腿臂间作痛者。

［方解］

风寒湿邪留滞经络，气血不得宣通，营卫失于流畅。方中制川乌、制草乌辛热有毒，温经散寒，祛风除湿，以通经络，共为君药；天南星苦辛温，有毒，祛络中风痰，且能燥湿，为臣药；乳香辛苦温、没药苦平，均能行气活血，化瘀定痛，为佐药；地龙咸寒，善通经络，有化瘀之功，且解草乌之毒，《蜀本草》[80]谓其"解射罔毒"（据《本草纲目》记载"草乌头取汁，晒为毒药，射禽兽，故有射罔之称"），酒则善行善散，引导诸药直达病所，共为使药。

诸药合用，使风寒湿邪、痰浊、瘀血尽祛，有活血通络之效，故方名"活络丹"。《素问·至真要大论》说"留者攻之""逸者行之"，此方是也。

[临床运用]

本方用治痹证肢体疼痛，或中风之后，手足不仁，腿臂作痛，审其确系风寒湿邪或湿痰死血凝滞经络，而体质尚属壮实者。

第二节　平熄内风

平熄内风剂，可治疗内脏病变所致的风病，以其临床症状有似风象的急骤、动摇和多变，故称之为内风。如猝然昏倒，口眼㖞斜，半身不遂，外无六经形证的"类中风"；神昏痉厥，四肢抽搐的"肝风"，皆属于内风的范畴。其发病机制，各有不同。如肝阳偏亢，肝风内动，血气逆乱，并走于上，常见头目眩晕，脑中热痛，面色如醉，甚则猝然昏倒，口眼㖞斜，半身不遂；或温病热邪久羁，热烁真阴，虚风内动，则见瘛疭，神倦，脉虚等症；如下元虚衰，虚阳浮越，痰浊上泛，则发为喑痱。亦有阳邪亢盛，热极动风，常见高热神昏，四肢抽搐，甚则痉厥。在治疗上，绝对禁用发散之品，因其非外来之邪，故无邪可散，只有采取平熄之法。应针对其致病之因，选用镇肝熄风、滋阴熄风或凉肝熄风等不同的方法治疗。由于内生之风多由阴虚不能制阳，阳亢生风所致，所谓"阴虚风动""木燥生风"，故滋阴是治疗内风的重要措施。滋阴可以润燥，可以柔肝，可以清热，可以潜阳，可以熄风。甚则加入重镇潜阳药。阴阳俱虚者可加入补阳药引火归源，不得妄投苦寒之品。阴虚有热，则必配伍清热之属，这些都是主要的配伍方法。内风与外风也有关系，"风气通于肝"（《素问·阴阳应象大论》），往往由于外风而引动内风，治疗时可在大量平熄内风之中佐以少量疏散外风之品，疗效往往比单纯用平熄内风之剂为好。

本节方剂常用平肝熄风药如羚羊角、天麻、钩藤、桑叶、滁菊、石决明、代赭石、龙骨、牡蛎等与滋阴养液药如生地黄、白芍、阿胶、鸡子黄、龟板、鳖甲、怀牛膝等组成。代表方有镇肝熄风汤、大定风珠、羚角钩藤汤、地黄饮子等。

镇肝熄风汤《医学衷中参西录》

[组成] 怀牛膝一两（30克） 生赭石一两，轧细（30克） 生龙骨五钱，捣碎（15克） 生牡蛎五钱，捣碎（15克） 生龟板五钱，捣碎（15克） 生杭芍五钱（15克） 玄参五钱（15克） 天冬五钱（15克） 川楝子二钱，捣碎（6克） 生麦芽二钱（6克） 茵陈二钱（6克） 甘草钱半（4.5克）

[用法] 原方未著用法。

现代用法：水煎服。

[功效] 镇肝熄风。

[主治] 内中风证，其脉弦长有力。或上盛下虚，头目时常眩晕，或脑中时常作疼发热，或目胀耳鸣，或心中烦热，或时常噫气，或肢体渐觉不利，或口眼渐形㖞斜，或面色如醉，甚或眩晕，至于颠仆，昏不知人，移时始醒，或醒后不能复原，精神短少，或肢体痿废，或成偏枯。

[方解]

内中风，亦名类中风，言风自内生，非外来之风也。方中重用怀牛膝引血下行，使阳不上亢，又能滋补肝肾之阴，以治其本，代赭石降胃镇肝以平气血之冲逆，二味共为君药；龙骨、牡蛎、龟板、芍药潜阳镇逆，柔肝熄风，玄参、天冬壮水涵肝，清金制木，正如张锡纯[81]所说："肺中清肃之气下行，自能镇制肝木"，以上诸药共助君药镇肝熄风，为臣药；肝为将军之官，内藏相火，性喜条达而恶抑郁，若单纯镇肝，势必影响其条达之性，激动其相火，反使肝阳更加上升，故以茵陈禀初春少阳升发之气，能清肝热而疏肝郁，生麦芽善舒肝气，顺肝木之性使不抑郁，川楝子疏肝理气，又能清泄肝阳，共为佐药；甘草甘缓柔肝，调和诸药，与麦芽相配，二药皆善和胃，以减少金石药物碍胃之弊，为使药。全方重用潜镇清降，在此前提下略用疏肝之品，有降有升，以降为主，成为一首很好的镇肝熄风之剂。

[临床运用]

本方是治疗类中风的常用方剂，无论在中风前或中风后，凡属肝阳化风者，均可用之。以头目眩晕，面色如醉，脉弦长有力为辨证要点。

大定风珠《温病条辨》

[组成] 生白芍六钱（18克） 阿胶三钱（9克） 生龟板四钱（12克） 干地黄六钱（18克） 麻仁二钱（6克） 五味子二钱（6克） 生牡蛎四钱（12克） 麦冬连心，六钱（18克） 炙甘草四钱（12克） 鸡子黄生，二枚（2枚） 鳖甲生，四钱（12克）

[用法] 原方水八杯，煮取三杯，去滓，再入鸡子黄，搅令相得，分三次服。

现代用法：水煎去渣，入阿胶烊化，再入鸡子黄搅匀，温服。

[功效] 滋阴熄风固脱。

[主治] 温病热邪久羁，热烁真阴，虚风内动，神倦瘈疭，脉气虚弱，舌绛苔少，时时欲脱者。

[方解]

本方证乃温邪久留，消烁真阴，或误汗或妄攻，重伤阴液所致。方中鸡子黄、阿胶滋阴养液以熄内风，为君药；白芍、甘草、五味子酸甘化阴，滋阴柔肝，生地、麦冬、麻仁滋阴润燥，共为臣药；龟板、鳖甲、牡蛎育阴潜阳熄风，其中牡蛎并有镇摄固脱之效，共为佐药；炙甘草又能调和诸药，为使药。诸药合用，滋阴熄风，且能固脱，为治疗虚风内动之良方。本方以大队滋阴药组成，君药鸡子黄宛如珠形，能熄内风，故名"大定风珠"。

[临床运用]

本方以滋阴熄风为主，凡真阴大伤，水不涵木，虚风内动，而致手足瘈疭者，均可使用。以神倦瘈疭，脉气虚弱，舌绛少苔为辨证要点。

羚角钩藤汤《重订通俗伤寒论》

[组成] 羚角片钱半，先煎（4.5克） 霜桑叶二钱（6克） 京川贝四钱，去心（12克） 鲜生地五钱（15克） 双钩藤三钱，后入（9克） 滁菊花三钱（9克） 茯神木三钱（9克） 生白芍三钱（9克） 生甘草八分（2.4克） 淡竹茹五钱，鲜刮，与羚角先煎代水（15克）

[用法] 原方未著用法。

现代用法：水煎服。

[功效] 凉肝熄风，增液化痰，舒筋通络。

[主治] 肝经热盛动风，壮热不退，烦闷躁扰，甚则神昏，手足抽搐，发为痉厥，舌绛而干，或舌焦起刺，脉弦而数。

[方解]

本方证乃温热病邪传入厥阴，阳热亢盛，热盛动风所致。方中羚羊角入肝经，凉肝熄风，钩藤清热平肝，熄风镇痉，共为君药。桑叶疏散肝热，菊花平肝熄风，助君药以清热熄风，共为臣药。火旺生风，风火相煽，最易耗伤阴液，故用鲜生地、生白芍、生甘草酸甘化阴，增液缓急；邪热亢盛，每易灼津为痰，故用川贝、竹茹清热化痰；风火相煽，必上薄于心，故又有茯神木平肝熄风，舒筋通络，宁心安神，以上共为佐药。生甘草又能调和诸药，兼以为使。诸药合用，共奏凉肝熄风，增液化痰、舒筋通络之效。

[临床运用]

本方为治疗热极动风的代表方剂。凡温热病邪传厥阴，出现壮热烦躁，手足抽搐，发为痉厥等症者，即可使用本方。若热邪内闭，神志昏迷，又当配合紫雪丹以凉开之。若大便闭结，须配合犀连承气汤（犀角汁，小川连，小枳实，鲜地汁，生绵纹，真金汁）凉血泻火，通腑泄热，始克有济。

地黄饮子《黄帝素问宣明论方》[82]

[组成] 熟干地黄　巴戟天去心　山茱萸　石斛　肉苁蓉酒浸，焙　附子炮　五味子　官桂　白茯苓　麦门冬去心　菖蒲　远志去心，等分

[用法] 原方为末，每服三钱，水一盏半，生姜五片，枣一枚，薄荷五七叶，同煎至八分，不计时候。

现代用法：加生姜、大枣、薄荷适量，水煎服，用量按原方比例酌情增减。

[功效] 滋肾阴，补肾阳，开窍化痰。

[主治] 喑痱，舌喑不能言，足废不能用，足冷面赤，脉沉细弱者。

[方解]

喑指语声不出，痱指足不履用。方中熟地黄滋补肾阴，为君药；山茱萸温肝固精，强阴助阳，肉苁蓉、巴戟天补肾壮阳，附子、肉桂温肾助阳，引火

归原，以上共为臣药；君臣相协，足以温养下元，摄纳浮阳。石斛、麦冬、五味子滋阴敛液，使阴阳相交，以济于平，又足以制桂、附之温燥；心火暴甚，肾水虚衰，水泛为痰，堵塞窍道，故用菖蒲、远志、茯苓交通心肾，开窍化痰，以上共为佐药。少量薄荷收其不尽之邪，使风无留着，生姜、大枣和其营卫，扶正可以祛邪，共为使药。综观全方，上下并治，标本兼顾，而以治下治本为主。诸药合用，补而不留邪，温而不刚燥，共奏滋肾阴，补肾阳，开窍化痰之功，使下元得以温养，浮阳得以摄纳，心肾交通，窍开痰化，喑痱自愈。本方以地黄为君药，药无过煎，数滚即服，不计时候，取其轻清之气，易为升降，迅达经络，流走四肢百骸，以交阴阳，故名之曰"地黄饮子"。

[临床运用]

1. 本方为治肾虚喑痱之主方，以语声不出，足废不用为辨证要点。若仅见足废不用之痱证，可以本方去菖蒲、远志、薄荷等宣通开窍之品。若仅见语声不出之喑证，即不宜使用本方。

2. 喑痱偏于阴虚而痰火盛者，可以本方去温燥之附、桂，加川贝、竹沥、胆星、天竺黄等以清化痰热。

第十二章

治燥剂

根据《素问·至真要大论》"燥淫于内，治以苦温，佐以甘辛""燥者润之""燥者濡之"的原则立法，凡用轻宣辛散或甘凉滋润的药物为主组成，具有轻宣外燥或滋阴润燥等作用，以治疗燥证的方剂，统称治燥剂。

第一节　轻宣外燥

轻宣外燥剂，适用于外感凉燥或温燥之证。凉燥多是深秋气凉，西风肃杀，骤凉束肺所致。凉燥犯肺，则肺气不宣，津液不布，聚而为痰，常见头痛恶寒，咳嗽痰稀，鼻塞嗌塞，舌苔薄白等症。治宜苦辛温润之剂以轻宣凉燥，常用杏仁、苏叶、前胡、桔梗等药物为主配伍成方，代表方有杏苏散。但凉燥虽属次寒，却易从火化，因此，用辛开温润之剂治疗凉燥，必须注意燥邪是否已从火化，不可过量。温燥则较凉燥为多见，且多发于初秋。因初秋承暑热之令，虽已入秋，其气尚温，若久晴无雨，秋阳燥热，此时人所感之者多病温燥。温燥伤肺，耗津灼液，则肺金清肃之令不行，常见头痛身热，干咳少痰，或气逆而喘，口渴鼻燥，舌边尖红，苔薄白而燥等症。治宜辛凉甘润之剂以清肺润燥，常用桑叶、杏仁、沙参、麦冬、石膏、阿胶等药物为主配伍成方，代表方有桑杏汤、清燥救肺汤等。

杏苏散《温病条辨》

[组成]　苏叶（9克）　杏仁（9克）　半夏（6克）　茯苓（9克）　橘皮（4.5克）前胡（6克）　苦桔梗（3克）　枳壳（4.5克）　甘草（3克）　生姜（3片）　大枣去核（3枚）[原方未著用量]

[用法]　原方未著用法。

现代用法：水煎服。

[功效]　轻宣凉燥，宣肺化痰。

[主治]　外感凉燥，头微痛，恶寒无汗，咳嗽稀痰，鼻塞嗌塞，脉弦，苔白。

[方解]

本方证乃凉燥外袭，肺气不宣，痰湿内阻所致。方中杏仁苦温而润，宣肺止咳化痰，《本经》谓其"主咳逆上气"，苏叶辛温，解肌发表，开宣肺气，使凉燥从表而解，二味共为君药；前胡苦辛微寒，疏风降气化痰，助杏、苏轻宣达表化痰，桔梗苦辛平，枳壳苦微寒，一升一降，助杏仁以宣肺气，共为臣药；半夏、橘皮、茯苓理气化痰，甘草合桔梗宣肺祛痰，为佐药；生姜、大枣调和营卫，为使药。诸药合用，共收发表宣化之功，以使表解痰化，肺畅气调。本方乃苦温甘辛之法，正合《素问·至真要大论》"燥淫于内，治以苦温，佐以甘辛"的理论。由此观之，凉燥之病，实乃秋令"小寒"为患，与寒邪所不同者，受邪较轻，且易于伤津化热耳。

[临床运用]

本方是治疗凉燥证的代表方剂，对秋季燥气流行所患的伤风咳嗽最为适合。

桑杏汤《温病条辨》

[组成]　桑叶一钱（3克）　杏仁一钱五分（4.5克）　沙参二钱（6克）　象贝一钱（3克）　香豉一钱（3克）　栀皮一钱（3克）　梨皮一钱（3克）

[用法]　原方水二杯，煮取一杯，顿服之，重者再作服。

现代用法：水煎服。

[功效]　轻宣燥热，凉润肺金。

[主治]　外感温燥，头痛身热，口渴咽干鼻燥，干咳无痰，或痰少而粘，舌边尖红，苔薄白而燥，右脉数大。

[方解]

本方证乃温燥外袭，肺阴受灼所致。方中桑叶轻宣燥热，杏仁润燥止咳，共为君药；香豉助桑叶轻宣透热，象贝助杏仁止咳化痰，沙参润肺止咳生津，共为臣；栀子皮质轻而入上焦，清泄肺热，梨皮清热润燥，止咳化痰，均为佐药。诸药合用，外以轻宣燥热，内以凉润肺金，乃辛凉之法，俾燥热除而肺津复，则诸症自愈。本方诸药用量较轻，吴氏认为："轻药不得重用，重用必过病所"，因"治上焦如羽，非轻不举"故也。

[临床运用]

本方有轻宣凉润之功，是治疗温燥外袭，肺燥咳嗽的代表方剂。据编者临床体会，若温燥伤肺而表热不甚，可将本方去香豉、栀子皮，加生玉竹、天花粉以养阴生津；若热伤阳络而致咳血，亦当用本方去香豉，加白茅根、茜草炭以凉血止血。

清燥救肺汤《医门法律》[83]

[组成] 桑叶经霜者，得金气而柔润不凋，取之为君，去枝梗，三钱（9克） 石膏煅，禀清肃之气，极清肺热，二钱五分（8克） 甘草和胃生金，一钱（3克） 人参生胃之津，养肺之气，七分（2克） 胡麻仁炒，研，一钱（3克） 真阿胶八分（3克） 麦门冬去心，一钱二分（4克） 杏仁泡，去皮、尖，炒黄，七分（2克） 枇杷叶一片，刷去毛，蜜涂，炙黄（3克）

[用法] 原方水一碗，煎六分，频频二三次滚热服。

现代用法：水煎服。

[功效] 清肺润燥。

[主治] 温燥伤肺，头痛身热，干咳无痰，气逆而喘，咽喉干燥，口渴鼻燥，胸满胁痛，舌苔薄白而燥，舌边尖红赤，脉虚大而数。

[方解]

秋令气候干燥，燥热伤肺。方中重用桑叶质轻性寒，宣透肺中燥热之邪，为君药。煅石膏辛甘而寒，极清肺热，助君药以治致病之源，为臣药。《难经·第十四难》说："损其肺者益其气。"而胃土又为肺金之母，故用甘草培土生金，人参生胃津，养肺气，又有麻仁、阿胶、麦冬润肺滋液，肺得滋润，则治节有权。《素问·藏气法时论》说"肺苦气上逆，急食苦以泄之"，故用杏仁、枇杷叶之苦以降泄肺气，气降则火降，而逆者不逆，咳者不咳，以上均为佐药。甘草又能调和诸药，以为使。如此，则肺金之燥热得以清润，肺气之上逆得以肃降，以救肺燥变生诸症，故名之曰"清燥救肺汤"。

[临床运用]

本方为治燥热伤肺的主要方剂。原方加减法："痰多加贝母、瓜蒌；血枯加生地黄；热甚加犀角、羚羊角，或加牛黄。"

第二节　滋润内燥

滋润内燥剂，适用于各种原因所致的脏腑津伤液耗的内燥证。其证或由汗、吐、下后重伤津液，或由久病精血内夺，或由感受温邪，化燥伤阴所致。由于发病部位的不同，因而见证与治法亦有差异。如燥在上者，多责之于肺，症见干咳少痰，咽燥咯血；燥在中者，多责之于胃，症见肌肉消瘦，口中燥渴，干呕食少；燥在下者，多责之于肾，症见下肢痿弱无力，消渴或津枯便秘等。

内燥的治疗原则，扼要言之，即上燥救（肺）津、中燥增（胃）液、下燥滋（阴）血。总之，治疗内燥必以甘寒滋润为要着，喜柔润而最忌苦燥。常用玄参、生地黄、麦冬、百合等药物为主组方，代表方有养阴清肺汤、百合固金汤、麦门冬汤、增液汤等。

养阴清肺汤《重楼玉钥》[84]

[组成]　大生地二钱（12克）　麦冬一钱二分（7克）　生甘草五分（3克）　玄参钱半（9克）　贝母八分，去心（4.5克）　丹皮八分（4.5克）　薄荷五分（3克）　炒白芍八分（4.5克）

[用法]　原方未著用法。

现代用法：水煎服。

[功效]　养阴清肺，解毒散邪。

[主治]　白喉，喉间起白如腐，不易拭去，咽喉肿痛，初起或发热或不发热，鼻干唇燥，或咳或不咳，呼吸有声，似喘非喘，脉数无力，或细数。

[方解]

白喉一证，多由患者素体阴虚蕴热，复感燥气疫毒，内燥与外燥相合而成。方中重用大生地养阴清热，为君；玄参养阴生津，泻火解毒，麦冬养阴清肺，《珍珠囊》谓其"治肺中伏火"，均为臣药；丹皮清热凉血，炒白芍益阴养血，贝母润肺化痰，清热散结，少量薄荷辛凉而散，疏表利咽，以上均为佐药；生甘草泻火解毒，调和诸药，为使药。合而成方，具有养阴清肺，解毒散邪之功。

[临床运用]

本方为治疗白喉的常用方。一般日服一剂，重证可以日服二剂。热毒重者，并可加入土牛膝泻火解毒，疗效尤佳。

百合固金汤《医方集解》引赵蕺庵方

[组成] 生地黄二钱（6克） 熟地黄三钱（9克） 麦冬钱半（4.5克） 百合 芍药炒 当归 贝母 生甘草各一钱（各3克） 元参 桔梗各八分（各2.4克）

[用法] 原方未著用法。

现代用法：水煎服。

[功效] 养阴清热，润肺化痰。

[主治] 肺肾阴亏，虚火上炎，咽喉燥痛，咳嗽气喘，痰中带血，五心烦热，舌红少苔，脉细数。

[方解]

本方证是肺肾阴亏所致。方中百合甘苦微寒，养阴清热，润肺止咳；生地黄甘苦寒，养阴清热；熟地黄甘微温，滋阴补血，以上共为君药。麦冬甘寒，助百合养阴清热，润肺止咳；玄参咸寒，助二地滋阴壮水，以制虚火，均为臣药。金虚不能制木，木火盛则刑金，故用当归、白芍养血和血兼以平肝；贝母润肺止咳化痰，均为佐药。生甘草清热泻火，调和诸药；少量桔梗合甘草清利咽喉，且载诸药上浮，为肺经引经药，共为使药。合而成方，滋阴润肺，金水并调，可使阴液渐充，虚火自清，以达到固护肺金之目的，故名曰"百合固金汤"。

[临床运用]

本方为治疗肺肾阴亏咳嗽的常用方。痰多者，可加瓜蒌皮以清金化痰；气喘甚，可去桔梗之升提；咳血者，亦去桔梗之升提，并加白及、茅根、仙鹤草以止血。

麦门冬汤《金匮要略》

[组成]　麦门冬七升（15克）　半夏一升（4.5克）　人参三两（9克）　甘草二两（6克）　粳米三合（15克）　大枣十二枚（四枚）

[用法]　原方六味，以水一斗二升，煮取六升，温服一升，日三夜一服。

现代用法：水煎服。

[功效]　润肺益胃，降逆下气。

[主治]　肺痿，咳唾涎沫，短气喘促，咽喉干燥，舌干红少苔，脉虚数。

[方解]

本方所治之肺痿，其病在肺，其源在胃，以土为金母，胃主津液。胃津不足，虚火上炎，灼伤肺阴。肺为娇脏，且为胃土之子，胃中津液不输于肺，肺失濡养，津枯肺燥，遂致肺叶日渐枯萎。方中重用麦门冬甘寒清润，入肺、胃经，养阴生津，滋液润燥，以清虚热，为君药；臣以人参、甘草、粳米、大枣益胃气，养胃阴，中气充盛，则津液自能上归于肺，于是肺得其养，即所谓"培土生金"；佐以少量半夏降逆下气，化其涎沫，虽属辛温之性，但与大量麦门冬配伍，则不嫌其燥，且麦门冬得半夏，则滋而不腻，相反相成；其中甘草并能润肺利咽，调和诸药，以为使。药仅六味，主从有序，润降得宜。合而成方，生胃津，润肺燥，下逆气，止浊唾，乃虚则补母之法也。

[临床运用]

1. 本方原治"大逆上气，咽喉不利"，后世医家皆谓是治疗虚热肺痿的主方。《肘后方》即有用本方治疗"肺痿咳唾涎沫不止"的记载。据编者临床体会，若肺痿津伤甚者，可加北沙参、玉竹；气虚甚者，可加生黄芪、山药；咳唾涎沫多者，可加茯苓。

2. 本方对于胃阴不足，胃失和降而致的呕吐、呃逆，颇有疗效。

增液汤《温病条辨》

[**组成**]　元参一两（30克）　麦冬连心，八钱（24克）　细生地八钱（24克）

[**用法**]　原方水八杯，煮取三杯，口干则与饮令尽。不便，再作服。

现代用法：水煎服。

[**功效**]　增液润燥。

[**主治**]　阳明温病，津液不足，数日不大便，口渴，舌干红，脉细微数或沉而无力。

[**方解**]

阳明包括胃肠。阳明温病不大便，不出热结、液干二途，须分虚实治疗。其偏于阳邪炽盛，热结之实证，则用承气汤急下存阴；其偏于热病耗损津液，液涸肠燥，传导失司，《温病条辨》所谓"液干多而热结少"，"水不足以行舟，而结粪不下者"，则不可用承气汤重竭其津。方中重用玄参苦咸寒，养阴清热，增液润燥，为君药；麦冬甘寒，增液润燥；细生地甘苦寒，养阴润燥，补而不腻，共为辅佐药。三药合用，养阴增液，使肠燥得润，大便自下，故名之曰"增液汤"。

本方乃咸寒苦甘法，为增水行舟之计，然非重用不为功。

[**临床运用**]

本方有增液润燥作用，临床上不仅用治热病伤津，肠燥便秘，而且多用于内伤阴虚之证，以便秘、口渴、舌干红，脉细微数或沉而无力为辨证要点。

第十三章

消导化积剂

凡是具有消食导滞、消癥化积的作用，以治疗食积脘痞、癥瘕积聚的方剂，统称消导化积剂，属于"八法"中的"消法"。

本章方剂常以山楂、神曲、麦芽、枳实、槟榔、鳖甲等药物为主组成，代表方有保和丸、枳术丸、木香槟榔丸、失笑丸、鳖甲煎丸等。

保和丸《丹溪心法》

[组成]　山楂六两（180克）　神曲二两（60克）　半夏　茯苓各三两（各90克）陈皮　连翘　莱菔子各一两（各30克）

[用法]　原方为末，炊饼丸如梧子大，每服七八十丸，食远白汤下。

现代用法：共为末，水泛为丸，每服6～9克，温开水或炒麦芽汤送下。亦可作汤剂，水煎服，用量按原方比例酌减。

[功效]　消食和胃。

[主治]　食积停滞，胸膈痞满，腹胀时痛，嗳腐吞酸，恶食呕吐，或大便泄泻，舌苔厚腻而黄，脉滑。

[方解]

"六腑者，传化物而不藏"（《素问·五藏别论》）。暴饮暴食，恣啖酒肉油腻面食之类，食积于中，而为伤食之证。故方中重用山楂酸甘微温，善消肉食油腻之积，《本草纲目》谓其"化饮食，消肉积"，故为君药。臣以神曲甘辛而温，消食和胃，能化酒食陈腐之积；莱菔子辛甘下气，长于消面食之积，宽畅胸膈，消除胀满。以上三药合用，可消化各种饮食积滞。食积中焦，生湿生痰，佐以半夏辛温，燥湿祛痰，下气散结；陈皮辛苦温，燥湿化痰，理气和

118

中；茯苓甘平，健脾和中，化痰利湿；食积停滞，郁而化热，又以连翘苦寒芳香，散结清热。诸药配伍，使食积消化，胃气因和。本方虽以消导为主，但药性平和，故以"保和"名之。

[临床运用]

本方为消食化积之平剂，宜于食停中脘而正气未虚者。若食积较甚，可加厚朴、枳实推荡积滞；食积化热甚者，宜加黄芩、黄连苦寒清热；大便秘结者，可加大黄通便导滞。

枳术丸《内外伤辨惑论》引张元素 [85] 方

[组成] 白术二两（60克） 枳实麸炒黄色，去穰，一两（30克）

[用法] 原方同为极细末，荷叶裹烧饭为丸，如梧桐子大。每服五十丸，多用白汤下无时。

现代用法：丸剂，每服 6～9 克，温开水送下。亦可作汤剂，水煎服，用量按原方比例酌减。

[功效] 健脾消痞。

[主治] 脾胃虚弱，饮食不消，心下痞闷。

[方解]

脾主运化，胃主受纳。方中白术苦甘温，健脾除湿，以助运化，为君药。臣以枳实苦微寒，下气化滞，散积消痞。白术用量重于枳实一倍，则以补为主，寓消于补之中，"本意不取其食速化，但令人胃气强实不复伤也"（《内外伤辨惑论》）。复以荷叶烧饭升养脾胃清气，以助白术健脾补胃；且与枳实相伍，一升清，一降浊，清升浊降，气机调畅，痞闷自消，正合"脾宜升则健，胃宜降则和"之理，为佐使药。本方消补兼施，以补为主；升降并用，以升为主，简当有法，切勿以其平易而忽之。

[临床运用]

本方系张元素从《金匮要略》枳术汤（枳实七枚，白术二两）变化而来的。枳术汤原治"心下坚，大如盘，边如旋盘，水饮所作"，因水饮停蓄于心下（胃），应当急去，故投以汤剂以荡涤之，而且重用枳实，取其攻逐停水，散结消痞，意在以消为主，再用白术培土制水，以补为辅。本方证则属脾不健运，饮食不消，当须缓除，故改汤为丸以缓消之，而且倍用白术健脾以助运化，意在以补为主，再用枳实散结消痞，以消为辅。一汤一丸，各有深意，临证之际，不得误用。

木香槟榔丸《儒门事亲》[86]

[组成] 木香　槟榔　青皮　陈皮　广茂（即莪术）烧　黄连麸炒，以上各一两（各30克）　黄柏　大黄各三两（各90克）　香附子炒　牵牛各四两（各120克）

[用法] 原方为细末，水丸如小豆大，每服三十丸，食后生姜汤送下。

现代用法：为细末，水泛为丸，每服6克，日服2～3次，生姜汤或温开水送下。

[功效] 行气导滞，攻积泄热。

[主治] 积滞内停，脘腹痞满胀痛，大便秘结，以及赤白痢疾，里急后重，舌苔黄腻，脉实者。

[方解]

饮食不节，积滞内停，气机壅阻，传化失常。方中木香辛苦温，乃三焦气分之药，能升降诸气，尤长于行肠胃滞气；槟榔苦辛温，入脾、胃、大肠经，下气最捷，二味合用，行气导滞，能消脘腹胀满，且除里急后重，共为君药。牵牛、大黄苦寒泄热，攻积导滞，泻下之力强大，共为臣药。青皮破气化滞，陈皮理气燥湿；香附理气，得木香则疏滞和中；莪术行气破血，消积止痛，善治饮食不消，脘腹疼痛；黄连、黄柏清热燥湿，且又止痢，以上均为佐药。综观全方，以木香槟榔为方名，且多用行气药物，立方之意，是以行气导滞为主，兼以攻积泄热。使气机通畅，积滞得下，湿清热化，诸症自除。

[临床运用]

本方行气攻积之力较强，宜于积滞内停，蕴为湿热，气机壅阻，邪正俱实者。

失笑丸（又名枳实消痞丸）《兰室秘藏》

[组成] 干生姜一钱（3克）　炙甘草　麦芽面　白茯苓　白术以上各二钱（各6克）　半夏曲　人参以上各三钱（各9克）　厚朴四钱，炙（12克）　枳实　黄连以上各五钱（各15克）

[**用法**] 原方为细末，汤浸蒸饼为丸，如梧桐子大，每服五七十丸，白汤下，食远服。

现代用法：水泛为丸或蒸饼糊丸，每服6～9克，日服二次，温开水送下；亦可作汤剂，水煎服，用量按原方比例酌情增减。

[**功效**] 消痞除满，健脾和胃。

[**主治**] 脾胃虚弱，寒热互结，心下痞满，不欲饮食，肢体困倦，苔腻而黄。

[**方解**]

脾胃素虚，升降失司，寒热互结，气壅湿聚，渐至痰食交阻。方中重用枳实苦微寒，入脾胃经，散积消痞，为君药。厚朴苦辛温，下气除满，为臣药。二味合用，针对主症心下痞满而设，以增强消痞除满之效。佐以黄连苦寒，清热燥湿，泻心除痞，半夏曲辛温，燥湿祛痰，消痞散结，少量干姜大辛大热，温中散寒，三味相伍，辛开苦降，共助枳、朴散结消痞；又有麦芽面咸平，消食和中；然而邪之所凑，其气必虚，故以人参、白术、茯苓、炙甘草补气健脾，扶正祛邪。其中炙甘草并能调和诸药，又为使药。用蒸饼糊丸，取其养脾胃，助消化。综观全方，以枳、朴、黄连的用量为最重，故着重于下气消痞，苦辛通降；至于参、术、苓、草仅为扶正祛邪而设，务使消不伤正，补不碍邪，共奏消痞除满，健脾和胃之功。

[**临床运用**]

本方系从半夏泻心汤和枳术汤化裁而成。本方所治之心下痞满，乃虚实相兼，寒热互结，热重于寒，实多虚少之证。若寒邪偏盛，舌苔白腻，当减少黄连用量，加重干姜用量，或再加入陈皮、木香、砂仁等理气温中。

鳖甲煎丸《金匮要略》

[**组成**] 鳖甲十二分，炙（90克） 乌扇（即射干）三分，烧（22.5克） 黄芩三分（22.5克） 柴胡六分（45克） 鼠妇（即地虱）三分，熬（22.5克） 干姜三分（22.5克） 大黄三分（22.5克） 芍药五分（37.5克） 桂枝三分（22.5克） 葶苈一分，熬（7.5克） 石韦三分，去毛（22.5克） 厚朴三分（22.5克） 牡丹五分，去心（37.5克） 瞿麦二分（15克） 紫葳（即凌霄花）三分（22.5克） 半夏一分（7.5克） 人参一分

（7.5克）　䗪虫五分，熬（37.5克）　阿胶三分，炙（22.5克）　蜂巢四分，炙（30克）
赤硝十二分（90克）　蜣螂六分，熬（45克）　桃仁二分（15克）

[用法]　原方二十三味，为末，取煅灶下灰一斗，清酒一斛五斗，浸灰，候酒尽一半，着鳖甲于中，煮令泛烂如胶漆，绞取汁，内诸药，煎为丸，如梧子大，空心服七丸，日三服。

现代用法：用黄酒适量，先煎鳖甲取汁，余药共研末，与药汁共煎为小丸，如梧桐子大，空腹每服3～6克，日服三次，温开水送下。

[功效]　消癥化积。

[主治]　疟疾日久不愈，左胁下结为癥瘕，名曰疟母。亦治癥积结于胁下，按之坚硬，推之不移，或时作疼痛，或时有寒热者。

[方解]

疟母之成，每因疟邪久踞少阳，正气渐衰，邪着不去所致。久疟不愈，寒热痰湿之邪与气血相搏，留于左胁之下，则结为癥瘕，名曰疟母。《素问·至真要大论》说："坚者削之，客者除之，结者散之，留者攻之。"方中重用鳖甲咸平，软坚散结消癥，《本经》谓其"主心腹癥瘕坚积，寒热"，故为君药。臣以大黄、芍药、䗪虫、桃仁、赤硝、牡丹、鼠妇、蜂巢、蜣螂、紫葳破血攻瘀，行其血分之瘀结。佐以厚朴、半夏、葶苈子、射干下气祛痰，行其气分之结滞；石韦、瞿麦利水导湿，从小便而出；柴胡、桂枝通达营卫，散结行瘀；干姜、黄芩和其阴阳，平调寒热；人参、阿胶益气养血，扶正固本。至于煅灶下灰性温走气，清酒性热走血，又能协同诸药共奏消癥化积之功，为使药。本方寒热并用，攻补兼施，理气理血，祛痰祛湿，诸法兼备，确为急治大方。原方"空心服七丸，日三服"，又取其缓而化之，徐除癥瘕。

[临床运用]

1.《千金方》所载鳖甲煎丸，用鳖甲十二片，又有海藻三分、大戟一分，无鼠妇、赤硝二味，以鳖甲煎和诸药为丸，其软坚逐水之力尤佳。

2. 本方运用范围并不局限于疟母，凡有形癥瘕，按之不移，气血凝滞，日久不消者，均可借此缓消渐散。

3. 本方虽有扶正之品，但仍以祛邪为主，对于久病体弱者，可与补益之剂结合使用。

第十四章

理气剂

凡以理气药物为主组成，具有行气或降气的作用，以治疗气滞、气逆等病证的方剂，统称理气剂。

第一节 行 气

行气剂，具有行气解郁作用，适用于气机郁滞的病证。由于气机郁滞，升降失常，常见胸闷、脘痛、呕吐、胁痛、梅核气等症。常用辛香理气药如香附、苏梗、木香、乌药，苦温破气药如青皮、槟榔、厚朴等为主组成方剂。由于气机郁滞所影响的脏腑不同，病情兼挟有异，因此在具体组方时还应注意灵活配伍。如气滞而兼痰，则行气中佐以化痰药，甚至还需用通阳散结祛痰之品。如气滞而兼寒，则行气与祛寒并用；气滞而兼热，则行气与清热并用；亦有气滞而兼血瘀者，则又当行气与化瘀合用。代表方有越鞠丸、良附丸、金铃子散、半夏厚朴汤、瓜蒌薤白白酒汤等。

越鞠丸（又名芎术丸）《丹溪心法》

[组成] 苍术　香附　川芎　神曲　栀子各等分（各9克）

[用法] 原方为末，水丸如绿豆大。

现代用法：水泛为丸，每服6克，日服2次，温水送下；或作汤剂，水煎服，用量按原方比例酌定。

[功效] 行气解郁。

[主治] 气、血、痰、火、湿、食六郁，胸膈痞闷，脘腹胀痛，吞酸呕吐，饮食不消，苔腻略黄。

[方解]

朱丹溪说："气血冲和，万病不生；一有怫郁，诸病生焉。"本方立意，重在行气解郁，使气行则血行，气畅则痰、火、湿、食诸郁亦易消解。方中香附行气解郁，以治气郁，故为君药；川芎活血行气，以治血郁，苍术燥湿运脾，以治湿郁，神曲消食和胃，以治食郁，栀子清热泻火，以治火郁，且能监制诸药温燥之性，使郁解而不助火热，均为辅佐药。气顺血和，湿火清而食滞化，痰郁亦因之而解，故不用化痰药物，乃治病求本之意。全方五味药物而能统治六郁，发越郁结之气、故方以"越鞠"名之。

[临床运用]

本方是治疗六郁的通治通用方，不过示人以治郁之大法，临床运用时，可根据六郁的偏重加减使用。如气郁者以香附为君药，血郁者以川芎为君药，湿郁者以苍术为君药，火郁者以栀子为君药，食郁者以神曲为君药。气郁可加木香、槟榔，血郁可加桃仁、红花，湿郁可加茯苓、白芷，火郁可加黄芩、青黛，痰郁可加海石、南星、瓜蒌，食郁可加山楂、麦芽。

金铃子散《素问病机气宜保命集》

[组成]　金铃子　延胡索各一两（各30克）

[用法]　原方为细末，每服三钱，酒调下。

现代用法：为末，每服9克，酒或温开水送下。亦可作汤剂，水煎服，用量按原方比例酌定。

[功效]　疏肝泄热，行气止痛。

[主治]　肝气郁滞，气郁化火，脘腹胁肋疼痛，或痛经，疝气痛，时发时止，烦躁，食热物而痛益甚，脉弦数，舌红苔黄。

[方解]

肝主疏泄，又为藏血之脏，其经脉过阴器，抵小腹，挟胃，属肝，络胆，上贯膈，布胁肋。金铃子又名川楝子，味苦性寒，疏肝泄热，理气止痛，为君药；延胡索味辛性温，活血行气止痛，为辅佐药。二药合用，为治疗肝郁化火，气滞血郁诸痛的常用方剂。

[临床运用]

1. 根据编者临证体验，治疗妇女痛经属肝郁气滞者，以本方合逍遥散疗效甚佳。并可加入香附、郁金、丹参等行气活血之品。

2. 本方加台乌药、荔枝核、橘核、小茴香、青皮等，可治气疝。偏寒者，可加吴萸、肉桂暖肝散寒。

半夏厚朴汤《金匮要略》

[组成] 半夏一升（12克） 厚朴三两（9克） 茯苓四两（12克） 生姜五两（15克）干苏叶二两（6克）

[用法] 原方五味，以水七升，煮取四升，分温四服，日三，夜一服。

现代用法：水煎服。

[功效] 行气开郁，降逆化痰。

[主治] 七情郁结，痰涎凝聚，咽中如有物阻，咯吐不出，吞咽不下，或胸闷气急，苔白润或白腻。

[方解]

人有郁气则津液不行，积为痰涎，与气相搏，逆于咽喉之间，遂致咽中如有物阻，吐之不出，吞之不下，即所谓梅核气。方中半夏降逆化痰，下气散结，厚朴下气燥湿，共为君药；茯苓化痰渗湿，苏叶行气散郁，生姜化痰降逆，且解半夏之毒，均为辅佐药。诸药合用，行气开郁，降逆化痰，则痰气郁结之证，自可消解。

[临床运用]

本方是治疗梅核气的常用方剂，宜于痰气交阻者。本方加大枣，名四七汤（《太平惠民和剂局方》引《易简方》[87]方），主治略同，而宜于痰湿不太甚者。

瓜蒌薤白白酒汤《金匮要略》

[组成] 瓜蒌实一枚，捣（15克） 薤白半升（9克） 白酒七升（适量）

[用法] 原方三味，同煮，取二升，分温再服。

现代用法：水煎服。

[功效]　通阳散结，行气祛痰。

[主治]　胸痹，喘息咳唾，胸背痛，短气，舌苔白腻，脉沉迟或紧。

[方解]

痹者，闭也。所谓胸痹，即胸中气机闭阻不行。所以然者，因诸阳受气于胸中而转行于背，胸阳不振，津液不能输布，凝滞为痰。方中瓜蒌甘寒，开胸散结，行气祛痰，《别录》谓其"治胸痹"，故为君药；薤白辛苦温，滑利通阳，下气散结，《本草纲目》谓其"治胸痹刺痛"，为臣药；白酒辛温，助药势上行，以增强瓜蒌、薤白通阳散结之效，为佐使药。诸药合用，使胸中阳气宣通，痰浊祛除，则胸痹自愈。

[临床运用]

本方为治疗胸痹证的主方。方中瓜蒌实即全瓜蒌。白酒即现在的米酒，黄酒亦可用，一般用30～60毫升。根据王绵之教授经验，亦可用生姜取代白酒。王老认为用鲜薤白比干薤白疗效好，鲜薤白有黏液，所谓辛通滑利之气即在于此。

第二节　降　气

降气剂，主要用于肺胃失降，气机上逆的病证。肺气宜肃降，胃气亦以下行为顺，故气机上逆，主要表现有肺气上逆与胃气上逆两方面。肺气上逆以气喘、咳嗽为主要症状，治宜降气平喘，常用苏子、杏仁、半夏、款冬花之类药物为主组成方剂。胃气上逆以噫气、呕吐、呃逆为主要症状，治宜和胃降逆，常用旋覆花、代赭石、半夏、橘皮、丁香、柿蒂之类药物为主组成方剂。

由于气逆之病有寒热虚实之分，因而降气法中就有各种不同的配伍。如气逆而又正虚，则降气与补虚并用；气逆而正不虚，则当以下气降逆为主，但也须随时注意，使降气而不致伤气。如气逆兼有虚热、虚寒，则降气须与清补或温补并用；气逆而兼有痰热或寒饮，则降气须与清化或温化并施。临床必须灵活化裁，务使切合病情。本类方剂的代表方有四磨汤、苏子降气汤、定喘汤、三子养亲汤、旋覆代赭汤、橘皮竹茹汤、丁香柿蒂汤等。

四磨汤《济生方》

[组成] 人参（9克） 槟榔（9克） 沉香（3克） 天台乌药各等分（9克）

[用法] 原方四味，各浓磨水，和作七分盏，煎三五沸，放温服。

现代用法：水煎服，用量按原方比例酌情增减。

[功效] 破滞降逆，兼以扶正。

[主治] 七情伤感，上气喘息，烦闷不食。

[方解]

七情伤感则肝气横逆，上犯肺脏则上气喘息，旁及脾胃则妨闷不食。其发病之标在肺与脾胃，发病之本则在于肝。本方用沉香为君药，温而不燥，行而不泄，既可降逆气，又可纳肾气，使气不复上逆；槟榔破气降逆，乌药顺气降逆，共助沉香以降逆气，共为臣药；但降气破气之品，每易耗损正气，故又佐以人参益气扶正，使逆气可降而正气不伤。原方四味均磨水煎服，则力专效速，故名之曰"四磨汤"。

[临床运用]

本方治疗因七情变动而致气逆不降，喘息不食等症。若体气壮实者，可以枳壳代人参，以增强降逆气的作用。

苏子降气汤《太平惠民和剂局方》

[组成] 紫苏子 半夏汤洗七次，各二两半（各9克） 川当归去芦，两半（6克） 甘草煅，二两（6克） 前胡去芦 厚朴去粗皮，姜汁拌炒，各一两（各4.5克） 肉桂去皮，一两半（3克）（一方有陈皮去白，一两半）

[用法] 原方为细末，每服二大钱，水一盏半，入生姜三片、枣子一个、苏五叶，同煮至八分，去滓热服，不拘时候。

现代用法：加生姜3片、大枣1枚、苏叶3克，水煎服。

[功效] 降气平喘化痰，温肾纳气归元。

[主治] 上盛下虚，痰涎壅盛，喘咳短气，胸膈满闷，大便不畅，腰疼脚弱，倦怠食少，舌苔白腻。

[方解]

本方证属肺有痰壅、肾不纳气的上盛下虚证。方中苏子温润下降，善于降气平喘消痰，且有利膈宽肠之效，故为君药；半夏下气化痰，厚朴下气平喘，前胡降气祛痰，共助君药加强降气平喘化痰之效，以治上盛，均为臣药；以其下虚，故用肉桂温肾纳气归元，使阳气充，气化行而痰饮去；当归之用有二：一则治咳嗽气逆，《本经》谓其"主咳逆上气"，二则本方辛燥之品居多，当归养血润燥，以防燥药伤阴耗血，且有润肠通便之功；阳气不足，极易感受风寒，又有姜、枣调和营卫，苏叶以散外寒，以上均为佐药。甘草调和诸药，为使药。诸药合用，有行有补，有燥有润，以降气平喘化痰为主，温肾纳气归元为辅，标本兼治，而以治上治标为主。本方以苏子为君药，以降气为主要目的，故方名苏子降气汤。

[临床运用]

本方主治上盛下虚之咳喘，据《医方集解》记载："一方无桂，有沉香。"则温肾之功略减而纳气平喘之力更强。根据编者临床体验，如肉桂、沉香同用则疗效更佳。

定喘汤《摄生众妙方》[88]

[组成]　白果二十一个，去壳，轧碎，炒黄色（12克）　麻黄三钱（9克）　苏子二钱（6克）　甘草一钱（3克）　款冬花三钱（9克）　杏仁一钱五分，去皮、尖（6克）桑白皮三钱，蜜炙（9克）　黄芩钱半，微炒（4.5克）　法半夏三钱（9克）

[用法]　原方水三盅，煎二盅，作二服，每服一盅，不用姜，不拘时，徐徐服。

现代用法：水煎服。

[功效]　宣肺降气，定喘化痰。

[主治]　风寒外束，痰热内蕴，痰多黄稠，咳嗽哮喘，或有恶寒发热，苔黄腻，脉滑数。

[方解]

平素肺有痰热胶固，又加外感风寒，郁而化热。方中麻黄宣肺定喘，发散风寒，白果敛肺定喘而祛痰浊，两药配伍，一散一收，既可增强平喘之效，又能防止麻黄耗散肺气之弊，共为君药；杏仁、苏子、半夏、款冬降气化痰，止咳平喘，为臣药；桑白皮配黄芩清泄肺热，下气平喘，为佐药；甘草调和诸药，为使药。诸药合用，共奏宣肺降气，化痰定喘之效。正如王旭高所谓："治之之法，表寒宜散，膈热宜清，气宜降，痰宜消，肺宜润，此方最为合度。"

[临床运用]

本方以三拗汤为基础，加桑白皮、黄芩、半夏、苏子、款冬、白果而成，用于风寒外束，痰热内蕴之哮喘。

三子养亲汤《韩氏医通》[89]

[组成]　紫苏子（9克）　白芥子（6克）　莱菔子（9克）[原方不著分量]

[用法]　原方三味各洗净，微炒击碎。看何症多，则以所主者为君，余次之。每剂不过三钱，用生绢小袋盛之，煮作汤饮，随甘旨，代茶饮水啜用，不宜煎熬太过。若大便素实者，临时加熟蜜少许；若冬寒，加生姜三片。

现代用法：水煎服。

[功效]　下气降逆，化痰消食。

[主治]　咳嗽气逆，痰多胸痞，食欲不振，舌苔白腻，脉滑者。

[方解]

本方原为高年咳嗽，气逆痰痞者而设。方中紫苏子下气消痰，止咳平喘；白芥子利气豁痰；莱菔子降气祛痰，行滞消食。三药合用，可使气顺痰化食消，咳逆自平。三子皆治痰之药，而又能于治痰之中各逞其长，临证当视气、痰、食三者之孰重孰轻，以定君药，余为辅佐药。原方三子，为事亲者设，故名"三子养亲汤"。

[临床运用]

1. 本方为治痰壅胸痞，咳嗽气逆的常用方。不分男女老幼，均可用之，尤以老年人为宜。然本方终属治标之剂，绝非治本之图，故气虚者非所宜也。因老人中虚，实为生痰之源，一俟症状缓解，即当改用补气健脾之剂。否则过事下气消导，更伤中气。

2. 据编者临床经验，对阳气虚弱，痰饮内生，咳嗽气逆者，以本方合苓桂术甘汤、二陈汤标本同治，收效颇捷。

旋覆代赭汤《伤寒论》

[组成] 旋覆花三两（9克） 人参二两（6克） 生姜五两（15克） 半夏半升，洗（9克） 代赭石一两（6克） 大枣十二枚，擘（4枚） 甘草三两，炙（9克）

[用法] 原方七味，以水一斗，煮取六升，去滓，再煎，取三升，温服一升，日三服。

现代用法：水煎服。

[功效] 降逆化痰，益气和胃。

[主治] 胃虚痰阻，胃气上逆。症见心下痞硬，噫气不除，或呃逆，反胃，呕吐涎沫，舌苔白滑，脉弦而虚。

[方解]

胃主受纳水谷，其气以下降为顺。胃气虚弱，则痰浊内阻，故心下痞硬；胃虚气逆，故噫气不除。气逆宜降，痰浊宜化，胃虚宜补。方中旋覆花下气消痰，降逆止噫，代赭石重以镇逆，能治噫气呕吐，二药配伍，善降逆气，故同为君药；半夏降逆祛痰，消痞散结，生姜下气祛痰，且解半夏之毒，二药配伍，则降逆祛痰之力更强，故为臣药；胃气虚弱，故用人参补益胃气，大枣益气补中，共为佐药；炙甘草益气补中，调和诸药，为使药。且参、枣、甘草同用，益气和胃之力更强。全方标本兼顾，以治标为主，治本为辅，使气逆得降，痰浊得化，胃气得和，诸症自解。

[临床运用]

凡因胃虚痰阻气逆所致的脘痞噫气、呃逆、反胃、呕吐等症，均可使用本方。如胃虚不甚，可减人参、大枣、甘草之甘壅；痰多可加茯苓、陈皮以化痰；心下痞硬甚者，可加砂仁下气和胃；呃逆甚者，可加丁香、柿蒂温胃降逆。

橘皮竹茹汤《金匮要略》

[组成] 橘皮二升（9克） 竹茹二升（9克） 大枣三十枚（5枚） 生姜半斤（9克） 甘草五两（6克） 人参一两（3克）

[用法] 原方六味，以水一斗，煮取三升，温服一升，日三服。

现代用法：水煎服。

[功效] 和胃降逆，清热益气。

［主治］ 胃虚有热，气逆不降，呃逆或干呕，舌苔薄白带黄，脉虚略数。

［方解］

久病胃虚，挟有胃热，以致胃失和降，气逆上冲，故见呃逆或干呕。方中橘皮理气和胃降逆，《本经》谓其善能"下气"，竹茹善清胃热，而无攻伐寒凉之弊，为治胃虚呕逆之要药，共为君药；人参补益胃气，与橘皮合用，则行中有补，生姜和胃降逆，与竹茹合用，则清中有温，共为臣药；大枣、甘草益气补中，且能缓和胃气之上逆，以为佐使药。本方清补降逆，但以降逆为主，清而不寒，补而不滞，使气顺热清，胃得和降，故对胃虚有热之呃逆干呕，最为适宜。

［临床运用］

本方为治胃虚有热，气逆不降而致呃逆干呕的常用方。若胃气不虚，可去人参、大枣、甘草；痰多者，可加半夏、茯苓；呕哕不止，可加枇杷叶；胃阴不足，舌红少苔，可加麦冬、石斛。

丁香柿蒂汤《症因脉治》[90]

［组成］ 丁香（3克） 柿蒂（6克） 人参（3克） 生姜（6克）[原方未著用量]

［用法］ 原方未著用法。

现代用法：水煎服。

［功效］ 温中益气、散寒降逆。

［主治］ 胃气虚寒，失于和降，呃逆、脘痞，舌淡苔白，脉沉迟。

［方解］

胃气虚弱，又为寒邪阻遏，失其通降之职，寒阻气逆，故呃逆作矣。方中丁香温中散寒，善于降逆，柿蒂降气止呃，两味均为治呃要药，故共为君药；臣以人参补中益气；佐以生姜温中散寒。四味合用，能使寒散气降，中阳健旺，呃逆自止。

［临床运用］

本方为治胃气虚寒，气逆不降而致呃逆的常用方。呃逆甚者，可加刀豆子以止呃逆；兼有气滞痰凝者，可加陈皮、半夏、沉香以理气化痰，降逆止呃。本方亦可用治胃寒气逆所致的呕吐。

理血剂

凡以理血药为主组成，具有活血祛瘀或止血作用，以治疗血瘀或出血证的方剂，统称理血剂。

第一节　活血祛瘀

活血祛瘀剂，适用于瘀血内停所致的一系列病症。由于瘀阻部位不同，发病原因有异，故出现的证候也各不相同。或下焦蓄血，少腹胀痛或硬满，小便自利，烦躁谵语，如狂发狂；或妇人经闭、痛经、瘀血崩漏，少腹疼痛拒按，脉沉涩有力；或产后恶露不行，小腹有块疼痛；或瘀血内停，头痛、胸痛、心腹疼痛；或因跌仆损伤，瘀积肿痛；或中风后气虚血瘀，而致半身不遂，口眼㖞斜。凡此种种，均应根据患者的具体病情，运用活血祛瘀之剂以消除或攻逐停滞于体内的瘀血。常用活血化瘀药物如大黄、桃红、红花、赤芍、川芎、五灵脂、丹皮、丹参等为主组成方剂，并常配伍理气的药物，以增强活血祛瘀的作用，因气为血之帅，气行则血行。此外，还应根据病情的寒热虚实，酌情配伍相应的药物。如兼寒者，配伍温经散寒药，以血得温则行，遇寒则凝；瘀热互结，配伍荡涤瘀热药，使瘀热下行，邪有出路；正虚有瘀者，又当与益气养血药同用，则祛邪而不伤正。至于孕妇有瘀血者，运用化瘀之剂，又当小量缓图，使瘀去而胎不伤，衰其大半而止，毋使过之。本节 代表方剂有桃核承气汤、桂枝茯苓丸、血府逐瘀汤、补阳还五汤、复元活血汤、温经汤、生化汤等。

桃核承气汤《伤寒论》

[组成] 桃核五十个，去皮、尖（12克） 桂枝二两，去皮（6克） 大黄四两（12克） 芒硝二两（6克） 甘草二两，炙（6克）

[用法] 原方五味，以水七升，煮取二升半，去滓，内芒硝，更上火微沸，下火。先食温服五合，日三服，当微利。

现代用法：水煎，去滓，冲入芒硝，温服。

[功效] 破血下瘀泻热。

[主治] 下焦蓄血，少腹急结，小便自利，烦躁谵语，其人如狂。以及妇女血瘀痛经，经闭不行，脉沉实者。

[方解]

伤寒邪热在太阳不解，传入下焦，与血相搏，瘀热互结，而致下焦蓄血证。本方即调胃承气汤加桃仁、桂枝而成。瘀热互结，故以桃仁苦甘平，破血祛瘀，《本经》记载"主瘀血血闭"，《珍珠囊》谓其"破蓄血"；大黄苦寒，下瘀泻热，《本经》记载"主下瘀血，血闭寒热"，《珍珠囊》谓其"泻诸实热不通"，两药同用，瘀热并治，共为君药。桂枝辛甘温，温通血脉，散下焦蓄血，助桃仁破血祛瘀；芒硝咸苦大寒，能入血分，软坚散结润燥，助大黄下瘀泻热，共为臣药。炙甘草调胃和中，缓和诸药峻烈之性，俾邪去而正不伤，为佐使药。诸药合用，寒温相配，共奏破血下瘀泻热之功，为治下焦蓄血之良方。原方先食温服，使药力下行，奏效尤速。药后微利，则仅通大便，不必定下血也。使邪有出路，诸症自解。

[临床运用]

本方为治疗瘀热互结，下焦蓄血的常用方剂。对于妇人瘀热经闭、痛经，常配合四物汤同用。若兼气滞者，可加香附、枳实、青皮以理气破滞。亦可用于产后恶露不下，少腹坚痛，喘胀欲死者，常配伍失笑散以活血祛瘀。

桂枝茯苓丸《金匮要略》

[组成] 桂枝 茯苓 牡丹去心 桃仁去皮、尖，熬 芍药各等分（各9克）

[用法] 原方五味末之，炼蜜和丸，如兔屎大，每日食前服一丸，不知，加至三丸。

现代用法：研末，炼蜜为丸，每服 1.5～6 克，每日二次，食前温开水送服。或作汤剂，各 9 克，水煎服，每日一剂。

[功效] 化瘀消癥。

[主治] 妇人宿有癥病，妊娠未及三月而得漏下不止，血色紫黑晦暗者。或妇人少腹癥块，按之痛甚，脉涩者。或妇人血瘀经闭，或经行腹痛，或难产，或死胎不下，或产后恶露不行而腹痛拒按者。

[方解]

癥者，有形可征，系指瘀血凝结成块在腹部的宿疾。癥之所由成，多因寒湿，方中桂枝辛甘而温，温通血脉，茯苓甘淡渗湿，且补正气，二味共为君药；瘀久则化热，又有丹皮、芍药凉血散血，化瘀消癥，桃仁性善破血，去瘀生新，共为辅佐药。合而成方，寒温并施，邪正兼顾，实为化瘀消癥之平剂。原方炼蜜和丸，目的在于缓和药力，使癥消而不伤胎。而其服法尤限以每日食前服兔屎大一丸，不知，加至三丸，正是刻刻以胎元为念。本方特点在于缓消癥块，因癥病痼疾，决非一时可去，自当缓缓消剥，使瘀去新生而胎有所养，自然安固。化瘀消癥而不嫌其伤胎者，有病则病当之，正如《素问·六元正纪大论》所谓："有故无殒，亦无殒也。""大积大聚，其可犯也，衰其大半而止。"

[临床运用]

本方为活血化瘀消癥之剂，用途甚广。除治癥病漏下外，并可用治癥块腹痛，瘀血经闭，痛经，难产，胞衣不下，死胎不下，产后恶露不行，腹痛拒按等症。亦治产后败血上攻，气促喘满。审属瘀血为患，均可用之。

血府逐瘀汤《医林改错》[91]

[组成] 当归三钱（9克） 生地三钱（9克） 桃仁四钱（12克） 红花三钱（9克） 枳壳二钱（6克） 赤芍二钱（6克） 柴胡一钱（3克） 甘草二钱（6克） 桔梗一钱半（4.5克） 川芎一钱半（4.5克） 牛膝三钱（9克）

[用法] 原方水煎服。

现代用法：与原方相同。

[功效] 活血化瘀，行气止痛。

[主治] 胸中瘀血而致头痛、胸痛，日久不愈，痛如针刺，且有定处，或呃逆干呕，或急躁易怒，或多梦失眠，或心悸怔忡，或入晚发热，舌质黯红，舌边有瘀斑瘀点，脉涩者。

[方解]

王清任[92]说："膈膜以上，满腔皆血，故名曰血府。"又说："血府即人胸下膈膜一片。"可见王氏所指的血府即是胸中。方中当归、桃仁、红花活血化瘀，为君药；赤芍、川芎助君药活血化瘀，生地配当归养血活血，使化瘀而不伤阴血，均为臣药；枳壳、桔梗一升一降，宽胸理气，使气行则血行，桔梗并能载药上行，使药力作用于胸中（血府），柴胡疏气解郁，升举清阳，与枳壳同用，尤善理气散结，牛膝破血逐瘀，善引瘀血下行，以上均为佐药；甘草缓急，利血气而调诸药，为使药。合而用之，活血而无耗血之虑，行气而无伤阴之弊，用治血府瘀血，俾血化下行，诸症可愈，故以"血府逐瘀汤"名之。

[临床运用]

本方为治疗血瘀胸中的常用方剂。根据王清任的临床经验，本方可用治头痛、胸痛、胸不任物、胸任重物、天亮出汗、食自胸后下、心里热（名曰灯笼病）、瞀闷、急躁、夜睡梦多、呃逆（俗名打咯忒）、饮水即呛、不眠、小儿夜啼、心跳心忙、夜不安、俗言肝气病、干呕、晚发一阵热等症，确有疗效。

复元活血汤《医学发明》[93]

[组成] 柴胡半两（15克） 瓜蒌根 当归各三钱（各9克） 红花 甘草 穿山甲炮,各二钱（各6克） 大黄酒浸,一两（30克） 桃仁酒浸,去皮、尖、研如泥,五十个（15克）

[用法] 原方除桃仁外，锉如麻豆大，每服一两，水一盏半，酒半盏，同煮至七分，去滓，大温服之，食前。以利为度，得利痛减，不尽服。

现代用法：加水四分之三、黄酒四分之一同煎，空腹温服，用量按原方比例酌减。

[功效] 活血祛瘀，通络散结。

[主治] 跌扑损伤，瘀血留于胁下，痛不可忍者。

[方解]

肝藏血，胁下为足厥阴肝经循行之处，或从高坠下，或跌仆斗殴，瘀血停留于胁下，血瘀气阻，以致痛不可忍。方中柴胡引诸药入于肝经，为君药；臣以当归活血，甘草缓急止痛，补气生血；佐以穿山甲破瘀通络，瓜蒌根润燥消瘀，《本经》谓其"续绝伤"，《日华子诸家本草》[94]记载"消扑损损瘀血"，桃仁、红花祛瘀生新；使以大量酒制大黄，荡涤凝瘀败血，导瘀下行，推陈致新，加酒同煮，取其善行药性，活血通络。诸药合用，使瘀祛新生，胁痛自平。正如张秉成所说："去者去，生者生，痛自舒而元自复。"故以"复元活血汤"名之。

[临床运用]

本方为伤科常用的内服方剂，主治跌仆损伤，瘀阻胁痛之症。若疼痛较剧，可加三七粉3～6克冲服，或酌加乳香、没药、延胡索等以增强活血止痛之效。惟跌仆损伤，不仅血瘀，其气亦滞，可酌加香附、郁金、橘络之属，使气行血活，疗效尤佳。

补阳还五汤《医林改错》

[组成]　黄芪生，四两（60克）　归尾二钱（6克）　赤芍一钱半（4.5克）　地龙去土，一钱（3克）　川芎一钱（3克）　桃仁一钱（3克）　红花一钱（3克）

[用法]　原方水煎服。

现代用法：与原方相同。

[功效]　补益元气，活血通络。

[主治]　中风后半身不遂，口眼㖞斜，语言謇涩，口角流涎，大便干燥，小便频数，遗尿不禁，舌淡苔白，脉缓无力。

[方解]

《灵枢·刺节真邪》说："虚邪偏客于身半，其入深，内居荣卫，荣卫稍衰则真气去，邪气独留，发为偏枯。"偏枯，即半身不遂之谓也。方中重用生黄芪补益元气，使气旺则血行，为君药；臣以归尾活血；佐以少量赤芍、川芎、桃仁、红花助归尾活血和营，地龙通经活络。诸药合用，共奏补益元气，活血通络之效。气属阳，本方善于补气，还其亏损的五成元气，以治疗半身不遂，故名之曰"补阳还五汤"。

[临床运用]

本方主要用治中风后半身不遂之症。气虚血瘀为其病机，舌淡舌白、脉缓无力，为其辨证要点。临床运用时黄芪用量宜重，活血通络药用量宜轻。重用补气药则有助于活血通络，少用活血通络药则祛邪而不伤正气，实为两全之计。

失笑散《太平惠民和剂局方》

[组成] 蒲黄炒香 五灵脂酒研，淘去砂土，各等分

[用法] 原方为末，先用酽醋调二钱，熬成膏，入水一盏，煎七分，食前热服。

现代用法：共为细末，每服 6 克，用黄酒或醋冲服；亦可每日用 6～12克，包煎，作汤剂。

[功效] 活血祛瘀止痛。

[主治] 瘀血停滞，妇女痛经、闭经，或崩漏色紫有块，小腹痛而拒按，或产后恶露不行，小腹剧痛，以及产后血晕。并治一切瘀血阻滞，心腹疼痛，脉涩等症。

[方解]

本方所治诸症，均由瘀血阻滞，血行不畅所致。方中蒲黄甘平，行血消瘀，《本经》谓其"消瘀血"，《本草纲目》谓其"凉血活血，止心腹诸痛"，炒用并能止血，以兼顾出血见症，使之攻而勿伐；五灵脂甘温，入肝经血分，通利血脉，散瘀止痛，二味相须为用，共为君药。调以米醋，味酸入肝，既助蒲黄、五灵脂散瘀活血，且制五灵脂气味之腥臊，陈藏器《本草拾遗》[95]谓其"治产后血运……杀恶毒"，故为佐使药。合而成方，共奏祛瘀止痛，推陈致新之功。前人运用本方，病者每于不觉中诸症悉除，不禁哑然而笑，故方以"失笑"名之。

[临床运用]

本方为治疗血瘀作痛的常用方剂，尤以肝经血瘀者为宜。若加当归、赤芍、川芎、生地、桃仁、红花、丹参等，则活血祛瘀之效更著；加乳香、没

药，则止痛之效益彰。兼气滞者，可加香附、郁金，或配合金铃子散，随证治之。

温经汤《金匮要略》

[组成]　吴茱萸三两（9克）　当归　川芎　芍药　人参　桂枝　阿胶　牡丹皮去心　生姜　甘草各二两（各6克）　半夏半升（9克）　麦冬去心，一升（12克）

[用法]　原方十二味，以水一斗，煮取三升，分温三服。

现代用法：水煎服。

[功效]　温经散寒，养血祛瘀。

[主治]　冲任虚寒，瘀血阻滞，月经不调，或经水过多，或至期不来，或崩漏下血不止，暮即发热，少腹冷痛，腹满，手掌烦热，唇口干燥。亦主妇人少腹寒冷，久不受胎。

[方解]

冲为血海，任主胞胎，二脉皆起于胞宫，循行于少腹。《素问·调经论》说："血气者，喜温而恶寒，寒则泣不能流，温则消而去之。"方中吴茱萸、桂枝温经散寒，且吴茱萸功擅暖肝止痛，桂枝长于温通血脉，共为君药。当归、川芎、芍药、阿胶养血调经，祛瘀生新，均为臣药。丹皮既助桂枝、当归、川芎活血祛瘀，并能清血分郁热，《本草纲目》谓其"治血中伏火，除烦热"；冲脉隶于阳明，故以人参、甘草、麦冬益胃气养胃阴，使中气充盛，自可化生血液；半夏降胃，即所以安冲；生姜暖肝和胃，且解半夏之毒，以上均为佐药。甘草又能调和诸药，以为使。诸药合用，有温有凉，有补有行，而又以温补为主，使血气得温则行，血行则自无瘀血停留之患，瘀去新生，诸症自愈，方名"温经汤"，其意即在于此。

[临床运用]

本方为妇科调经之祖方，主要用于冲任虚寒，瘀血阻滞所致的月经不调、少腹冷痛、崩漏下血等症。

生化汤《景岳全书》引会稽钱氏世传方

[组成]　当归五钱（15克）　川芎二钱（6克）　桃仁十粒，去皮、尖、双仁（4.5克）

焦姜三分（1克） 甘草炙，五分（1.5克）

　　[**用法**] 原方㕮咀，水二钟，枣二枚，煎八分温服。

　　现代用法：水煎服。

　　[**功效**] 温经活血，化瘀生新。

　　[**主治**] 产后恶露不行，瘀血内阻，小腹疼痛。

　　[**方解**]

　　所谓恶露，乃指产妇分娩后，胞宫内遗留的余血和浊液，理应排出体外。方中重用当归补血活血，化瘀生新，为君药；川芎辛散温通，活血行气，为臣药；佐以少量桃仁化瘀生新，炮姜温经散寒，既助当归以生新，又助芎、桃而化瘀，盖血得温则行，《素问·调经论》所谓"寒则泣不能流，温则消而去之"；使以炙甘草、大枣甘以缓之，使活血化瘀药的作用更为持续而缓和，且能补虚扶脾，调和诸药。合而成方，共奏温经活血，化瘀生新之效，正如《血证论》[96]所说："血瘀能化之，则所以生之，产后多用。"故以"生化"名之。

　　[**临床运用**]

　　本方为产后常用方，但药性偏温，以产后寒凝血瘀者为宜。若血热而有瘀滞者，究非本方之所宜。

第二节 止 血

　　止血剂，适用于血溢脉外，离经妄行而出现的吐血、衄血、咳血、便血、尿血、崩漏等各种出血症，常用止血药如大蓟、小蓟、侧柏叶、茅根、槐花或灶中黄土、阿胶、艾叶等为主组成方剂。但出血病情颇为复杂，病因有寒热虚实的不同，病位有上下内外的区别，病势有轻重缓急的差异。所以止血剂的运用，应随具体证情而异。一般来说，如因于血热妄行者，治宜凉血止血；因于阳虚不能摄血者，治宜温阳止血；因于冲任虚损者，治宜补冲止血。如突然大出血，则采用急则治标之法，着重止血；气随血脱，又急需大补元气，使阳生阴长，补气摄血；慢性出血，应着重治本，或标本兼顾。代表方有十灰散、槐花散、黄土汤、小蓟饮子、胶艾汤等。

十灰散《十药神书》[97]

[组成]　大蓟　小蓟　荷叶　侧柏叶　白茅根　茜草　山栀　大黄　牡丹皮　棕榈皮各等分

[用法]　原方各烧灰存性，研极细末，用纸包，碗盖于地上一夕，出火毒，用时将白藕捣汁或萝卜汁磨真京墨半碗，调服五钱，食后服下。

现代用法：各药烧炭存性，为末，藕汁或萝卜汁磨京墨适量，调服9～15克；亦可作汤剂，水煎服，用量按原方比例酌定。

[功效]　凉血止血。

[主治]　血热妄行，吐血、咯血。

[方解]

吐血、咯血，多由火热炽盛，损伤血络，离经妄行所致。血得热则妄行，方中大蓟、小蓟、侧柏叶、茅根、茜草、山栀皆为凉血止血之品，益以棕榈皮收涩止血，荷叶散瘀止血，大黄下行，能泻血分实热，兼以祛瘀。合而成方，以凉血止血为主，同时配伍化瘀之品，使血止而不留瘀。方中诸药均烧炭存性，以加强收涩止血作用，正如葛可久所谓："大抵血热则行，血冷则凝，见黑则止，此定理也。"用藕汁或萝卜汁磨京墨调服，其意亦在增强清热降气止血之效。本方十味药物，均烧灰存性，研为散剂备用，故名"十灰散"。又本方为《十药神书》中的第一方，故原书又名"甲字十灰散"。

[临床运用]

本方主治血热妄行所致的吐血、咯血，乃急则治标之剂。血止之后，还当随证调理，方能巩固疗效。

槐花散《普济本事方》[98]

[组成]　槐花炒　柏叶烂杵，焙　荆芥穗　枳壳去穰，细切，麸炒黄，等分

[用法]　原方细末，用清米饮调下二钱，空心食前服。

现代用法：为细末，每服6克，开水或米汤调下；亦可作汤剂，水煎服，用量按原方比例酌定。

[功效]　清肠止血，疏风行气。

[主治]　肠风脏毒，大便下血，血色鲜红或紫暗，舌红苔黄，脉数者。

[方解]

前人认为，大便下血，色鲜红者为肠风，紫暗者为脏毒。究其病因，乃由风热或湿热壅遏大肠血分，热伤阴络而成，正如《医宗金鉴·杂病心法要诀》所说："便血二证，肠风、脏毒。其本皆热伤阴络，热与风合为肠风，下血多清；热与湿合为脏毒，下血多浊。"方中槐花专清大肠，凉血止血，为君药；柏叶燥湿清热，助君药凉血止血，为臣药；荆芥穗疏风理血，枳壳宽肠行气，共为佐药。诸药合用，既能凉血止血，又清大肠湿热，疏风行气，使血止而无留瘀之弊。用药虽少，配伍得宜，故用治肠风脏毒下血，确有良效。原方以米饮调服，取其兼顾脾胃，使寒凉而不伤中气。

[临床运用]

本方为治肠风、脏毒下血的常用方剂，亦可用治痔疮出血。如大肠热盛，可加黄芩、黄连、大黄以清泄大肠实热；下血较多，方中荆芥穗可炒炭用，并加地榆炭以加强清热止血作用；若便血日久不止，导致血虚者，当加入养血之品，如《济生方》加减四物汤，即四物汤去芍药与本方合用，以治疗肠风下血而阴血不足者。

黄土汤《金匮要略》

[组成] 甘草 干地黄 白术 附子炮 阿胶 黄芩各三两（各9克）灶中黄土半斤（30克）

[用法] 原方七味，以水八升，煮取三升，分温二服。

现代用法：先煎灶中黄土，澄清取汁，代水再煎余药，再取汁，入阿胶烊化后温服。

[功效] 温阳健脾，养血止血。

[主治] 脾气虚寒，不能统血，大便下血，或吐血、衄血，血色紫暗，四肢不温，面色萎黄，舌淡苔白，脉沉细无力者。

[方解]

脾为统血之脏，脾气虚寒，不能统血。方中重用灶中黄土，又名伏龙肝，味辛微温，温中止血，为君药；配合白术、附子健脾温阳，以复脾土统血之权，为臣药；出血量多，阴血亏耗，佐以生地、阿胶、甘草滋阴养血止血；又有黄芩苦寒止血,《本草纲目》载其治"诸失血",且能协助生地、阿胶共同制约黄土、白术、附子温燥之性,恐其耗血动血,以为反佐;甘草并能调中和药,以为使。诸药合用,刚柔相济,温凉并进,使温阳健脾而不致伤阴动血,滋阴养血而不致妨碍脾阳。吴鞠通称本方为"甘苦合用,刚柔互济法",可谓配伍得宜。

[临床运用]

本方主要用于脾气虚寒,不能统血所致的大便下血或吐血、衄血。但目前药铺多不备灶中黄土,可以赤石脂代之。如胃纳差者,阿胶可改为阿胶珠,以减其滋腻之性;气虚甚者,可加人参或党参以补气摄血;出血多者,亦可酌加三七等止血药;脾胃虚寒较甚者,可加炮姜炭以温中止血。

小蓟饮子《济生方》

[组成]　生地黄洗,四两(24克)　小蓟根(12克)　滑石(12克)　木通(6克)蒲黄炒(6克)　淡竹叶(9克)　藕节(12克)　当归去芦,酒浸(6克)　山栀子仁(9克)甘草炙,各半两(6克)

[用法]　原方㕮咀,每服四钱,水一盏半,煎至八分,去滓,温服,空心食前。

现代用法:水煎服。

[功效]　凉血止血,利水通淋。

[主治]　下焦结热,血淋,小便频数,赤涩热痛或尿血,舌红,脉数者。

[方解]

《素问·气厥论》说:"胞移热于膀胱,则癃溺血。"下焦结热,损伤阴络,迫血下溢,渗入膀胱,与小便俱出,其痛者为血淋,若不痛者为尿血。方中小蓟凉血止血,祛瘀生新;大量生地黄清热凉血,止血消瘀,二味共为君药。臣以炒蒲黄凉血止血,且利水道;藕节收涩止血,兼能化瘀,君臣相配,使血止而不留瘀。《素问·阴阳应象大论》说:"其下者,引而竭之。"热在下焦,宜因势利导,故佐以滑石、木通、淡竹叶清热利水通淋,栀子仁清泄下焦结热,从小便而出;又有当归祛瘀生新,引血归经,配伍生地,使清热利水而不伤阴血。使以炙甘草缓急止痛,调和诸药。合而成方,共奏凉血止血,利水通淋之效。

[临床运用]

本方止血之中兼以化瘀，清利之中寓以养阴，是治疗下焦结热，血淋、尿血的常用方剂。方中炙甘草一般可改为甘草梢，取其直达茎中，清热止痛。若血淋疼痛剧烈，可加入琥珀末 1.5 克吞服，取其利水通淋，止血消瘀。若血淋、尿血不止，可加入白茅根（鲜者尤良），取其凉血止血，且利小便。

胶艾汤《金匮要略》

[组成] 芎蒌　阿胶　甘草各二两（各6克）　艾叶　当归各三两（各9克）芍药四两（12克）　干地黄四两（12克）[干地黄原书未著分量，此据《千金方》补入]

[用法] 原方七味，以水五升，清酒三升，合煮，取三升，去滓，内胶，令消尽，温服一升，日三服。不差更服。

现代用法：以水三分之二，黄酒三分之一，同煎，去滓，加入阿胶烊化，温服。

[功效] 养血调经，安胎止漏。

[主治] 妇人冲任虚损，崩中漏下，或月经过多，淋漓不断，或半产后下血不绝，或妊娠下血，腹中痛者。

[方解]

冲为血海，任主胞胎，冲任虚损，不能统摄血脉。方中阿胶甘平，养血止血，《本经》谓其主"女子下血，安胎"；艾叶苦辛温，温经止血，《别录》谓其治"妇人漏血"，二者皆为调经安胎，治崩止漏之要药，故共为君药。干地黄、芍药、当归、川芎养血调经，化瘀生新，以防止血留瘀，均为辅佐药。血不自生，生于阳明水谷之海，甘草补土，即所以养血，且能调和诸药，甘草配阿胶则善于止血，配芍药则酸甘化阴，缓急止痛；加入清酒同煮，引药入于血脉，并使血止而不留瘀，均为使药。诸药合用，标本兼顾，塞流澄源，共奏养血调经，安胎止漏之效。

[临床运用]

本方止血安胎，为治疗妇女崩漏，月经过多，半产下血，妊娠胞阻的要方。亦可用治妊娠跌仆损伤，而致胎动不安，下血腹痛者。

第十六章

祛湿剂

凡以祛湿药为主组成，具有化湿利水，通淋泄浊的作用，以治疗湿邪为病的方剂，统称祛湿剂。其中大多数方剂属于"十剂"中"燥可去湿，通可去滞"的范围。

第一节　芳香化湿

芳香化湿剂具有芳香化湿，辟秽去浊的作用，适用于湿浊内盛，困阻脾胃所致的脘腹胀满，嗳气吞酸，呕吐泄泻，食少体倦，舌苔浊腻等症。湿为重浊黏腻之邪，治疗当选用芳香化湿、苦温燥湿之品，使湿去浊化，气机通畅。常用藿香、苍术、厚朴、陈皮、半夏等为主组成方剂，代表方有平胃散、藿香正气散等。

平胃散《医方类聚》引《简要济众方》

[组成]　苍术去黑皮，捣为粗末，炒黄色，四两（120克）　厚朴去粗皮，涂生姜汁，炙令香熟，三两（90克）　陈橘皮洗令净，焙干，二两（60克）　甘草炙黄，二两（60克）

[用法]　原方四味，捣罗为散，每服二钱，水一中盏，入姜二片、枣二枚，同煎至六分，去滓，食前温服。

现代用法：共为细末，每服6克，水煎服。亦可作汤剂，水煎服，用量按原方比例酌情增减。

[功效]　燥湿运脾，行气和胃。

[主治] 湿阻脾胃，脘腹胀满，不思饮食，口腻无味，呕哕恶心，嗳气反酸，怠惰嗜卧，体重节痛，常多自利，苔白厚腻，脉缓。

[方解]

脾主运化，喜燥恶湿，若吸受湿浊之气或过食生冷、油腻之物，均能导致湿困脾胃。方中重用苍术苦温辛烈，燥湿运脾，为君药；臣以厚朴苦辛温，行气化湿，消胀除满；佐以陈皮辛苦温，理气和胃，燥湿健脾；使以甘草补益脾胃，调和诸药，生姜、大枣益胃和中。本方以治湿为主，佐以行气，气行则有助于湿化。如此则脾运复常，胃气和降，诸症自愈。方名"平胃"，正如张景岳说："平胃者，欲平治其不平也……为胃强邪实者设，故其性味从辛、从燥、从苦，而能消、能散，惟有滞、有湿、有积者宜之。"

[临床运用]

1. 本方为燥湿运脾的常用方，以脘腹胀满，不思饮食，苔白厚腻，脉缓为辨证要点。若食少而呆滞不化，或因食作泻，宜加炒楂肉、炒神曲、鸡内金以消食化滞，此为《时病论》[99]楂曲平胃法。若兼热象，苔腻而黄，口苦咽干而不甚欲饮，此为湿热合邪，宜加入黄芩、黄连等苦寒药以清热燥湿，始合病情。

2. 本方用甘草、姜、枣，以示中和之意，实际上以少用或不用为好。恐其助湿满中，反使湿邪不化。

藿香正气散《太平惠民和剂局方》

[组成] 藿香去土，三两（90克） 大腹皮 白芷 紫苏 茯苓去皮，各一两（各30克） 半夏曲 白术 陈皮去白 厚朴去粗皮，姜汁炙 苦桔梗各二两（各60克）甘草炙，二两半（75克）

[用法] 原方为细末，每服二钱，水一盏，姜钱三片，枣一枚，同煎至七分，热服，如欲出汗，衣被盖，再煎并服。

现代用法：为散剂，每服6～9克，日服二次，加生姜3片，大枣1枚，水煎服。或作丸剂，每服6～9克，日服二次，温开水送下。亦可作汤剂，水煎服，用量按原方比例酌减。

[功效] 解表化湿，理气和中。

[主治]　外感风寒，内伤湿滞，恶寒发热，头疼，胸膈满闷，脘腹疼痛，恶心呕吐，肠鸣泄泻，舌苔白腻，脉濡。

[方解]

本方证乃外感风寒，内伤湿滞所致。方中重用藿香辛温芳香，外解表邪，内化湿浊，理气和中，辟秽止呕，为君药。紫苏、白芷助君药解表散寒，且有芳香化湿之功；半夏曲、陈皮燥湿祛痰，和胃降逆；厚朴、大腹皮化湿散满，下气宽中，使气行则湿浊易去，以上均为臣药。湿滞之成，由于脾不健运，故又以白术、茯苓健脾化湿；桔梗宣肺利膈，以通调水道，排除湿邪，均为佐药。炙甘草益气健脾，调和诸药；生姜、大枣益胃和中，共为使药。综观全方，解表疏里，升清降浊，扶正祛邪，使风寒外散，湿浊内化，气机通畅，脾胃调和，则诸症自愈。本方以藿香为君药，能正不正之气，故方名"藿香正气散"。

[临床运用]

本方为芳香化湿的代表方剂，又兼有解表作用，所治之证，乃外感风寒，内伤湿滞，而以湿滞脾胃为主者。尤其对夏月内受湿浊，外客风寒，肠胃不和者，每每采用本方。对于山岚瘴气，水土不服所致的呕吐泻利，运用本方，亦有一定的疗效。

第二节　清热祛湿

清热祛湿剂具有湿热两清的作用，适用于湿热俱盛（包括湿从热化及湿热下注）所致的湿温、黄疸、热淋、痿痹等症。热为阳邪，湿为阴邪，清热多用苦寒药，祛湿多用苦温或淡渗药。常用苦寒清热药如栀子、大黄、黄芩、黄连、黄柏、连翘等与苦温燥湿药如厚朴、半夏、藿香、蔻仁、苍术，淡渗利湿药如滑石、薏苡仁、通草等配伍成方。代表方有茵陈蒿汤、三仁汤、甘露消毒丹、八正散、二妙散等。

茵陈蒿汤《伤寒论》

[组成]　茵陈六两（18克）　栀子十四枚，擘（9克）　大黄二两，去皮（6克）

[**用法**]　原方三味，以水一斗二升，先煮茵陈，减六升，内二味，煮取三升，去滓，分温三服。

现代用法：水煎服。

[**功效**]　清热利湿退黄。

[**主治**]　湿热黄疸，一身面目俱黄，黄色鲜明如橘子色，但头汗出，身无汗，小便不利，腹微满，口渴，舌苔黄腻，脉沉实或滑数。

[**方解**]

湿邪与瘀热相合，蕴结于里，热不得外越，湿不得下泄，湿热郁蒸，发为阳黄。方中重用茵陈蒿苦泄下降，功专除湿清热退黄，《本经》谓其主"热结黄疸"，《别录》谓其"主通身发黄，小便不利"，以其善清肝胆之热，兼理肝胆之郁，故为君药；臣以栀子苦寒，泻火除烦，清热利湿，使湿热从小便而出；佐以少量大黄，通泄瘀热，且利湿热从小便而出，故《本草纲目》谓其治"小便淋沥……黄疸"；《温热经纬》引徐灵胎说："先煮茵陈，则大黄从小便出，此秘法也。"是以原方后注："小便当利，尿如皂荚汁状，色正赤，一宿腹减，黄从小便去也。"三药配伍，苦泄下降，清热利湿，使邪有去路，则黄疸自退。

[**临床运用**]

本方为治疗阳黄热重于湿的主方。以一身面目俱黄，黄色鲜明，小便不利，舌苔黄腻为辨证要点。若小便黄赤短涩甚者，可加车前子、泽泻、碧玉散以清热利湿；若大便秘结，可重用大黄以泻热通便；若大便较溏，可去大黄加黄连，《医方集解》名之曰"茵陈三物汤"；若脘腹胀满较甚，可加制香附、广郁金、山楂炭、鸡内金以行气活血，消导积滞。

三仁汤《温病条辨》

[**组成**]　杏仁五钱（15克）　飞滑石六钱（18克）　白通草二钱（6克）　白蔻仁二钱（6克）　竹叶二钱（6克）　厚朴二钱（6克）　生薏仁六钱（18克）　半夏五钱（15克）

[**用法**]　原方以甘澜水八碗，煮取三碗，每服一碗，日三服。

现代用法：水煎服。

[**功效**]　宣畅气机，清利湿热。

[主治]　湿温初起，邪在气分，头痛恶寒，身重疼痛，面色淡黄，胸闷不饥，午后身热，舌白不渴，脉弦细而濡。

[方解]

湿温初起，邪气逗留气分，湿重热轻。方中杏仁苦温，善开上焦，宣降肺气，以通调水道。盖肺主一身之气，气化则湿亦化；白蔻仁芳香辛温，行气化湿，作用于上中二焦；生苡仁甘淡微寒，渗利湿热，以其色白入肺，味甘入脾，味淡渗湿，性寒泄热。三仁均为君药。半夏、厚朴苦温燥湿，助杏仁、蔻仁宣上畅中；滑石、通草甘淡而寒，助薏仁清利湿热；竹叶辛淡甘寒，轻清透热，淡渗利湿，均为辅佐药。诸药相合，宣上畅中渗下，以治弥漫之湿，其中尤以宣上为主，使气机宣畅，湿祛热清，诸症自解。原方用甘澜水煮，取其甘淡质轻，不致助湿。

[临床运用]

本方是治疗湿温初起，邪在气分，湿重于热的常用方剂。此时若仅与苦辛温燥以化湿，则热益炽；若单用苦寒直折其热，则湿仍留，用本方宣畅三焦，分消湿热，最为恰当。

甘露消毒丹（又名普济解毒丹）《续名医类案》引叶天士方

[组成]　飞滑石十五两（450克）　淡黄芩十两（300克）　茵陈十一两（330克）石菖蒲六两（180克）　川贝母　木通各五两（各150克）　藿香　射干　连翘　薄荷　白蔻仁各四两（各120克）

[用法]　原方生晒研末。每服三钱，开水调下，或神曲糊丸，如弹子大，开水化服亦可。

现代用法：各药生晒，共研细末，作丸剂或散剂，每服9克，日服二次；亦可作汤剂，水煎服，用量按原方比例酌减。

[功效]　清热解毒、利湿化浊。

[主治]　湿温时疫，邪在气分，发热倦怠，胸闷腹胀，肢酸咽肿，周身发黄，颐肿口渴，小便短赤，吐泻疟痢，淋浊疮疡，舌苔淡白，或厚腻、或干黄者。

[方解]

本方证乃感受湿温时疫，邪在气分，湿热并重，郁阻气机，蕴蒸不解之候。方中重用飞滑石甘淡而寒，祛暑清热，利水除湿，为君药。黄芩苦寒，清热燥湿，茵陈苦平微寒，清利湿热，共为臣药。连翘、射干苦寒，清热解毒，木通苦寒，清热利湿；石菖蒲、藿香、白蔻仁辛温芳香，化湿辟秽，宣畅气机，气化则湿易化；湿热蕴蒸，易生痰浊，川贝母苦甘微寒，清化痰热；薄荷辛凉，轻清宣透，使热邪从里外达，以上均为佐药。诸药配伍，寒凉清热解毒，淡渗分利湿热，芳香化湿辟秽，三法齐备。而三法之中，又以清热为主，渗湿为辅，芳化为佐，主次分明，用治湿热秽浊之邪，多获良效。本方清热于湿中，渗湿于热下，以消除湿热毒邪，一若甘露降而暑气潜消，故名之曰"甘露消毒丹"。

[临床运用]

本方在夏令暑湿季节最为常用。凡湿温、暑温、时疫之属湿热并重，邪留气分者，皆可以本方主治之，故王孟英推崇本方为"治湿温时疫之主方。"

八正散《太平惠民和剂局方》

[组成] 车前子　瞿麦　萹蓄　滑石　山栀子仁　甘草炙　木通　大黄面裹煨，去面，切，焙，各一斤（各500克）

[用法] 原方为散，每服二钱，水一盏，入灯心煎至七分，去滓温服，食后临卧。小儿量力少少与之。

现代用法：水煎服，用量按原方比例酌减。

[功效] 清热泻火，利水通淋。

[主治] 湿热下注，发为热淋、血淋、石淋，尿频涩痛，淋漓不畅，小便黄赤，甚或癃闭不通，小腹胀满，咽干口燥，舌质红苔黄腻，脉数实者。

[方解]

湿热下注，蓄于膀胱，则水道不利，发为热淋。方中瞿麦苦寒沉降，清热泻火，利水通淋，《本经》谓其"主关格，诸癃结，小便不通"，《本草备要》谓其"逐膀胱邪热，为治淋要药"，故为君药；萹蓄苦平，清热利水通淋，《本草纲目》谓其"利小便"，为臣药；木通苦寒，车前子、滑石甘寒，均能清热利水通淋，山栀苦寒泻热，清利三焦，导湿热从小便而去，煨大黄苦寒下达，泻火凉血，除湿热，利小便，《珍珠囊》谓其"除下焦湿热"，《本草纲目》谓其"治小便淋沥"，以上均为佐药；炙甘草调和诸药，以防苦寒太过，损伤胃气，且能缓急止痛，为使药。以上八味，清热泻火，利水通淋，以治湿热下注之淋证，"热者寒之"，为正治之法，又制成散剂煎服，故名之曰"八正散"。原方入灯心煎，取其味淡气轻，有清热利水之效，因其专入心肺二经，清肺热而降心火，肺为气化之源，心为小肠之合也。

[临床运用]

本方苦寒通利，为治疗热淋的常用方剂。凡属湿热下注，小便淋漓不畅，尿频涩痛，甚或癃闭不通，小腹胀满，证属实热，皆可以本方主治之。若血淋者，可酌加小蓟、白茅根以凉血止血；石淋者，可酌加金钱草、海金沙、石韦、鸡内金以化石通淋。

二妙散《丹溪心法》

[组成]　黄柏炒　苍术米泔浸炒（各等分）[原方未著分量]

[用法]　原方二味为末，沸汤，入姜汁调服。二物皆有雄壮之气，表实气实者，加酒少许佐之。

现代用法：作散剂，或作丸剂，每服6克，日服两次，白开水或生姜汤送下。亦可作汤剂，水煎服，用量根据病情酌定。

[功效]　清热燥湿。

[主治]　湿热下注，下肢痿软无力，或足膝红肿疼痛，带下淋浊，或下部湿疮，舌苔黄腻。

[方解]

久居湿地或冒雨涉水，湿热郁蒸，浸淫筋脉，以致筋脉弛缓不用，故下肢痿软无力，乃成痿证。方中黄柏苦寒，清热燥湿，苍术苦温燥湿，两味合用，具有清热燥湿之效，对于湿热下注而正气未虚者，最为合拍。正如王晋三所说："此偶方之小制也……治阴分之湿热，有如鼓应桴之妙。"故以"二妙"名之。

[临床运用]

本方为治疗湿热下注的常用方剂。一般来说，方中黄柏、苍术用量可以相等。若热重湿轻者，可加重黄柏用量；湿重热轻者，可加重苍术用量。根据临床症状的不同，还可适当加味治之。如本方加川牛膝，作丸剂，名三妙丸（《医学正传》[100]），治湿热下流，两脚麻木，或如火烙之热者；若湿热下注，两足麻痿肿痛，小便不利，可再加薏苡仁淡渗利湿，使湿热从小便而去，名四妙丸（《成方便读》[101]）。本方加槟榔，各等分，为细末，名三妙散（《医宗金鉴》），外用于脐中出水及湿癣，有清热燥湿止痒之效。

第三节 利水渗湿

利水渗湿剂，适用于水湿壅盛，小便不利，或为水肿、癃闭、泄泻等症。采用本节方剂，可使水湿从小便排泄。常用利水渗湿药如茯苓、猪苓、泽泻、滑石等为主组成方剂，代表方有五苓散、猪苓汤、五皮散等。

五苓散《伤寒论》

[组成] 猪苓十八铢，去皮（9克） 泽泻一两六铢（15克） 茯苓十八铢（9克）
桂枝半两，去皮（6克） 白术十八铢（9克）

[用法] 原方五味捣为散，以白饮和服方寸匕，日三服，多饮暖水，汗出愈，如法将息。

现代用法：作散剂，每服6～9克，日服二次，空腹以温水或米汤送服。或作汤剂，水煎服。

[功效] 化气利水。

[主治]

1.外有表证，内有蓄水，头痛微热，渴欲饮水，或水入则吐，心下痞满，小便不利，少腹急迫不舒，舌苔白腻，脉浮。

2.水湿内停所致的水肿、身重、泄泻、小便不利，以及霍乱吐泻等症。

3.痰饮，脐下动悸，吐涎沫而巅眩者。

[方解]

太阳经表邪未解，外邪循经内传太阳之腑膀胱，以致膀胱气化不利，水蓄下焦。方中重用泽泻甘淡而寒，入膀胱经，利水渗湿，为君药；臣以茯苓、猪苓甘淡渗湿，通利水道；佐以白术苦甘而温，健脾燥湿利水，乃培土以制水也；使以少量桂枝，辛甘而温，既能外解太阳之表，又能温化膀胱之气。五药相合，以令气化水行。原方捣为散，以白饮（即米汤）和服，并多饮暖水，助药力以发汗，令其汗出尿通，则表里双解矣。

[临床运用]

1. 本方具有化气利水之功，凡水饮内停，或为膀胱蓄水，或为水逆，或为痰饮，或为水肿，或为泄泻，均可以本方加减治之。

2. 根据前人经验，外有表证，欲其发散，则用桂枝；若无表证，可用肉桂易桂枝，则温阳化气之功更胜。

猪苓汤《伤寒论》

[组成] 猪苓去皮　茯苓　阿胶　滑石碎　泽泻各一两（各9克）

[用法] 原方五味，以水四升，先煮四味，取二升，去滓，内阿胶烊消，温服七合，日三服。

现代用法：水煎服。

[功效] 利水清热养阴。

[主治] 阴虚水热互结，小便不利，发热，渴欲饮水，或心烦不得眠，或兼下利、咳嗽、呕吐者。

[方解]

伤寒之邪传入阳明或少阴，化而为热。邪热伤阴，水热互结。方中猪苓甘平，以淡渗见长，《本经》载其"利水道"，故为君药；茯苓甘平，淡渗利水，泽泻甘淡利水，性寒又能泻膀胱之热，共为臣药；滑石甘寒而滑，寒能清热，滑利水道，使水热俱从小便而去，阿胶甘平，滋阴润燥，且防诸药渗利伤阴之弊，共为佐药。五药合而成方，利水而不伤阴，滋阴而不敛邪，使水去而热解，阴复则烦除，而成利水清热养阴之剂，但总以利水为主，清热养阴次之。

[临床运用]

本方主治阴虚水热互结，小便不利，乃虚实参半之证。若热淋、血淋、血尿之属于阴虚水热互结者，亦可用本方加减治之，乃标本兼顾之法。

五皮散（又名五皮饮）《华氏中藏经》[102]

[组成]　生姜皮　桑白皮　陈橘皮　大腹皮　茯苓皮各等分

[用法]　原方为粗末，每服三钱，水一盏半，煎至八分，去滓，不计时候温服，忌生冷油腻硬物。

现代用法：水煎服，用量按原方比例酌定。

[功效]　利水消肿，理气健脾。

[主治]　水肿，头面四肢悉肿，肢体沉重，心腹胀满，上气促急，小便不利，舌苔白腻者。

[方解]

脾属土，气化水。方中陈橘皮辛苦温，理气化湿和中，为宣通疏利之品，茯苓皮甘平，利水渗湿消肿，专治水肿肤胀，两药相配，使气行湿化，土能制水，共为君药；桑白皮甘寒，泻肺降气，行水消肿，使肺气清肃，水自下趋。大腹皮辛微温，下气利水，生姜皮辛凉，利水消肿，共为辅佐药。五药相合，体现了行气与利水同用的配伍方法，使气行则水行，共奏疏理脾气，利湿消肿之效。本方五药皆用其皮，取以皮行皮之意，且作散剂煎服，故名曰"五皮散"。

[临床运用]

本方为治疗水肿的通用方。以头面四肢皮肤肿胀，腹胀气急，小便不利为辨证要点。其病位在脾、肺二脏。若腰以上肿甚，兼挟风邪者，可加苏叶、秦艽、荆芥、防风等；腰以下肿甚，水湿下注者，可加赤小豆、苡仁、防己、车前子、泽泻等；大小便不通，可加杏仁、葶苈：审是阴水，可加附子、桂枝；审是阳水，可加木通、滑石。

防己黄芪汤《金匮要略》

[组成]　防己一两（12克）　黄芪一两一分，去芦（15克）　白术三分（9克）甘草半两，炙（6克）

[用法] 原方锉，每服五钱匕，生姜四片，枣一枚，水盏半，煎取八分，去滓温服，良久再服。

现代用法：加姜、枣适量，水煎服。

[功效] 益气祛风，健脾利水。

[主治] 风水或风湿，脉浮身重，汗出恶风，小便不利者。

[方解]

本方所治之风水、风湿，乃由表气不固，外受风邪，水湿郁于肌腠所致。方中重用生黄芪甘微温，益气固表，且能利水，《药征》[103]谓其"主治肌表之水"，防己大苦辛寒，祛风利水，与黄芪相配，利水力强而不伤正，共为君药；臣以白术苦甘温，健脾燥湿，既助防己以利水，又助黄芪固表止汗；佐以甘草益气健脾，使脾胃健运，水湿自去，且能调和诸药，缓和防己大苦辛寒之性，又为使药；生姜、大枣辛甘发散，调和营卫，亦为使药。全方药仅六味，扶正祛邪，相得益彰，使卫强表固，则风邪去而不致复入；脾气健运，则水湿去而不致复聚。表虚风水、风湿诸症，自可向愈。原方后云："服后当如虫行皮中。"即是卫阳复振，风湿欲解之验。又云："从腰下如冰，后坐被上，又以一被绕腰以下，温令微汗差。"此为外护之法，以通阳气。

[临床运用]

本方为治疗表虚风水、风湿证的常用方剂。以水肿或四肢麻木，腰髋疼痛为主症；以脉浮身重，汗出恶风，小便不利为兼症。

第四节　温化水湿

温化水湿剂，具有温阳化湿的作用，适用于湿从寒化所致的肾著、脚气和阳虚气不化水所致的痰饮、阴水等。常用温阳药物如干姜、桂枝、附子等配合利水药物如白术、茯苓等为主组成方剂。代表方有实脾散、苓桂术甘汤、鸡鸣散等。

实脾散《济生方》

[组成] 厚朴去皮，姜制，炒　白术　木瓜去瓤　木香不见火　草果仁　大

腹子 附子炮，去皮、脐 白茯苓去皮 干姜炮，各一两（各30克） 甘草炙，半两（15克）

[用法] 原方㕮咀，每服四钱，水一盏半，生姜五片，枣子一枚，煎至七分，去滓，温服，不拘时候。

现代用法：加生姜5片，大枣1枚，水煎服，用量按原方比例酌减。

[功效] 温阳健脾，行气利水。

[主治] 阴水，肢体浮肿，尤以身半以下肿甚，胸腹胀满，身重食少，手足不温，口中不渴，小便短少而清白，大便溏薄，舌淡苔腻，脉沉迟或沉细者。

[方解]

阴水缘于脾肾阳虚，气不化水，水湿内停所致。方中附子、干姜大辛大热，温壮脾肾，扶阳抑阴，为君药；白术、茯苓健脾益气，渗湿利水，为臣药；佐以厚朴散满，木香行气，大腹子（即槟榔）行气利水，草果仁温中燥湿，尤妙在木瓜一味，酸以收敛阴津，温以去湿和中，既可监制辛热之品，以免伤阴，且使水去而津不伤；使以甘草、生姜、大枣和诸药而调营卫，其中生姜用量较多，亦有温散水气之功。诸药合用，温阳健脾，行气利水，诚如《医宗金鉴》所说："气者水之母也，土者水之防也。气行则水行，土实则水治，故名曰'实脾'也。"

[临床运用]

本方是治疗阴水的重要方剂。但方中温阳行气之品有余，扶正益气之力不足，若见气少声微，正气大虚者，须加减运用。《医宗金鉴》主张："以理中汤加附子，数倍茯苓以君之，温补元气以行水，为万当也。"

苓桂术甘汤《金匮要略》

[组成] 茯苓四两（12克） 桂枝三两（9克） 白术三两（9克） 甘草二两（6克）

[用法] 原方上四味，以水六升，煮取三升，去滓，分温三服。

现代用法：水煎服。

[功效] 温阳化饮，健脾化饮。

[主治]　痰饮，胸胁支满，目眩心悸，短气而咳，舌苔白滑，脉弦滑或沉紧。

[方解]

中焦阳虚，脾失健运，气不化水，聚湿生痰成饮。方中重用茯苓健脾渗湿利水，《本经》谓其"主胸胁逆气……利小便"，故为君药；桂枝温阳化气利水，为臣药；白术健脾燥湿利水，为佐药；炙甘草调和诸药，且配茯苓、白术补脾益气，伍以桂枝辛甘化阳，为使药。四药合用，使中阳复而气化行，脾运健而饮邪去，实为治本之法。亦是《金匮要略》"病痰饮者，当以温药和之""夫短气有微饮，当从小便去之"的具体方剂。可见和以温药，利其小便，为治疗痰饮病的重要方法。

[临床运用]

本方为温阳化饮的主要方剂。若痰多者，可加制半夏、陈皮以燥湿化痰；若脾虚甚者，当再加党参以益气补脾。

鸡鸣散《类编朱氏集验方》[104] 引淮头老兵方

[组成]　槟榔七枚（12克）　陈皮　木瓜各一两（9克）　吴茱萸二钱（3克）桔梗半两（4.5克）　生姜和皮，半两（4.5克）　紫苏茎叶三钱（6克）

[用法]　原方为粗末，分作八服，隔宿用水三大碗，慢火煎，留半碗；去滓，留水二碗，煎滓，取一小碗，两次以煎汁相和，安顿床头，次日五更分二三次服，只是冷服，冬月略温亦得，服了用饼饵压下，如服不尽，留次日渐渐吃亦可。服此药至天明，大便当下一碗许黑粪水，即是原肾家感寒湿毒气下来也。至早饭前后痛住肿消，但只是放迟迟吃物，候药力过，此药不是宣药，并无所忌。

现代用法：作汤剂，水煎，晨起空腹分2～3次冷服。用量按原方比例酌情增减。

[功效]　下气降浊，温化寒湿。

[主治]　湿脚气。足胫肿重无力，行动不便，麻木冷痛，甚则胸闷泛恶；亦治风湿流注脚足，痛不可忍，筋脉肿大者。

[方解]

《灵枢·百病始生》说："清湿袭虚，则病起于下。"《外台秘要》说："夫脚气者，壅疾也。"惟宣通可去壅滞。方中重用槟榔辛苦而温，下气逐湿，为君药；臣以陈皮辛苦而温，理气燥湿，木瓜酸温，舒筋活络，和胃化湿，《医宗必读》记载"脚气惟兹最妙"；佐以吴茱萸辛苦大热，下气散寒，生姜辛温，散寒化湿，紫苏叶辛温香窜，香能透表，温可散寒，且其同陈皮则行气，配木瓜则散湿；使以桔梗宣开上焦肺气，使气化则湿化，升清有利于降浊。诸药配伍，开上、导下、疏中，共奏下气降浊，温化寒湿之效，俾久着之寒湿从大便而出，用治湿脚气颇有良效。原方于五更时服用，五更鸡鸣乃阳升之时，阳升则阴降，使寒湿阴邪随阳气升发而散之，取其空腹服，则药力专行，故方名"鸡鸣散"。药取冷服，以寒湿为阴邪，冷服则以阴从阴，可以避免格拒之弊，有助于提高疗效，正如《素问·五常政大论》所说："治寒以热，凉而行之。"亦为从治之法。

[临床运用]

本方用治湿脚气，足胫肿重无力，行动不便，麻木冷痛者，疗效较好。可以遏其病势，避免冲心之变。

第五节　祛风胜湿

祛风胜湿剂，适用于风寒湿邪在表所致的恶寒微热，头身痛重；或风湿着于筋骨，腰膝顽麻痛痹等症。常用祛风湿药如羌活、独活、防风、秦艽等为主组成方剂。对于风湿痹痛，常须配伍养血活血的药物，如当归、川芎、地黄、芍药等，取"治风先治血，血行风自灭"之意。若久病肝肾两亏，正气不足，还当酌加补益之品，以期祛邪不伤正，扶正以祛邪。代表方有羌活胜湿汤、独活寄生汤等。

羌活胜湿汤《内外伤辨惑论》

[组成]　羌活　独活各一钱（各3克）　藁本　防风　甘草　川芎各五分（各1.5克）　蔓荆子三分（1克）

[**用法**]　原方㕮咀，都作一服，水二盏，煎至一盏，去滓，大温服，空心食前。

现代用法：水煎服。

[**功效**]　祛风胜湿。

[**主治**]　风湿在表，头痛头重，腰脊重痛，或一身尽痛，难以转侧，恶寒微热，苔白腻，脉浮缓。

[**方解**]

太阳主一身之表，《灵枢·经脉》说："膀胱足太阳之脉……从巅入络脑，还出，别下项……挟脊，抵腰中。"方中羌活辛苦而温，味薄气雄，功专上升，《本经逢原》谓其"治足太阳风湿相搏，一身尽痛"，有祛风胜湿止痛之效，为君药。臣以独活辛苦微温，助羌活通达周身，祛风胜湿止痛，《本经逢原》谓其"升中有降，能通达周身而散风胜湿"。佐以藁本辛温升散，善达巅顶，祛风胜湿，《珍珠囊》谓其"治太阳头痛，巅顶痛"；防风辛甘微温，善祛风邪，胜湿止痛；川芎辛温升散，升清阳，祛风湿，为治头痛要药，配羌活尤善治太阳头痛；蔓荆子苦辛平，体轻而浮，上升而散，祛风除湿以止头痛。使以炙甘草调和诸药，甘以缓之，使诸风药不致发散太过，令湿着之邪能从微汗而去。原方剂量较轻，取"轻可去实"之意，服本方发汗，当以微汗为佳，使风湿之邪得以并去，若大发其汗，但风气去而湿不去，病必不除。

[**临床运用**]

本方不但用治风湿在表，头痛头重，腰脊重痛等症，且对伤风头痛疗效亦好。《医方集解》按："此汤虽名胜湿，实伤风头痛通用之方。"

独活寄生汤《备急千金要方》

[**组成**]　独活三两（9克）　寄生　杜仲　牛膝　细辛　秦艽　茯苓　桂心防风　芎䓖　人参　甘草　当归　芍药　干地黄各二两（各6克）

[**用法**]　原方十五味药，㕮咀，以水一斗，煮取三升，分三服，温身勿冷也。

现代用法：水煎服。

[**功效**]　益肝肾，补气血，祛风湿，止痹痛。

[**主治**]　肝肾两虚，风寒湿痹，腰膝冷痛，腿足屈伸不利，或麻木不仁，畏寒喜温，舌淡苔白，脉象细弱。

[**方解**]

腰为肾之府，膝为筋之府。肝肾两虚，则风寒湿邪乘虚客于腰膝。方中重用独活辛苦微温，入足少阴肾经，祛风胜湿，蠲痹止痛；桑寄生苦平，入肝肾经，补肝肾，强筋骨，除风湿，《本经》谓其"主腰痛"，《别录》谓其"去痹"，以上二味共为君药。臣以杜仲甘辛温，滋补肝肾，强筋健骨；《本经》谓其"主腰脊痛……坚筋骨"；牛膝苦酸平，补肝肾，强腰膝，且能活血，通利关节，《本经》谓其"主寒湿痿痹，四肢拘挛，膝痛不可屈伸"。佐以人参、茯苓、甘草益气扶正，所谓"祛邪先补正，正旺邪自除"；川芎、当归、芍药、地黄养血和营，所谓"治风先治血，血行风自灭"；又有细辛发散少阴经风寒，使邪外出；桂心入肝肾血分，以祛阴寒；秦艽、防风祛风胜湿，蠲痹止痛。独活为少阴引经药，故又兼使药。诸药合用，标本兼顾，扶正祛邪，使血气足而风湿除，肝肾强而痹痛愈，立方用意颇为周到。

[**临床运用**]

本方用治肝肾两虚，风寒湿痹的本虚标实证；或风寒湿痹日久，导致肝肾不足，气血两虚者。若痹证疼痛较甚，可加丹参；肾阳虚衰，可加附子、鹿角片。

第十七章

祛痰剂

凡以祛痰药为主组成，具有排除或消解痰涎的作用，以治疗各种痰病的方剂，统称祛痰剂。属于"八法"中的"消法"。

第一节　燥湿化痰

燥湿化痰剂，适用于湿痰为病。湿痰的生成，由于脾阳不振，运化失司，水湿停留，凝聚为痰。症见咳嗽痰多色白，胸脘痞闷，呕吐恶心，肢体困倦，或头眩心悸，舌苔白润或白腻。常用燥湿化痰药如半夏、橘红等为主组成方剂，代表方有二陈汤等。

二陈汤《太平惠民和剂局方》

[组成]　半夏汤洗七次　橘红各五两（各9克）　白茯苓三两（6克）　甘草炙，一两半（3克）

[用法]　原方㕮咀，每服四钱，用水一盏，生姜七片，乌梅一个，同煎六分，去滓，热服，不拘时候。

现代用法：加生姜3片，乌梅1个，水煎服，用量按原方比例酌减。或作丸剂，取前四味为末，用生姜汤，或水泛为丸，每服6～9克，日服二次，温开水送下。

[功效]　燥湿化痰，理气和中。

[主治]　湿痰，咳嗽痰多色白，胸脘胀满，呕吐恶心，头眩心悸，舌苔白润或白腻，脉滑。

160

[方解]

饮食不节，脾胃不和，健运失常，水湿内停，则湿聚为痰。方中半夏辛温，入脾胃经，功专燥湿化痰，降逆止呕；气机不畅则痰凝，痰凝则气机更为阻滞，故用橘红辛苦温，理气燥湿化痰，使气顺则痰降，二味共为君药。痰从湿生，脾健则湿去，湿去则痰消，故以茯苓甘平，健脾渗湿化痰，为臣药。佐以生姜辛温，祛痰下气，降逆止呕，既可制约半夏之毒，又能助半夏、橘红下气化痰；复用少量乌梅酸平，收敛肺气，且以生津，与半夏、橘红配伍，则散中有收，使痰去而肺气不伤，燥湿而不耗津液，有相得益彰之妙。使以甘草调和诸药，且助茯苓补土和中，俾脾健则湿化痰消。全方配伍严谨，具有燥湿化痰，理气和中之效。方中君药半夏、橘红，贵其陈久，则少燥散之性，故以"二陈"名之。

[临床运用]

本方是祛痰剂的一个基础方、通治方。随症加减，可广泛运用于各种痰证。《医方集解》载其加减法："治痰通用二陈，风痰加南星、白附、皂角、竹沥；寒痰加半夏、姜汁；火痰加石膏、青黛；湿痰加苍术、白术；燥痰加瓜蒌、杏仁；食加山楂、麦芽、神曲；老痰加枳实、海石、芒硝；气痰加香附、枳壳；胁痰在皮里膜外，加白芥子；四肢痰加竹沥。"

第二节　清热化痰

清热化痰剂，适用于热痰为病。热痰的生成，多因热淫于内，灼津成痰，或痰郁化火。症见咳嗽痰黄，黏稠难咯，舌苔黄腻，脉滑数，或癫狂、惊悸、瘰疬等。常用苦寒清热药如黄芩、黄连、大黄等与化痰药如竹茹、瓜蒌、胆南星、贝母、礞石等配伍组成方剂。代表方有温胆汤、小陷胸汤、滚痰丸、消瘰丸等。

温胆汤《备急千金要方》

[组成]　生姜四两（12克）　半夏二两，洗（6克）　橘皮三两（9克）　竹茹二两（6克）　枳实二枚，炙（6克）　甘草一两，炙（3克）

[**用法**] 原方六味切，以水八升，煮取二升，去滓，分三服。忌羊肉、海藻、菘菜、饧。

现代用法：水煎服。

[**功效**] 清胆和胃，化湿祛痰。

[**主治**]

1.胆虚痰热不眠，惊悸不安，口苦呕涎，苔腻。

2.湿热邪留三焦气分，寒热起伏，胸痞腹胀，小便短赤，苔腻而黄。

[**方解**]

本方证多由情志郁结，气郁痰生，痰热内扰，胆失疏泄，胃失和降所致。方中半夏辛温，和胃降逆，燥湿祛痰，为君药；橘皮辛苦温，理气和胃，化湿祛痰，大量生姜辛温，祛痰和胃，且制半夏之毒，均为臣药；竹茹甘寒，涤痰开郁，清热止呕，枳实苦微寒，下气行痰，其性甚速，均为佐药；少量甘草调和诸药，以为使。诸药合用，化痰而不燥，清热而不寒，使痰热尽去，胆腑自然恢复其少阳温和之气，故以"温胆"名之。

[**临床运用**]

1.《三因方》[105]《济生方》之温胆汤，即本方加茯苓、大枣而成，用治惊悸不眠等症。验之临床，加入茯苓，确实疗效更好。但大枣则不必加入，恐其甘腻壅滞，反而助长痰湿。

2.若心胆虚怯，触事易惊，夜多恶梦，或短气心悸乏力，或复自汗，四肢浮肿，饮食无味，心虚烦闷，坐卧不安者，可以本方去竹茹，加人参、熟地、枣仁、远志、五味子、白茯苓，名十味温胆汤（《世医得效方》[106]）。若烦热甚者，可以本方加黄连、白茯苓，名黄连温胆汤（《医方证治汇编歌诀》[107]）。

小陷胸汤《伤寒论》

[**组成**] 黄连一两（3克） 半夏半升，洗（9克） 瓜蒌实大者一枚（18克）

[**用法**] 原方三味，以水六升，先煮瓜蒌，取三升，去滓，内诸药，煮取二升，去滓，分温三服。

现代用法：水煎服。

[**功效**] 清热涤痰，宽胸散结。

［主治］ 痰热互结心下，按之则痛，苔黄滑或黄浊，脉浮滑者。

［方解］

本方原治伤寒表证误下，邪热内陷，与痰浊互结于心下而致的小结胸病。方中瓜蒌实甘寒，清热涤痰，宽胸散结，且利大肠，使痰热下行，为君药；臣以黄连苦寒泄热；佐以半夏辛温祛痰，下气散结，与黄连合用，辛开苦降，能清化痰浊。三药合用，诚为清热涤痰，宽胸散结之良剂。本方治疗小结胸病，攻虽不峻，但能蠲除胸中痰热互结之邪，如同陷阵，故名之曰"小陷胸汤"。

［临床运用］

本方用治痰热互结心下（胸膈）的小结胸病，以心下按之痛，苔黄滑或黄浊，脉浮滑为辨证要点。若痛甚者，加入枳壳、桔梗升降气机，疗效更佳。

礞石滚痰丸《泰定养生主论》[108]

［组成］ 青礞石一两（30克） 沉香五钱（15克） 大黄 黄芩各八两（各250克）

［用法］ 原方将礞石打碎，用朴硝一两同入瓦罐，盐泥固济，晒干火煅，石色如金为度，研末，和诸药，水丸……大抵服药，必须临睡就床，用热水一口许，只送过咽，即使仰卧，令药在咽膈间徐徐而下……多半日不可饮食汤水，及不可起身坐行言语，直候药丸除逐上焦痰滞恶物，过膈入腹，然后动作，方能中病。每次须连进两夜，先夜所服，次日痰物即下三五次，次夜减十丸。下一二次者，仍服前数。下五七次，或只二三次，而病势顿已者，次夜减二十丸。头夜所服，并不下恶物者，次夜加十丸。壮人病实者，多至百丸。大抵服罢仰卧，咽喉稠涎壅塞不利者，乃痰气泛上，药物相攻之故也。少顷药力既胜，自然宁贴。大抵次早先去大便一次，其余遍次，皆是痰涕恶物，亦有看是溏粪，用水搅之，尽系痰片粘液……此药并不洞泄刮肠大泄，但能取痰积恶物，自胃肠次第穿凿而下，腹中糟粕并不相伤。

现代用法：为细末，水泛为丸，如梧桐子大，每服9～12克，临卧时用温开水送下。

［功效］ 降火逐痰。

［主治］ 实热老痰，发为癫狂惊悸，或怔忡昏迷，或咳喘痰稠，或胸脘痞闷，或眩晕耳鸣，大便秘结，苔黄厚腻，脉滑数有力。

[方解]

实热老痰，久积不去，变幻多端。方中青礞石甘咸平，其性下行，功专镇坠，善能攻逐陈积伏匿之老痰，为君药；臣以大黄苦寒，荡涤实热，以开痰火下行之路；佐以黄芩苦寒，清热泻火，《别录》谓其"疗痰热"，大黄、黄芩用量独重，此治痰必须清火也；使以少量沉香辛苦温，降泄下气，助诸药攻逐积痰，此治痰必须利气也。四药合用，确具降火逐痰之效，因其攻逐实热顽痰之力峻猛，服后其痰下滚，从大便而出，故名之曰"滚痰丸"。

[临床运用]

本方专治实热老痰为病。凡癫狂惊悸，怔忡昏迷，咳喘痰稠，或眩晕耳鸣，种种怪症。若见大便干燥，苔黄厚腻，脉滑数有力，即可运用本方降火逐痰，使痰积恶物自肠道而下。

消瘰丸《医学心悟》[109]

[组成]　玄参蒸　牡蛎煅，锉研　贝母去心，蒸，各四两（各125克）

[用法]　原方共为细末，炼蜜为丸，每服三钱，开水下，日二服。

现代用法：共为细末，炼蜜为丸，每服9克，日服二次，温开水送下。亦可作汤剂，水煎服，用量按原方比例酌减。

[功效]　清热化痰，软坚散结。

[主治]　瘰疬，痰核，瘿瘤。兼见咽干，舌红，脉弦滑略数者。

[方解]

本方所治之瘰疬、痰核、瘿瘤，由于肝肾阴亏，肝经血燥有火，灼津为痰，痰火凝聚而成。方中玄参苦咸寒，滋阴降火，能散瘰疬、痰核、瘿瘤，《别录》记载"散颈下核"，《本草纲目》谓其"消瘰疬亦是散火"，故为君药；牡蛎咸平微寒，化痰软坚散结，为臣药；贝母苦寒，清热化痰散结，为佐药。三药合用，标本兼顾，使液增痰化结散，瘰疬、痰核、瘿瘤自消。

[临床运用]

1. 本方主治瘰疬、痰核、瘿瘤属痰火凝聚者。若肿块大而坚硬，宜重用牡蛎，酌加海藻、昆布、夏枯草以软坚散结；痰火盛者，宜重用贝母，酌加瓜蒌皮、海蛤粉、海浮石以清热化痰散结；阴虚甚者，宜重用玄参，酌加生地、麦冬以滋阴养液；肝火旺者，酌加丹皮、山栀、连翘以清泄肝火；兼肝郁气滞者，宜加柴胡、香附、郁金、青皮以疏肝理气解郁，或配合逍遥散同用。

2. 原方用煅牡蛎，若作汤剂，当用生牡蛎，疗效更好。

第三节　润燥化痰

润燥化痰剂，适用于燥痰为病。燥痰的生成，由于燥热伤肺，灼津为痰。症见咳呛气促，痰稠而粘，咯之不爽，咽喉干燥，声音嘶哑等。常用润燥化痰药如贝母、瓜蒌等为主组成方剂。代表方有贝母瓜蒌散。

贝母瓜蒌散《医学心悟》

[组成]　贝母一钱五分（4.5克）　瓜蒌一钱（3克）　花粉　茯苓　橘红　桔梗各八分（各2.4克）

[用法]　原方水煎服。

现代用法：与原方相同。

[功效]　润肺清热，化痰止咳。

[主治]　肺燥有痰，咳呛。咯痰不爽，涩而难出，咽喉干燥哽痛，舌干少苔者。

[方解]

湿痰多生于脾，燥痰多生于肺。方中重用贝母苦甘微寒，润肺清热，化痰止咳，瓜蒌甘寒，润燥清热化痰，二味共为君药；臣以花粉甘寒，润肺化痰止咳；佐以茯苓甘平，能化痰涎，橘红辛苦温，理气化痰；使以桔梗辛散苦泄，宣肺祛痰，且为肺经引经药。诸药合用，使肺润则气肃，热清则痰消，宜于肺燥有痰之证。

[临床运用]

本方用治肺经燥热有痰而致的咳呛。如喉中作痒，可加前胡、牛蒡子以宣肺利咽；咽干燥痛甚者，可加玄参、麦冬以清热润燥；声音嘶哑，痰中带血者，可去橘红，加沙参、阿胶以养阴止血。

第四节　温化寒痰

温化寒痰剂，适用于寒痰为病。寒痰的生成，由于脾胃阳虚，寒饮内停。症见吐痰清稀，咳逆胸满，手足不温，舌淡苔白滑，脉沉。常用辛热药如干姜、细辛等与化痰药如茯苓、半夏等配合组成方剂。代表方有苓甘五味姜辛汤。

苓甘五味姜辛汤《金匮要略》

[组成]　茯苓四两(12克)　甘草三两(9克)　干姜三两(9克)　细辛三两(9克)
五味子半升(6克)

[用法]　原方五味，以水八升，煮取三升，去滓，温服半升，日三。
现代用法：水煎服。

[功效]　温肺化饮。

[主治]　寒饮内停，咳逆痰稀，多唾胸满，舌苔白滑，脉沉弦。

[方解]

本方证乃因阳虚阴盛，寒饮内停所致。方中重用茯苓甘平，健脾渗湿，化饮利水，一以导既聚之饮从小便而去，一以杜其生痰之源，使脾运健而湿无由聚，故为君药；干姜大辛大热，既能温肺以散寒，又能燥湿以化饮；细辛辛温，温肺散寒且化痰饮，共为臣药；为防干姜、细辛耗散肺气，故又以五味子酸温，敛肺止咳，使散不伤正，敛不留邪，为佐药，亦即《素问·藏气法时论》"肺欲收，急食酸以收之，用酸补之，辛泻之"之意；甘草温中，调和诸药，为使药。全方药仅五味，配伍严谨，散中有敛，开中有阖，标本兼顾，实为温肺化饮之良剂。

[临床运用]

本方主治寒饮内停，咳逆痰稀，多唾等症。据《金匮要略》法，若并见眩晕呕吐，可加制半夏燥湿化痰，降逆止呕；若其人形肿，可加杏仁宣利肺气，气化则饮消，形肿亦随之而减；若面热如醉，可加大黄利大便以泄胃热。

第五节 治风化痰

治风化痰剂，适用于风痰为病。风痰的生成，有内外二端。外风挟痰，由外感风邪，肺气不宣所致，可见恶风发热，咳嗽有痰等症。内风挟痰，多由脾湿生痰，肝风内动，风痰上扰所致，可见眩晕头痛，甚则昏厥等症。外风挟痰，治宜疏风化痰，常用宣散外邪与止嗽化痰之品，如荆芥、紫菀、桔梗、橘红等为主组成方剂，代表方有止嗽散。内风挟痰，治宜熄风化痰，常用平熄内风与燥湿化痰之品，如天麻、半夏、白术、茯苓等为主组成方剂，代表方有半夏白术天麻汤。

止嗽散《医学心悟》

[组成] 桔梗炒　荆芥　紫菀蒸　百部蒸　白前蒸，各二斤（1000克）　甘草炒，十二两（375克）　陈皮水洗，去白，一斤（500克）

[用法] 原方为末，每服三钱，开水调下，食后临卧服。初感风寒，生姜汤调下。

现代用法：共为细末，每服9克，日服二次，温开水或生姜汤送下。亦可作汤剂，水煎服，用量按原方比例酌减。

[功效] 止嗽化痰，解表宣肺。

[主治] 风邪犯肺，咳嗽咽痒，或微有恶风发热，舌苔薄白。

[方解]

肺为娇脏，外合皮毛，最易受邪。方中紫菀辛苦温，下气止嗽化痰，为君药；百部甘苦微温，润肺止咳，白前辛甘微温，降气下痰止嗽，共为臣药；荆芥辛温，祛风解表，且利咽喉，桔梗苦辛平，宣肺祛痰，橘红辛苦温，理气化痰，以上共为佐药；少量甘草调和诸药，与桔梗同用，又能清利咽喉，为使药。诸药合用，温润和平，不寒不热，重在止嗽化痰，兼以解表宣肺，对于外感咳嗽较久，表邪未尽，咽痒而咯痰不畅者，疗效显著，故名之曰"止嗽散"。

[临床运用]

本方是治疗外感咳嗽的常用方剂。若风寒表证较重者，可加苏叶、防风、生姜以解表散寒；若咳嗽痰多色白，舌苔白腻者，可加制半夏、茯苓以燥湿化痰。

半夏白术天麻汤《医学心悟》

[组成]　半夏一钱五分（4.5克）　天麻　茯苓　橘红各一钱（各3克）　白术三钱（9克）　甘草五分（1.5克）

[用法]　原方生姜一片，大枣一枚，水煎服。

现代用法：与原方相同。

[功效]　健脾燥湿，化痰熄风。

[主治]　风痰上扰，眩晕头痛，胸闷呕恶，舌苔白腻，脉弦滑。

[方解]

本方证乃脾湿生痰，肝风内动所致。方中半夏辛温，燥湿化痰，天麻甘微温，平熄内风，二味合用，为治风痰眩晕头痛的要药，正如《脾胃论》所说："足太阴痰厥头痛，非半夏不能疗；眼黑头旋，风虚内作，非天麻不能除。"故共为君药；臣以白术苦甘温，健脾燥湿，《珍珠囊》谓其"除湿益气……消痰逐水"，与君药配伍，燥湿祛痰，止眩之功益佳；佐以茯苓甘平，健脾渗湿，与白术相合，以治生痰之源，橘红辛苦温，理气燥湿化痰，使气顺则痰消；甘草、生姜、大枣健脾和中，为使药。诸药合用，共奏健脾燥湿，化痰熄风之效。

[临床运用]

本方为治风痰上扰，眩晕头痛的常用方剂。若眩晕较甚，可加钩藤、桑叶、菊花、南星以熄风化痰；头痛较甚，可加蔓荆子以止痛；气虚者，可加党参以补气。

第十八章

驱虫剂

凡以安蛔、驱虫药物为主组成，用于治疗人体消化道寄生虫病的方剂，统称驱虫剂。

乌梅丸《伤寒论》

[**组成**] 乌梅三百枚（500克） 细辛六两（180克） 干姜十两（300克） 黄连十六两（500克） 当归四两（120克） 附子六两，炮，去皮（180克） 蜀椒四两，出汗（120克） 桂枝六两，去皮（180克） 人参六两（180克） 黄柏六两（180克）

[**用法**] 原方十味，异捣筛，合治之。以苦酒渍乌梅一宿，去核，蒸之五斗米下，饭熟，捣成泥，和药令相得，内臼中，与蜜杵二千下，丸如梧桐子大，先食饮，服十丸，日三服，稍加至二十丸。禁生冷、滑物、臭食等。

现代用法：乌梅用50%醋浸一宿，去核捣烂，和入余药捣匀，炼蜜制丸，每服9克，日服2～3次，空腹温开水送下。亦可作汤剂，水煎服，用量按原方比例酌减。

[**功效**] 温脏安蛔，泄肝安胃。

[**主治**]

1.蛔厥，腹痛时作，手足厥冷，时静时烦，时发时止，得食而呕，常自吐蛔。兼治久利。

2.厥阴病，消渴，气上撞心，心中疼热，饥不欲食，食则吐蛔，下之利不止。

[**方解**]

《医宗金鉴》说："蛔厥者，谓蛔痛手足厥冷也。"蛔厥之症，是因患者素有蛔虫，复由阳明肠胃虚寒，蛔上入膈所致，从而形成上热下寒，寒热错杂的局面。方中重用乌梅酸平，收敛肝气，生津止渴，和胃安蛔，《本经》谓其"主下气，除热烦满"，《本草纲目》谓其主"蛔厥吐利"，故可用治厥阴病"消渴，气上撞心，心中疼热"之症，且治蛔厥，尤以苦酒（醋）渍之，益增其效，为君药。臣以蜀椒辛热下气，温脏驱蛔；黄连苦寒下蛔，清泄肝胆。君臣相配，正如柯琴所说："蛔得酸则静，得辛则伏，得苦则下。"然而蛔厥之所以产生，是因内脏虚寒，蛔动不安，故又以细辛、桂枝、干姜、附子大队辛热之品佐蜀椒温脏祛寒，使蛔虫能安居肠内，不致上窜，其中细辛、桂枝又能入厥阴经辛散下气，"肝欲散，急食辛以散之"（《素问·藏气法时论》）；且干姜、附子能入阳明经鼓舞胃阳。黄柏苦寒，佐黄连清泄肝胆相火，且能监制大队辛热之品，以免引动相火，消铄津液。肝主藏血，佐以当归甘辛苦温，补养肝血。如此寒热互用，苦辛酸并投，则药味错杂，气味不和，故又佐以人参甘温，调其中气。加蜜为丸，以蛔得甘则动，略用甘味，从虫所好以引蛔，使之更好地发挥药效，是为反佐药；蜜能调和诸药，又为使药。合而成方，共奏温脏安蛔，泄肝安胃之效，对于蛔厥、久利、厥阴病属寒热错杂而气血不足者，极为适宜。

[临床运用]

本方为治疗蛔厥证的主方，亦为治疗厥阴病寒热错杂证的主方，寒热并用，土木两调，不但安蛔，亦能安胃，故一名乌梅安蛔丸，又名乌梅安胃丸。

布袋丸《补要袖珍小儿方论》[110]

[组成] 夜明砂拣净 芜荑炒，去皮 使君子肥白者，微炒，去皮，各二两（各60克） 白茯苓去皮 白术无油者，去芦 人参去芦 甘草 芦荟研细，各半两（各15克）

[用法] 原方为细末，汤浸蒸饼和丸，如弹子大，每服一丸，以生绢袋盛之，次用精猪肉二两，同药一处煮，候肉熟烂，提取药于当风处悬挂，将所煮肉并汁令小儿食之。所悬之药，第二日仍依前法煮食，只待药尽为度。

现代用法：按原方比例，将诸药研为细末，作散剂，每服6～9克，以布袋盛之，再用精猪肉30～60克，与药同煮，待肉熟透，去袋，将肉与药汁令小儿空腹时一次服尽。

[功效]　杀虫消疳，补气健脾。

[主治]　小儿虫疳，面色萎黄，肚腹胀大，日见羸瘦，发焦目暗，舌质淡，脉细弱。

[方解]

小儿饮食不洁，生虫成积，损伤脾胃，消耗气血，久乃成疳。不杀虫则病邪不除，不补虚则正气不复。方中重用夜明砂辛寒，治疳明目，芜荑辛苦温、使君子甘温，消疳杀虫，共为君药；芦荟苦寒，既助君药消疳杀虫，又能泻下以排除虫体，为臣药；因虫致虚，佐以少量人参、白术、茯苓、甘草补气健脾；甘草又能调和诸药，兼为使药。原方与精猪肉同煮，取其丰肌泽肤之效。全方攻补兼施，使虫驱疳消而正气不伤，乃治小儿虫疳之妙方。以布袋盛丸煮汁服，故名之曰"布袋丸"。

[临床运用]

本方既能杀虫消疳，又能补气健脾，宜用于小儿虫疳而脾胃虚弱者。

肥儿丸《太平惠民和剂局方》

[组成]　神曲炒　黄连去须，各十两（各300克）　肉豆蔻面裹煨　使君子去皮　麦芽炒，各五两（各150克）　槟榔不见火，细锉，晒，二十个（150克）　木香二两（60克）

[用法]　原方为细末，猪胆汁为丸，如粟米大，每服三十丸，量岁数加减，热水下，空心服。

现代用法：诸药为细末，取猪胆汁和丸，每丸重3克。三岁以上者每服二丸，二岁者每服一丸，周岁以内者每服半丸，空腹时以温开水化服。

[功效]　杀虫消积，健脾清热。

[主治]　小儿疳积，消化不良，面黄形瘦，肚腹胀满，口臭发热，舌苔黄腻。

[方解]

小儿虫积成疳，食不消化，郁热内生。方中使君子甘温，杀虫消疳，槟榔苦辛温，杀虫消积，共为君药；臣以神曲、麦芽以消食积，黄连以清郁热；

佐以肉豆蔻健脾消食，木香调气行滞；更以猪胆汁和丸，与黄连相合，清泄郁热。服用本方，使虫驱积消，脾健热清，儿体自然肥壮，故方以"肥儿"名之。

[临床运用]

本方能杀灭多种肠寄生虫，而以杀蛔虫、绦虫为最效。若无郁热，可去黄连、猪胆汁，用面糊丸即可。脾气虚弱者，可酌加党参、白术、茯苓；大便秘结者，可加大黄、枳实。服后虫积得去，便当调补脾胃，使正气恢复。

注　释

[1]《伤寒论》: 东汉张仲景所著医学经典著作, 是一部阐述外感病治疗规律的专著, 全书 12 卷。现今遗存 10 卷 22 篇。张仲景原著《伤寒杂病论》在流传的过程中, 经后人整理编纂将其中外感热病内容结集为《伤寒论》, 另一部分主要论述内科杂病, 名为《金匮要略方论》。

[2]《神农本草经》: 又称《本草经》或《本经》, 托名 "神农" 所作, 实成书于汉代, 是中医四大经典著作之一, 是现存最早的药物学著作。

[3]《医宗金鉴》: 是清政府组织太医院院判吴谦等编撰的一部大型医学丛书, 90 卷, 成书于 1742 年。全书采集了上自战国秦汉, 下至明清时期历代医书的精华。

[4]《伤寒明理论》: 是宋金时期著名医学家成无己编撰的中医伤寒病著作。

[5] 王叔和 (210—280): 晋代医学家, 名熙, 高平 (今属山东) 人。在中医学发展史上, 他做出了两大重要贡献, 一是整理《伤寒论》, 一是著述《脉经》。

[6] 李时珍 (1518—1593): 字东璧, 晚年自号濒湖山人, 明代著名医药学家。完成了 192 万字的巨著《本草纲目》, 被后世尊为 "药圣"。著述还有《奇经八脉考》《濒湖脉学》等多种。

[7] 王旭高 (1798—1862): 名泰林, 以字行, 晚号退思居士, 江苏无锡人。起初从事外科, 后来专力于内科杂病, 且对温病尤多关注, 临证审证用药甚为精当。王氏学术代表著作为《西溪书屋夜话录》, 书成后惜多散佚, 仅存治肝三十法。

[8]《肘后备急方》: 简称《肘后方》, 8 卷, 70 篇, 东晋时期葛洪著。古代中医方剂著作, 是中国第一部临床急救手册。

[9]《太平惠民和剂局方》: 为宋代太平惠民和剂局编写, 是全世界第一部由官方主持编撰的成药标准。

[10]《温病条辨》：清代吴瑭（鞠通）著，为温病通论著作。该书在清代众多温病学家成就的基础上，进一步建立了完全独立于伤寒的温病学说体系，创立了三焦辨证纲领，被称为清代温病学说标志性著作。

[11]《小儿药证直诀》：北宋钱乙的弟子阎孝忠收集钱乙的临证经验编成的中医儿科学专著。

[12]喻嘉言（1585—1670）：本名喻昌，字嘉言，明末清初著名医学家。医名卓著，冠绝一时，与张路玉、吴谦齐名，号称清初三大名医。

[13]《重订通俗伤寒论》：清代绍兴名医俞根初原著；后经何秀山撰按、何廉臣校勘；再经近人曹炳章增订，徐荣斋重订而成的版本。是一部博采历代各家之长、理法方药齐全的外感热病专著。

[14]《本草纲目》：明代李时珍（东璧）著，52 卷。作者用了近 30 年时间编成，收载药物 1892 种，附药图 1000 余幅，阐发药物的性味、主治、用药法则、产地、形态、采集、炮制、方剂配伍等，并载附方 10000 余首。集我国 16 世纪之前药学成就之大成，被国外学者誉为中国之百科全书。

[15]《小品方》：12 卷，东晋陈延之撰。本书早佚，其佚文散见于《外台秘要》《医心方》中。

[16]《素问》：即《黄帝内经素问》，9 卷，81 篇。与《黄帝内经灵枢》（即《灵枢经》）为姊妹篇，合之而为《黄帝内经》。

[17]《金匮要略》：是我国东汉著名医学家张仲景所著《伤寒杂病论》的杂病部分，也是我国现存最早的一部论述杂病诊治的专书。所述病证以内科杂病为主，兼及外科、妇科疾病及急救猝死、饮食禁忌等内容。被后世誉为"方书之祖"。

[18]《先醒斋医学广笔记》：4 卷，明代缪希雍撰。

[19]《医方论》：清代费伯雄编撰的医方著作，刊于 1865 年。

[20]《丹溪心法》：元代朱震亨著述、明代程充校订的一部综合性医书，共 5 卷，刊于 1481 年。该书并非朱氏自撰，由他的学生根据其学术经验和平素所述纂辑而成。

[21]《证治准绳》：本书由明代著名医学家王肯堂撰，刊于 1602 年。所述以证候治法尤详，故名《证治准绳》。又因所论内容为 6 种，故又有《六科证

治准绳》《六科准绳》之称。

[22] 刘河间（约 1110—1200）：名完素，字守真，河间（今河北河间）人，故后世又称其为刘河间。是中医历史上著名的"金元四大家"之一"寒凉派"的创始人。

[23]《伤寒六书》：又名《陶氏伤寒全书》，6 卷，明代陶华（节庵）撰，成书于 1445 年，伤寒著作。本书为陶氏所撰 6 种伤寒著作之合订本，包括《伤寒琐言》《伤寒家秘的本》《伤寒杀车槌法》《伤寒一提金》《伤寒截江网》《伤寒明理续论》等六书。

[24] 柯琴（1662—1735）：字韵伯，号似峰，浙江慈溪人，清代伤寒学家。他的以方名证、因方类证的做法较切临床实用，对后世研究《伤寒论》颇有影响。

[25] 汪昂（1615—1694）：清初医家，字讱庵，初名恒，安徽休宁县城西门人，新安医学名家。编著有《素问灵枢类纂约注》《医方集解》《本草备要》《汤头歌诀》等。

[26]《通俗伤寒论》：清代俞根初著，12 卷。该书融合了古今有关论著，结合个人临证心得，对伤寒的证治规律进行了深入阐述。

[27]《景岳全书》：明代张景岳晚年集自己的学术思想、临床各科、方药针灸之大成，辑成《景岳全书》。书中内容丰富，囊括理论、本草、成方、临床各科疾病，是一部全面而系统的临床参考书。

[28] 刘草窗：即刘溥，明代太医，字元博，号草窗，长洲（今江苏苏州）人。"景泰十才子"之首。

[29]《名医别录》：简称《别录》，辑者佚名（一作陶宏景），约成书于汉末，药学著作，3 卷。是汉末医家对《神农本草经》一书药物的药性功用主治等内容有所补充之外，又补记 365 种新药物。

[30]《珍珠囊》：金代张元素撰著的一部本草类中医著作，约成书于 1234 年。

[31]《济生续方》：宋代严用和撰著的一部方书类中医著作，8 卷，附补遗 1 卷，约成书于 1267 年。

[32] 王绵之（1923—2009）：北京中医药大学终身教授、博士生导师，首

届国医大师，我国著名的中医学家，是现代中医方剂学的创始人之一。

[33] 张景岳（1563—1640）：名介宾，字会卿，号景岳，别号通一子，因善用熟地黄，人称"张熟地"，绍兴府山阴（今浙江绍兴）人。明代杰出医学家，温补学派的代表人物。

[34]《外科证治全生集》：清王洪绪（字维德）撰，刊于1740年。外科著作。王氏是在秉承家学的基础上，积40年临证实践经验撰著而成此书。

[35]《本草求真》：清代黄宫绣，字锦芳撰，刊于1769年，12卷。一作10卷。本书载药520味，分上、下两编，上编对药物的形态、性味、功能、主治以及禁忌记载甚详，下编分列脏腑病证主药、六淫病证主药和药物总义三部分。

[36] 叶天士（1666—1745）：即叶桂，字天士，号香岩，别号南阳先生，江苏吴县（今江苏苏州）人。清代著名医学家，温病四大家之一。

[37]《备急千金要方》：又称《千金要方》《千金方》，唐代孙思邈所著，约成书于652年，共30卷，综合性临床医著。该书集唐代以前诊治经验之大成，对后世医家影响极大，被誉为中国最早的临床百科全书。

[38]《外台秘要》：又名《外台秘要方》，40卷，是由唐代王焘辑录唐以前的许多医药著作而成的综合性医书。

[39]《疫疹一得》：清代余师愚撰于1794年，2卷，全书重点论述疫疹证治。

[40]《东垣试效方》：是金代李杲撰写的一本方书类中医文献，9卷，成书于1266年。是书所涉病种较广，但重点为脾胃病证用方，反映了脾胃学派的特色。

[41]《校注妇人良方》：系明代著名医学家薛己，号立斋，以宋代陈自明《妇人大全良方》为蓝本校注编著而成，全书共24卷。

[42] 岳美中（1900—1982）：当代著名中医学家、临床家、教育家，我国中医研究生教育的奠基人。较早地提出了专病、专方、专药与辨证论治相结合的原则，善用经方治大病。

[43] 大塚敬节（1900—1980）：日本医家，研究汉方医学。1972年9月，日本医师会授予大塚敬节"最高功勋奖"，奖励其为汉方医学发展做出的卓越贡献。

[44]《医方集解》：系我国清代著名医家汪昂搜罗古今名方，精心整理编撰而成，书成于 1682 年。全书共分 3 卷，以正方及附方的形式选录古今临床常用方剂 700 余首，其中正方 388 首。

[45]《兰室秘藏》：元代李杲撰，刊于公元 1276 年，3 卷。全书分 21 门，包括内、外、妇、儿临床各科。本书为李东垣代表作之一。

[46]《素问病机气宜保命集》：金代刘完素撰于 1186 年，综合性医书，共 3 卷，为作者于晚年总结其毕生医药理论和临床心得之作。

[47]《明医杂著》：该书由明代王纶撰于 1502 年，薛己注，刊于 1549 年。综合性医书，共 6 卷。

[48]《伤寒直格》：金代刘完素撰，葛雍编，成书于 1186 年，共 3 卷（原为 6 卷）。全书仅 17009 字，从热病证治角度发挥伤寒蕴义。

[49]《温热经纬》：清代王士雄（孟英）纂于 1852 年，5 卷，为温病通论类著作。本书"以轩岐仲景之文为经，叶薛诸家之辨为纬"，故以"经纬"名书。

[50] 吴鞠通（1758—1836）：名塘，字配珩，鞠通乃其号，江苏淮阴人。清代杰出的中医温病学家，山阳医派创始人。

[51]《本草经疏》：又名《神农本草经疏》，明代缪希雍著。共 30 卷，药学著作。

[52] 苏恭：即苏敬，中国唐代药学家，宋时因避讳，改为苏恭或苏鉴，陈州淮阳（今河南省周口市淮阳区）人。主持编撰世界上第一部由国家正式颁布的药典《新修本草》（又名《唐本草》）。

[53]《广济方》：为唐玄宗组织编撰。全书包括内、外、妇各科病症 60 余种，收方 104 首。

[54]《本经逢原》：清代著名医家张璐著，成书于 1695 年，药物学著作，全书 4 卷。

[55]《鸡峰普济方》：南宋张锐撰，成书于 1133 年，方书，30 卷。

[56] 黄宫绣（1720—1817）：字锦芳，江西省宜黄县棠阴君山人，清代著名医学家，乾隆时代宫廷御医。

[57] 张秉成（生卒年未详）：清代医家，字兆嘉，江苏武进人。

[58]《脾胃论》：撰于公元 1249 年，3 卷，是李东垣创导脾胃学说的代表著作。

[59]李东垣（1180—1251）：名杲，字明之，号东垣老人，真定（今河北正定）人。他是中国医学史上"金元四大家"之一，是中医"脾胃学说"的创始人。

[60]《内外伤辨惑论》：3 卷，李东垣撰于 1247 年。书中主要讨论内伤和外感两大病类的病因、病状、脉象、治法等问题。

[61]《本草备要》：清代汪昂于 1694 年创作的药物学著作，共 8 卷。本书可视为临床药物手册，亦为医学门径书。

[62]《济生方》：又名《严氏济生方》，南宋严用和（子礼）撰，1253 年成书。方书，共 10 卷。

[63]《正体类要》：明代薛己著，成书于 1529 年，2 卷。本书以论述一般性软组织损伤的证治经验为主，每一病证后均有临证医案。

[64]《千金翼方》：唐代医学家孙思邈撰，约成书于 682 年，共 30 卷。系作者集晚年近三十年之经验，以补早期巨著《备急千金要方》之不足，故名"翼方"。

[65]钱乙（约 1032—1113）：字仲阳，东平人。是我国宋代著名的儿科医家，别称"儿科之圣""幼科之鼻祖"。

[66]朱丹溪（1281—1358）：字彦修，元代著名医学家，婺州义乌（今浙江金华义乌）人，"滋阴派"的创始人。与刘完素、张从正、李东垣并列为"金元四大家"。

[67]《续名医类案》：清代魏之琇（玉璜）编，原 60 卷，经王孟英新增重编为 36 卷。分 345 门，集录清以前历代名医的验案，包括临床各科，尤以温热病更突出，某些病案有王孟英按语。

[68]魏玉璜（生卒年未详）：清良医，号柳州，浙江杭州人。

[69]《医方类聚》：朝鲜金礼蒙等撰于 1443 年，原刊 365 卷。它汇辑了 152 部中国唐、宋、元、明初的著名医书及一部朝鲜本国医书《御医撮要》，共计 153 部。为中国明代以前医方的集大成著作。

[70]《究原方》：南宋医家张松撰写的一部临证集验方书，已佚。

[71]《本草衍义》：北宋寇宗奭撰，刊于公元 1116 年，为药论性本草著作，共 20 卷。

[72] 王晋三（生卒年未详）：清代名医。

[73]《内科摘要》：明代薛己撰著，成书于 1529 年，2 卷。本书为薛氏诊治内科杂病的经验实录，从《薛氏医案》中选摘而成。

[74]《医学衷中参西录》：近代名医张锡纯撰，系作者多年治学临证经验和汇通中西体会之总结。

[75]《傅青主女科》：清代傅山著，刊于 1827 年，妇科著作，2 卷。

[76]《本草从新》：清代吴仪洛撰，成书于 1757 年，18 卷，为清代流传较广的临床实用本草著作。

[77]《成方切用》：清代名医吴仪洛编著，秉"医贵通变，药在合宜"之旨，收录古今医方 1102 首，是继明《医方考》、清《医方集解》后又一部较为著名的方论类著作。

[78]《难经》：关于《难经》的作者与成书年代历来有不同的看法，一般认为其成书不晚于东汉，内容可能与秦越人（扁鹊）有一定关系。"难"是"问难"之义，或作"疑难"解。"经"或是指《内经》，即问难《内经》。作者把自己认为难点和疑点提出，然后逐一解释阐发，部分问题做出了发挥性阐解。全书共分八十一节，对人体腑脏功能形态、诊法脉象、经脉针法等诸多问题逐一论述。

[79]《杨氏家藏方》：南宋杨倓（子靖）辑，刊于 1178 年，方书，20 卷。

[80]《蜀本草》：本书是五代后蜀之主孟昶命翰林学士韩保昇等将《新修本草》增补注释，尤其是对药物图形的解说，更详于以前的本草著作。计 20 卷。

[81] 张锡纯（1860—1933）：字寿甫，祖籍山东诸城，河北盐山人，中西医汇通学派的代表人物之一，近现代中国中医学界的泰斗人物。

[82]《黄帝素问宣明论方》：又名《宣明论方》，金代刘完素撰，成书于 1172 年，15 卷。《宣明论方》是一部很有临床价值的著作，金元时期盛行于北方，与南宋的《和剂局方》形成了南北对峙的局面，后人称之为"南局北宣"。

[83]《医门法律》：清代喻昌（嘉言）著，6 卷。依风、寒、暑、湿、燥、

火六气及诸杂证而分门别类。每门分论、法、律三项，"论"是总论病证，"法"是治疗法则，"律"是指出医生在治疗上的过失。

[84]《重楼玉钥》：清代郑梅涧（宏纲）约撰于乾隆年间，后其子郑承瀚加以补充，初刊于1838年。喉科著作，2卷。

[85] 张元素（1131—1234）：字洁古，金代易水（今河北易县）人，中医易水学派创始人。洁古重视脏腑辨证及扶养胃气的思想，对李杲创立以"补土"为特色的系统的脾胃理论有重要影响，并最终成为"易水学派"最突出的理论特色。

[86]《儒门事亲》：金代张从正编撰的中医著作，共15卷，成书于1228年。秉承张氏"唯儒者能明其理，而事亲者当知医"之思想，故命名为《儒门事亲》。

[87]《易简方》：宋代王硕撰，约刊于12世纪末期，医方著作，1卷。

[88]《摄生众妙方》：明代张时彻辑，刊于1550年，11卷，医方著作。

[89]《韩氏医通》：明代韩懋撰于1522年，2卷，综合性医书。

[90]《症因脉治》：明代秦景明撰，清代秦皇士补辑，刊于1706年，4卷。

[91]《医林改错》：清代王清任撰，刊行于1830年。全书分为上、下两卷，记载了王氏的气血脏腑学说的立论，对古医籍中脏腑错误的纠正，以及杂症辨治，尤其是气虚血瘀的辨证论治。

[92] 王清任（1768—1831）：字勋臣，直隶玉田（今属河北）人，清代医学家。

[93]《医学发明》：元代李东垣撰，其弟子罗谦甫刊行于1315年。每篇均以经文的论点为标题，并注明出处，如《针经》《素问》《难经》等，而后探本求源，加以论证，发挥经义，并列方70余首，总以温补脾胃为指归。本书充分体现了东垣学说的成就。

[94]《日华子诸家本草》：简称《日华子本草》或《日华本草》，著作年代、作者不详。本书内容丰富、实用，是研究中药和五代药学史的重要文献。

[95]《本草拾遗》：一名《陈藏器本草》，唐代陈藏器撰于739年，10卷。陈藏器以收集《新修本草》遗漏的药物为主，著成《本草拾遗》一书，对《新修本草》做了补充。

[96]《血证论》：清代唐宗海著，8 卷，成书于 1884 年，是我国第一部有关血证治疗的专著。

[97]《十药神书》：元代葛可久撰，刊于 1348 年。本书收载了十个治疗虚劳吐血的经验方，分别以甲、乙、丙、丁等天干次序排列。治疗方剂奇而不离于正，实用有效。

[98]《普济本事方》：宋代许叔微撰，约刊于 1132 年，10 卷。本书是许氏集平生所验效方，附以医案，并记其事实之书。

[99]《时病论》：清代雷丰（少逸）1882 年著成，为时病通论著作，该书为首部关于时病的专著。

[100]《医学正传》：明代虞抟继承祖父医业，私淑丹溪遗风，经 40 年对《素问》《难经》等古医籍之钻研，参考历代医家所述，并结合本人临床经验，于 1515 年编撰成本书。

[101]《成方便读》：清代张秉成撰，刊于 1904 年。本书汇编古今常用成方 290 余首。

[102]《华氏中藏经》：又名《中藏经》，综合性临床医著，分 3 卷，传说为华佗所作，具体成书年代不详。《中藏经》较早地提出了以形色脉证相结合、以脉证为中心分述五脏六腑寒热虚实的辨证方法。

[103]《药征》：日本吉益东洞撰，成书于 1771 年，3 卷。本书是吉益氏毕生研究《伤寒论》用药规律的一部著作。

[104]《类编朱氏集验方》：宋代朱佐撰，刊于 1266 年，医方著作。本书收集宋代医家常用的方剂和单方 1000 余首。

[105]《三因极一病证方论》：简称《三因方》，南宋陈言撰著，成书于 1174 年。该书 18 卷，分为 180 门，收方 1050 余首。

[106]《世医得效方》：元代危亦林编撰，19 卷。以"依按古方，参以家传"的编辑方法撰称，故名。为危氏五世家传经验医方。

[107]《医方证治汇编歌诀》：是清代王泰林编著的一部方书类中医著作，不分卷，成书于 1897 年，系《王旭高医书六种》之一。

[108]《泰定养生主论》：元代王珪，号中阳撰，撰年不详，16 卷，养生著作。

[109]《医学心悟》: 清代程国彭（钟龄）撰，成书于1732年，5卷。总结了辨证施治的八纲、八法、因证立方，条分缕析，多为临床心得之语。末附《外科十法》。

[110]《补要袖珍小儿方论》: 明代庄应祺补要，祝大年、孟继孔校正，刊于1574年。儿科著作，10卷。

方名索引

Essential Famous Formula

of

Past Dynasties

Editor-in-Chief   Lian Jian-wei

Deputy Editor   Shen Shu-hua   Zhu Wen-pei

ZHEJIANG UNIVERSITY PRESS

浙江大学出版社

·杭州·

Abstract

Essential Famous Formula of Past Dynasties (*Chinese and English Versions*) contains 175 famous representative formulas of traditional Chinese medicine commonly applied in clinical practice with definite curative effects, which are systematically introduced in 18 chapters. Each prescription is divided into 6 items: Ingredient, usage, action, indication, formula analysis, and clinical application.

The book is practical and easy both for Chinese and foreign readers to learn and master the clinical application rules of famous formulas in past dynasties, so as to meet the needs of current clinical practice.

The book is suitable for Chinese and foreign medical workers, teachers and students of medical colleges, traditional Chinese medicine enthusiasts for clinical and learning reference.

Description

Chinese medicine is a great treasure house that should be explored, improved, inherited, maintained and innovated. Therefore, *Essential Famous Formula of Past Dynasties (Chinese and English Versions)* was compiled to promote Chinese medicine and benefit the people of the world.

1. This book aims to clarify the clinical application rules of famous formulas in past dynasties of traditional Chinese medicine. A total of 175 famous formulas were selected, all of which were typical famous formulas of past dynasties commonly applied in modern times and have exact curative effects. According to the different treatment methods and effects, the formulas are divided into several chapters as: Exterior-Releasing Formulas, Emetic Formulas, Purgative Formulas, Harmonizing Formulas, Warming Interior Formulas, Heat-Clearing Formulas, Resuscitative Formulas, Tonifying and Replenishing Formulas, Astringent Formulas, Tranquilizing Formulas, Wind Relieving Formulas, Dryness Relieving Formulas, Digestive and Evacuative Formulas, Qi Regulating Formulas, Blood Regulating Formulas, Dampness Dispelling Formulas, Phlegm Expelling Formulas, and Worm-Expelling Formulas, *etc.*

2. Each chapter has an overview of all the formulas, including the concept, classification, *etc.* The indications, commonly used medicines, compatibility characteristics and representative formulas are introduced in the openings of each section, which is helpful for scholars to have a general understanding of each kind of formula.

3. The content of each formula is divided into six items: ingredient, usage, action, indication, formula analysis, clinical application.

4. To maintain the original appearance of the famous formulas in past dynasties, the composition and usage of the formula are marked with the original dosage and usage in Chinese *pinyin*, the modern dosage (in brackets) and usage are separately

noted. Among them, the modern dose is generally converted according to the proportion of the original one. If the original dose is inconsistent with modern clinical practice, the dose shall be determined according to the standard dosage of modern Chinese medicine. Modern doses are measured in "grams". If the dose of the original formula recorded as "equal dose", the morden dose will generally not marked. Readers can flexibly regulate the dose according to the real situations.

5. The indication item mainly narrates the original formula's primary treatment syndrome, and adds more mature treatment experience in ancient and modern medical records.

6. The formula analysis item makes an in-depth and strightforward analysis and explanation on the principle of *Jun-Chen-Zuo-Shi* (Chief, Deputy, Assistant, Envoy), explaining the characteristics of its formula medication, so as guiding clinical practice.

7. The clinical application item focus on the clinical practice, clarifying the application experience of the formula in ancient and modern medical cases, expounding the chief editor's clinical experience, usage considerations and taboos, *etc.*

8. The formula name index, the annotation is attached to the end of the book for scholars to consult.

Lian Jian-wei in Zhejiang Chinese Medical University

September 1st, 2022

CONTENTS

Chapter 1

Exterior-Releasing Formulas

These formulas mainly consist of exterior-releasing medicine that induces sweating, releases the exterior (muscle layer), and promots the eruption of papules, which can scatter and dissipate external pathogens, release exterior syndrome. They are collectively called Exterior-Releasing Formula, belonging to the "sweat promotion" of "eight methods".

Section 1   Formulas that releases the exterior with acrid-warm

Formulas that can release the exterior with acrid-warm medicine are used for exterior syndromes caused by contracting external wind-cold. The syndromes include aversion to cold with fever, headache and painful and stiff nape, aching pain of the limbs, no thirst, absence of sweating or abnormal sweating, thin and white coating on the tongue, floating and tight pulse or floating and moderate pulse, *etc.* Acrid flavors of medicine can disperse; warm flavors of medicine can remove the cold, so the main constituent of exterior-releasing is acrid-warm medicines such as *má huáng*, *guì zhī*, *sū yè* and *cōng bái* to form a formula. According to the patient's condition, sometimes acrid-cool or heat-clearing medicines can be added, but the acrid-warm medicines still take the lead; their property of releasing the exterior will not change. The representative' releasing the exterior with acrid-warm medicine' formulas include *Má Huáng Tāng* (Ephedra Decoction, 麻黄汤), *Guì Zhī Tāng* (Cinnamon Twig Decoction, 桂枝汤), *Dà Qīng Lóng Tāng* (Major Green Dragon Decoction, 大青龙汤), *Xiǎo Qīng Lóng Tāng* (Minor Green Dragon Decoction, 小青龙汤), *Cōng Chǐ Tāng*

(Scallion and Fermented Soybean Decoction, 葱豉汤), *Xiāng Sū Sǎn* (Cyperus and Perilla Powder, 香苏散), *Xiāng Rú Sǎn* (Mosla Powder, 香薷散), *etc.*

Má Huáng Tāng (Ephedra Decoction, 麻黄汤)
Treatise on Cold Damage (*Shāng Hán Lùn,* 伤寒论)[1]

[Ingredient]

Má Huáng (Herba Ephedrae)　3 *liang*, remove stemnodes (9 g)

Guì Zhī (Ramulus Cinnamomi)　2 *liang*, remove peel (6 g)

Xìng Rén (Semen Armeniacae Amarum)　70 pcs, remove peel and tip (9 g)

Gān Cǎo (Licorice)　1 *liang*, dry-fried with liquid adjuvant (3 g)

[Usage]　There are four medicines in the original formula, decoct *má huáng* with 9 *sheng* (1800 ml) of water first, then subtract 2 *sheng* of water, remove the froth on the surface and add other medicines, boil into 2.5 *sheng* of the decoction, remove the sediment, drink 0.8 *sheng* decoction, if [patient] sweating emerges after covering with a quilt, then don't have to eat porridge. Take the rest of the decoction in the same usage as *Guì Zhī Tāng* (cinnamon twig decoction).

Modern usage: Decoct the medicines with water and covers with a quilt until slightly sweating.

[Action]　Induce sweating to release the exterior, diffuse the lung and calm panting.

[Indication]　Exterior excessive syndrome caused by externally-contracted wind-cold. The patient will have the symptoms such as aversion to cold with fever, headache, aches in joints, lumbago, panting with the absence of sweating, thin and white coating, floating and tight pulse.

[Formula Analysis]　This syndrome is caused by wind-cold restricting the exterior. In this formula, *má huáng* is mainly used, for its acrid-warm flavor, capable of inducing sweating to dispel exogenous pathogenic factors and dispersing the lung-qi, so cough and panting will be relieved. *Shen Nong's Classic of the Materia Medica* (*Shén Nóng Běn Cǎo Jīng,* 神农本草经)[2] says, "inducing sweating to release the exterior, to remove the pathogenic and hot qi so the cough with counterflow qi ascent

can be relieved". Hence, *má huáng* is the chief medicine. *Guì zhī* is acrid-warm with a dispersing effect, the combination of *guì zhī* and *má huáng* can diffuse *wei* yang, vent *ying* qi. After combining with the chief herb, it strengthens the sweating effect and disperses the pathogen, so *guì zhī i*s the deputy medicine. *Xìng rén* is bitter and slightly warm; it can diffuse and govern the descent of lung-qi, and help the chief medicines to relieve panting, so it is the assistant medicine. *Gān cǎo* can harmonize the actions of all medicines in a formula, making *má huáng* which works on the *wei* level cooperated with *guì zhī*, which works on the *ying* level, promote the ascending *má huáng* to cooperate with the bitter and descending *xìng rén*. The envoy medicine, *gān cǎo* can also moderate the acrid quality of the two main sweating herbs, *má huáng* and *guì zhī*, which protect the patient from sweating too much. The compatibility of these four medicines can remove the cold pathogen on the exterior, open the blocked and constraint lung-qi, so the exterior pathogen will be dispersed, the lung-qi will be diffused and the patient will recover.

[Clinical Application] This formula is a drastic one which releases the exterior with acrid-warm medicine; *Treatise on Cold Damage* (*Shāng Hán Lùn*, 伤寒论) uses this formula to treat cold damage on *Taiyang*. The cold damage on *Taiyang* is exterior excess caused by wind-cold, so *Golden Mirror of the Medical Tradition* (*Yī Zōng Jīn Jiàn*, 医宗金鉴)[3] says, "This formula is the most drastic one to open the exterior, disperse pathogen and induce sweating by Zhang Zhong-jing."

Guì Zhī Tāng (Cinnamon Twig Decoction, 桂枝汤)
Treatise on Cold Damage (*Shāng Hán Lùn*, 伤寒论)

[Ingredient]

Guì Zhī (Ramulus Cinnamomi)　3 *liang*, remove peel (9 g)

Sháo Yào (Radix Paeoniae)　3 *liang* (9 g)

Gān Cǎo (Licorice)　2 *liang*, dry-fried with liquid adjuvant (6 g)

Shēng Jiāng (Fresh Ginger)　3 *liang*, cut (9 g)

Dà Zǎo (Fructus Jujubae)　12 pcs, broken (4 pcs)

[Usage]　In the original formula, the five medicines should be cut[bit] into

pieces, decoct with 7 *sheng* of water, remove the froth and use low fire to decoct until 3 *sheng* is left, then removethe sediment. When the temperature is appropriate, take 1 *sheng*. After taking the decoction, ask the patient to eat a bowl of hot porridge to help strengthen the effect, also tell the patient to cover himself with a quilt for 2 hours until they lightly perspire but avoid profuse sweating. If the patient recovers after taking one intake of decoction, he can stop taking it; if he's not recovered and without sweating, then the patient should continue to take the decoction one more time in the same way; if still has no sweats after two formula intake, then [he] should shorten the decoction intake time, taking three times in half a day. If the patient's situation is urgent, the decoction should be taken daily and kept in observation. If the patient has not recovered with no perspiring after one intake, take one more. If no perspiration is occurring, then keep drinking the decoction two to three more times. No raw or cold, spoiled and viscous food, or foul-smelling food, [he] should not eat spicy food, like onion, garlic, scallions, leeks, or shallots.

Modern usage: Decocted by water, eats a small amout of hot porridge after taking the decoction, and then cover with a quilt until the patient is slightly perspiring.

[Action]　Resolve muscle and release exterior, harmonize *ying* and *wei* levels.

[Indication]　Externally-contracted wind pathogen, fever and headache, aversion to wind after sweating, snoring and retching, thin and white coating, floating and moderate pulse.

[Formula Analysis]　In this formula, the syndromes are caused by externally-contracted wind pathogens, disharmony between *ying* and *wei* qi. *Guì zhī* is acrid-warm, it can warm the channels and dissipate cold, resolve muscle and release exterior, enter *ying* and promote *wei*, so it's the chief medicine. *Sháo yào* is sour, bitter and a little cold, can astringe yin, supplement and nourish *ying*-yin, it acts as the deputy medicine. *Guì zhī* and *sháo yào* combine together, one is contractive, the other is dissipative, they simultaneously enhance the ability of the protective qi to dispel pathogenic influences while strengthening the nutritive qi, they can resolve muscle and release exterior but help *ying*-yin stay inside, meanwhile harmonize *ying* and *wei* levels. *Gān cǎo* combined with *guì zhī*, the acrid flavor meets with a sweet flavor to

act on the yang aspect and enhance the effect of inducing perspiration and resolving muscles. *Gān căo* combined with *sháo yào*, sour and sweet acts on the yin aspect, which can enhance the effect of restraining fluid and boosting yin, so *gān căo* is the assistant medicine. *Shēng jiāng* and *dà zăo* can supplement and nourish the spleen and stomach, and harmonize *ying* and *wei* levels. *Concise Supplementary Exposition On Cold Damage (Shāng Hán Míng Lǐ Lùn,* 伤寒明理论)[4] says, "The purpose of using *shēng jiāng* and *dà zăo* is to help produce fluid so that *ying* and *wei* can be in harmony", so these two are the envoy medicines. Sweat is produced by essential qi, water, and engendered by grain, so nourishing the spleen and stomach can help enrich the origin of sweat.

[Clinical Application]

1. In *Treatise on Cold Damage (Shāng Hán Lùn,* 伤寒论), the formula is used for treating *Taiyang* wind-invasion syndrome. This syndrome is actually a wind-cold syndrome of exterior-deficiency type, which is described as "*Taiyang* syndrome, fever, sweating, aversion to wind, a moderate pulse is called wind-strike (*zhòng fēng,* 中风). But clinically, the formula can also be used for miscellaneous diseases, such as for postpartum women and disharmony between *ying* and *wei* manifesting with a slight aversion to wind-cold, intermittent fever, sweating, moderate pulse.

2. The externally-contracted wind-cold, exterior excess with an absence of sweating, or exterior constraint with interior heat, vexation and agitation with an absence of sweating or newly-contracted warm disease which presents interior heat and thirst, red tongue and rapid pulse, or damp-heat inside the person who consumes alcohol CANNOT uses this formula. Wang Shu-he[5] said, "If a person is yang exuberance, and he takes the *Guì Zhī Tāng,* there will be severe consequences", Li Shi-zhen[6] said, "*Guì Zhī Tāng* is forbidden if there is no sweating." These words indeed have some clinical values.

Dà Qīng Lóng Tāng (Major Green Dragon Decoction, 大青龙汤)
Treatise on Cold Damage (*Shāng Hán Lùn*, 伤寒论)

[Ingredient]

Má Huáng (Herba Ephedrae) 6 *liang*, remove stem nodes (18 g)

Guì Zhī (Ramulus Cinnamomi) 2 *liang*, skin removed (6 g)

Gān Cǎo (Radix Et Rhizoma Glycyrrhizae) 2 *liang*, honey-fired (6 g)

Xìng Rén (Semen Armeniacae Dulce) 40 pcs, skin and tip removed (6 g)

Shēng Jiāng (Rhizoma Zingiberis Recen) 3 *liang*, cut (9 g)

Dà Zǎo (Fructus Jujubae) 12 *mei* [①], split (4 pcs)

Shí Gāo (Gypsum Fibrosum Praeparatum) as big as an egg, break into small pieces (30 g)

[Usage] First, using 9 *sheng* water boil *má huáng* to 7 *sheng*, remove the froth. Add other medicines and boil until 3 *sheng* is left. Abandon the sediment and take 1 *sheng* of the decoction, drink it. Slight perspiration is appropriate. If the perspiration is profuse, take the *warm powder* (fired rice flour) to cover the body. If sweating is induced by 1 potion, stop taking it. If more decoctions are taken, there will be profuse perspiration which leads to yang depletion, manifests as the aversion to wind, vexation and insomnia.

Modern Usage: Decocted by water.

[Action] Relive exterior syndrome by sweating, clear heat and reliev vexation.

[Indication] External wind and cold, severe fever and chill, floating and tight pulse, body aches, none-sweating and vexation.

[Formula Analysis] The pulse in this syndrome is floating and tight. Floating pertains to wind evil which will damage the defensive yang, and tight pulse pertains to cold evil which will damage nutrient yin. The damage to nutrient yin and defensive yang will lead to severe fever, chills and body aches. This is achieved by an ingenious modification of *Má Huáng Tāng*. The dosages of *má huáng* and *guì zhī* have been doubled, while that of *xìng rén* has been reduced. In this formula, *má huáng*, the chief

---

① *Mei* (*méi*, 枚): Chinese medicine noun. An evaluative unit of measurement for a drug. It can be used to calculate fruit or root block drugs, such as jujube, aconite, *etc.*

herb, is taken in a large dosage to enhance the sweating function of relieving exterior syndrome. *Guì zhī*, the deputy herb, promotes the sweating-inducing function of *má huáng*. *Xìng rén* can disperse lung qi and assist *má huáng and guì zhī* to relieve the external by sweating. *Shēng jiāng* and *dà zǎo* can regulate *ying* and *wei* and promote the circulation of fluids. *Shí gāo*, acrid, sweet in taste and cold in nature, is added to clear heat and relieve vexation, restrict the pungent warm nature of *má huáng* and *guì zhī* without the risk of giving rise to internal heat. The above medicines are all assistants. *Gān cǎo*, the envoy medicine, is applied to harmonize all herbs and restrict the fierce nature of *má huáng* and *guì zhī* to prevent profuse sweating. Meanwhile, the combination of *gān cǎo* and *shí gāo* will clear the heat better by engendering liquid with sweet-cold medicine. This formula can induce sweating and clear pathogenic heat, all symptoms will be cured.

[Clinical Application] Wang Xu-gao[7] said, "The key indexes (symptoms) of *Dà Qīng Lóng Tāng* are fever, aversion to cold, none-sweating, vexation and agitation." It means the external cold syndrome manifesting fever and aversion to cold without sweats, combined with the internal heat syndrome manifesting vexation are the necessary indications for the application of this formula. Stop taking it if the exterior pathogen and vexation are relieved with sweating.

Xiǎo Qīng Lóng Tāng (Minor Green Dragon Decoction, 小青龙汤)
Treatment on Febrile Disease caused by Cold (*Shāng Hán Lù*, 伤寒论)

[Ingredient]
Má Huáng (Herba Ephedrae)   3 *liang*, remove stem nodes (9 g)

Sháo Yào (Radix Paeoniae)   3 *liang* (9 g)

Wǔ Wèi Zǐ (Fructus Schisandrae Chinensis)   half *sheng* (9 g)

Gān Jiāng (Rhizoma Zingiberis)   3 *liang* (9 g)

Gān Cǎo (Radix et Rhizoma Glycyrrhizae)   3 *liang*, honey-fired (9 g)

Guì Zhī (Ramulus Cinnamomi)   3 *liang*, skin removed (9 g)

Bàn Xià (Rhizoma Pinelliae)   half *sheng*, washed (9 g)

Xì Xīn (Herba Erigerontis)   3 *liang* (9 g)

[Usage]   Firstly, add 1 *dou* (2000 ml) water to decoct *má huáng* until 2 *sheng* reduced, and remove the froth. Put the rest of the herbs into the decoction and simmer it until 3 *sheng* left. Abandon the sediment and take 1 *sheng* of the decoction, drink when it is warm.

Modern Usage: Decoct with water.

[Action]   Release the exterior and dissipate cold, warm the lung and reduce fluid retention.

[Indication]   External wind and cold invasion, internal retention of water fluid, fever and aversion to cold without sweating, cough and panting, copious sputum, retching without thirst, white, moisten and slippery coating, floating pulse. Or subcutaneous fluid retention which leads to edema around four limbs, body aches.

[Formula Analysis]   Restricted exterior by wind-cold leads to the obstruction of pores, resulting in fever and aversion to cold but without sweats. In this formula, *má huáng*, the chief herb, relieves the exterior by sweating, diffuses the lung and relieves panting. *Guì zhī, as* the deputy, promotes the exterior-relieving function of *má huáng. Bàn xià* dries dampness and dissolves phlegm, alleviate water-rheum and directs qi downward. *Gān jiāng* warms the spleen and lung yang, dissolves fluid. *Xì xīn* can dissipate wind-cold externally, warm lung and reduce fluid retention. However, *gān jiāng* and *xì xīn* are pungent, warm and hot, which easily injure the lung qi. Thus, *wǔ wèi zǐ*, which can prevent the leakage of lung qi and astringes fluid was added. *Wǔ wèi zǐ, gān jiāng* and *xì xīn* act in restricting and dispersing, also playing a good role in warming lung and relieving cough. *Sháo yào* nourishes and generates yin and blood. All herbs mentioned above are assistant medicines. *Gān cǎo*, the envoy medicine, is used to harmonize all medicines. *Gān cǎo* plus *sháo yào* are sour and sweet can generate yin, which can restrict the sweating-inducing function of *má huáng* and *guì zhī* to prevent qi and yin consumption. All these eight herbs are composed scrupulously to play a role in releasing the exterior and dissipating cold, warming the lung and dissolving fluid retention. It was named *Minor Green Dragon Decoction* for its function in inducing perspiration was not as strong as *Major Green Dragon Decoction*.

[Clinical Application]　This formula is created for external cold and internal fluid retention. If the external cold is relieved, treatment principle should be switched to the harmonizing method by warm medicines. Apply *Líng Guì Zhú Gān Tāng* and the likes to cope with the condition as it is. If one takes Minor Green Dragon Decoction for a long time, it will damage lung qi, worsen the deficiency.

Cōng Chǐ Tāng (Scallion and Fermented Soybean Decoction, 葱豉汤)
Emergency Formulas to Keep Up One's Sleeve (Zhǒu Hòu Bèi Jí Fang, 肘后备急方[8])

[Ingredient]

Cōng Bái (Bulbus Allii Fistulosi)　1 *hu kou*[①] (5 twig)

Dòu Chǐ (Semen Sojae Praeparatum)　1 *sheng* (15 g)

[Usage]　Put 3 *sheng* water to decoct the herbs until 1 *sheng* is left. Take it in one draft to achieve sweating. If no sweating and the symptoms are aggravated, add *gé gēn* 2 *liang*, *shēng má* 3 *liang* then decoct with 5 *sheng* water until 2 *sheng* left. There must be sweating after finishing the decoction. If there is still no sweating, add *shēng má* 2 *liang* and shallot soup with ground rice 2 *he*[②], boiling them with 1 *sheng* water. Then add salty *dòu chǐ* and *cōng bái* separately and stew them until 3 *sheng* left. Take the decoction in one draft to achieve sweating.

Modern Usage: Decocted by water.

[Action]　Induce sweating and dissipate cold.

[Indication]　Slight external wind and cold syndrome, slight aversion to wind and cold, fever, headache without sweating, nose obstruction with discharge, sneezing, thin and white tongue coating, floating pulse.

[Formula Analysis]　The fever and chills are not severe for the slight external wind and cold syndrome. In this formula, *cōng bái*, the chief medicine, is pungent and warm which can disperse the external pathogenic factor, unblock yang and induce

---

① 　*hu kou* (*hú kǒu*, 虎口): tiger' mouth, circle your thumb and index finger into a round shape, for measuring the twig of *cōng bái* (onion stalk).

② 　*he* (*hé*, 合): 20 ml.

sweating. *Dòu chǐ*, the assistant medicine, is pungent, sweet and slight warm, which can relieve exterior syndrome by diaphoresis. The combination of *cōng bái* and *dòu chǐ* can remove the excess mildly by inducing sweating and dispersing cold evil.

[Clinical Application]   The nature of this formula is mild. It is pungent and warm but not dry, dispersing but not violent. It has no disadvantage of damaging fluids by over-sweating, attracting the attention of doctors of all dynasties.

Xiāng Sū Sǎn (Cyperus and Perilla Powder, 香苏散)
Formulary of the Pharmacy Service for Benefiting the People in the Taiping Era (Tài Píng Huì Mín Hé Jì Jú Fāng, 太平惠民和剂局方)[9]

[Ingredient]

Xiāng Fù (Rhizoma Cyperi)   4 *liang* (120 g) fired and fur-removed

Zǐ Sū Yè (Folium Perillae)   4 *liang* (120 g)

Chén Pí (Pericarpium Citri Reticulatae)   2 *liang*, white part preserved (60 g)

Gān Cǎo (Radix et Rhizoma Glycyrrhizae)   1 *liang*, honey-fired (30 g)

[Usage]   The dosage form of the original formula is for a coarse powder. Take 3 *qian*[①] with 1 cup water each time and decoct until seven-tenths left. Discard the sediment. Take the decoction 3 times a day or whenever it is warm. Take 2 *qian* with salt when it is a powder dosage form.

Modern Usage: Take 6 g when it's a powder, 2–3 times a day. Or decoct it by water, and then slightly decrease the dosage according to the original proportion.

[Action]   Scatter and dissipate wind cold, regulate qi and harmonize the middle warmer.

[Indication]   External wind and cold with internal qi stagnation, chill and fever, headache without sweating, chest fullness, poor appetite, thin and white coating, floating pulse.

[Formula Analysis]   The symptoms are caused by wind-cold attacking the exterior with liver and stomach qi stagnation. In this formula, *xiāng fù* can regulate qi to resolve constraints and disperse the exterior evil. *Zǐ sū yè* can disperse wind cold,

---

① *Qian* (*qián*, 钱): 1.5–1.8 g.

regulate qi and harmonize the middle warmer. These two herbs are chief medicines. *Chén pí*, the assistant medicine, can regulate and harmonize middle qi. *Gān cǎo*, the envoy medicine, can harmonize all medicines. Combining these four herbs can eliminate wind cold externally and regulate liver and stomach qi internally.

[Clinical Application]   The formula is appropriate for the external wind cold and internal qi stagnation syndrome. It can also be applied to the patient who has liver qi stagnation accompanied by external wind cold. Female patients are susceptible to this kind of disease.

Xiāng Rú Sǎn (Mosla Beverage, 香薷散)
Formulary of the Pharmacy Service for Benefiting the People in the Taiping Era (*Tài Píng Huì Mín Hé Jì Jú Fāng*, 太平惠民和剂局方)

[Ingredient]

Xiāng Rú (Herba Moslae Diantherae)   impurities removed, 1 *jin* (500 g)

Bái Biǎn Dòu (Semen Lablab Album)   fired slightly, half *jin* (250 g)

Hòu Pò (Cortex Magnoliae Officinalis)   rough skin removed, fired with ginger juice half *jin* (250 g)

[Usage]   The dosage forms of the original formula are coarse powder. Take 3 *qian* every time and apply water 1 cup and wine [one-tenth of the water volume], decoct until seven-tenths is left. Deposit in cold water after discarding the sediment. It will have a miraculous effect after taking 2 close continuously.

Modern Usage: Decoct in water, and take when it is cold, the dosage is reduced according to the original proportion.

[Action]   Release the exterior and dissipate cold, remove dampness and harmonize the middle.

[Indication]   Excessive intake of cold water in summer, [attacked by] external cold and internal dampness, [leads to] the heaviness of the head and headache, no sweating, chest fullness, or weak four limbs, abdominal pain, vomiting and diarrhea, white and greasy tongue coating.

[Formula Analysis]   Laying in a cool or cold place in summer [which] leads

to cold pathogenic factors invading the exterior. This formula takes *xiāng rú*, which is pungent, warm, and good at dispersing, relieving exterior syndrome by sweating and remove dampness and harmonize the spleen. Li Shi-zhen said, "*Xiāng rú*, the exterior-relieving herb in summer, is like its counterpart *má huáng* in winter." Thus, it is the chief medicine. *Hòu pò*, the deputy medicine, is bitter, pungent and warm, successfully removing dampness and harmonizing the middle. *Biǎn dòu*, the assistant medicine, is sweet and neutral to invigorate the spleen and dissolve dampness. Wine, which can warm the blood vessels to eliminate cold dampness, is the envoy medicine. The compatibility can relieve the depressed exterior and harmonize the spleen and stomach.

[Clinical Application] This formula is also called *Sān Wù Xiāng Rú Yǐn* in later times. It can disperse cold to relieve the exterior and dissolve dampness to harmonize the stomach. Thus, it is a standard formula to treat cool-coveting in summer for those who are attacked by cold and dampness.

Section 2　Formulas that releases the exterior with acrid-cool

The formulas that release exterior with acrid-cool medicines are suitable for the exterior syndromes externally contracted by wind-heat. The symptoms are fever, slight aversion to wind and cold, headache, thirst, sore throat, red tongue tip with thin white or thin yellow coating and floating pulse, *etc.* Concerning acrid [natures] medicines releasing the exterior and the cool [natures] clearing the heat, the acrid-cool medicines like *niú bàng zǐ, sāng yè, jú huā and lián qiào* are usually used as the main ingredients in the formulas. Depending on the disease conditions, some practitioners combine acrid-warm medicines with cold ones in treatment formulations as the acrid warm releases the exterior. However, the dosage of acrid-warm is not supposed to be higher than that of acrid-cool medicines. The typical formulas are *Yín Qiào Sǎn* (Lonicera and Forsythia Powder, 银翘散), *Sāng Jú Yǐn* (Mulberry Leaf and Chrysanthemum Beverage, 桑菊饮) and *Má Huáng Xìng Rén Shí Gāo Gān Cǎo Tāng* (Ephedra, Apricot Kernel, Gypsum and Licorice Decoction, 麻黄杏仁石膏甘草汤), *etc.*

Yín Qiào Sǎn (Lonicera and Forsythia Powder, 银翘散)
Systematic Differentiation of Warm Diseases (*Wēn Bìng Tiáo Biàn*, 温病条辨)[10]

[Ingredient]

Lián Qiào (Fructus Forsythiae) 1 *liang* (30 g)

Jīn Yín Huā (Flos Lonicerae Japonicae) 1 *liang* (30 g)

Jié Gěng (Radix Platycodonis) 6 *qian* (18 g)

Bò He (Herba Menthae) 6 *qian* (18 g)

Zhú Yè (Folium Phyllostachydis Henonis) 4 *qian* (12 g)

Gān Cǎo (Radix et Rhizoma Glycyrrhizae) 5 *qian* (15 g)

Jīng Jiè (Herba Schizonepetae) 4 *qian* (12 g)

Dàn Dòu Chǐ (Semen Sojae Praeparatum) 5 *qian* (15 g)

Niú Bàng Zǐ (Fructus Arctii) 6 *qian* (18 g)

[Usage] The original formula is ground into a powder, every time the patient takes the dosage of 6 *qian*, boiled with *Wěi Jīng Tāng*, which is cooked just long enough for the aroma to become strong, but do not overdo it. The medicines that go to the upper *jiao* [lung] are light; over-boiling will make the flavor thick and enter the middle *jiao*. For patients with serious conditions, they should take the decoction every four hours, three times a day and one dose at night; patients with mild conditions should take the decoction every six hours, twice during the day and once at night; after that, if symptoms still exist, continue taking the medicine.

Modern usage: Add a moderate quantity of *lú gēn*, decocted by water, and adjust the proportion according to the original formula.

[Action] Acrid-cool to vent the exterior, clear the heat and resolve toxin.

[Indication] At the beginning of the warm disease, [patient manifesting] fever, slight aversion to wind and cold, no sweat or difficulty sweating, headache, thirst, cough, sore throat, red tongue tip with thin white or thin yellow coating and floating pulse.

[Formula Analysis] "When the warm pathogen invades the upper *iiao*, the lung will be disturbed first", "the lung governs qi and is ascribed to the *wei* level", and the lung is connected to the skin and body hair, governs the exterior of the whole body. In the formula, a large dosage of sweet, cold and aromatic *jīn yín huā* is used

13

to clear the heat and resolve toxins, dispel filth and remove turbidity, bitter *lián qiào* is used to clear the heat and dissolve the toxins and diffuse the exterior, which serves as the chief medicine with *jīn yín huā, bò he* is acrid and cool to induce sweating, eliminate the wind-heat, and refresh the mind and vision. *Jīng jiè* and *dàn dòu chǐ* are acrid and warm, but not dry; combined with *bò he*, they serve as deputy medicines. *Niú bàng zǐ, jié gěng* and *gān cǎo* diffuse the lung and dispel phlegm, dissolve the toxin and relieve sorethroat. *Zhú yè* and *lú gēn* are sweet, cold and light to vent the heat and promote fluid production; those five herbs are all assistant medicines. *Gān cǎo* can act as the envoy medicine. Combine all those medicines to dispel heattoxins and dissipate the wind-heat.

[Clinical Application]

1. This formula is called "pungent, cool and moderate formula" in the *Systematic Differentiation of Warm Diseases* (*Wēn Bìng Tiáo Biàn*, 温病条辨), suitable for the first stage of warm disease and exterior syndrome externally-contracted by wind-heat.

2. According to the editor's clinical experience, this formula is used for wind-heat exterior syndrome when the fever is gone. However, the pathogen remains, and *Sāng Jú Yǐn* can be used to treat patients with cough.

Sāng Jú Yǐn (Mulberry Leaf and Chrysanthemum Beverage, 桑菊饮)
Systematic Differentiation of Warm Diseases (*Wēn Bìng Tiáo Biàn*, 温病条辨)

[Ingredient]

Xìng Rén (Semen Armeniacae Amarum) 2 *qian* (6 g)

Lián Qiào (Fructus Forsythiae) 1 *qian* 5 *fen* (4.5 g)

Bò He (Herba Menthae) 8 *fen* (2.4 g)

Sāng Yè (Folium Mori) 2 *qian* 5 *fen* (7.5 g)

Jú Huā (Flos Chrysanthemi) 1 *qian* (3 g)

Kǔ Jié Gěng (Radix Platycodonis) 2 *qian* (6 g)

Gān Cǎo (Radix et Rhizoma Glycyrrhizae) 8 *fen* (4.2 g)

Weǐ Gēn 2 *qian* (6 g)

[Usage] The original formula is cooked into one cup from two water, and

after boiled, drink one cup twice a day.

Modern usage: Decocted by water.

[Action] Dispersing the wind-heat, facilitating the lung and relieving cough.

[Indication] Wind-warm in *taiyin*, cough, moderate fever, mild thirst.

[Formula Analysis] This syndrome was caused by wind-warm invading the hand *taiyin* lung channel. With sweet, bitter tastes and slightly cold nature, *sāng yè* and *jú huā* scatter the wind-heat in the upper *jiao*; they are the chief medicines. The acrid cool *bò he* releases the exterior, helps the chief medicines to scatter the wind and discharges heat from the skin. *Xìng rén* has a descending action, while *jié gěng* has the ascending action, they assist the chief herbs by facilitating the flow of lung qi to stop coughing, also release the exterior, both serving as deputy medicines. The bitter cold *lián qiào*, strengthens the exterior-releasing properties. Sweet cold *lú gēn* clears heat and generates fluids; it is an assistant medicine. *Gān cǎo* combined with *jié gěng* clears the throat and harmonizes the actions of all medicines in the formula. It serves as the envoy medicine. All the combined medicines scatter wind-heat in the upper *jiao* and diffuse lung qi, dispelling the pathogen and relieving cough.

[Clinical Application]

1. This formula is called "pungent, cool and mild formula" in the *Systematic Differentiation of Warm Diseases* (*Wēn Bìng Tiáo Biàn*, 温病条辨), suitable for patients with invasion by the wind-heat and have cough as the main symptoms.

2. According to the clinical experience of the editor, patients who have a wind-warmth cough with sticky phlegm can be treated with this formula, adding *guā lóu pí*, *zhè bèi mǔ* to clear the phlegm.

Má Huáng Xìng Rén Shí Gāo Gān Cǎo Tāng (Ephedra, Apricot Kernel, Gypsum, and Licorice Decoction, 麻黄杏仁石膏甘草汤) *Treatise on Cold Damage* (*Shāng Hán Lùn*, 伤寒论)

[Ingredient]

Má Huáng (Herba Ephedrae)   4 *liang*, remove branch knots (12 g)

Xìng Rén (Semen Armeniacae Amarum)   50 pcs, remove skin (9 g)

Gān Cǎo (Radix et Rhizoma Glycyrrhizae)   2 *liang*, liquid-fried (6 g)

Shí Gāo (Gypsum Fibrosum)   0.5 *jin*, crushed, wrapped with cotton cloth (24 g)

[Usage]   In the original book, firstly, boil *má huáng* with 7 *sheng* of water and decoct into 2 *sheng*, remove the foam and add the other ingredients into the decoction and continue boiling, then take 2 *sheng* out and filter it, keep 1 *sheng* for drinking.

Modern usage: Decocted by water.

[Action]   Diffuse and discharge with acrid and cool medicines, clear the lung and calm wheezing by directing qi downward.

[Indication]   Externally-contracted wind pathogen, persistent fever, sweat or no sweat, cough, panting [caused by] qi counterflow, or even flaring of the nostrils, thirst, red tongue, thin white or thin yellow coating, floating, slippery and rapid pulse.

[Formula Analysis]   This syndrome is caused by the exterior pathogen [enter inside and] transforming into internal heat and obstructing the lung. *Má huáng* is acrid, bitter, good at facilitating the circulation of lung qi and stops wheezing. Li Shi-zhen said, "*Má huáng* is the specialized medicine for lung meridians, though it is the significant herb of releasing the *Taiyang*, but also adept in releasing the constrained heat in the lung meridian." A large quantity of *shí gāo* is used. It is acrid, sweet and very cold and helps to discharge lung heat, drains heat from the lung and controls the sweating action of *má huáng*. They are both serving as chief medicines. *Xìng rén*, assists *má huáng* in facilitating the flow of lung qi, relieving cough and wheezing, serving as assistant medicine; *gān cǎo* harmonizes the actions of all medicines in the formula, not only by preserving the stomach qi from the cold nature of *shí gāo*, but also by engendering fluids with its sweet and cold nature. Due to "sweating leads to wheezing", the lung heat consumes the fluids, *gān cǎo* is also an envoy medicine. There are only four medicines, but the combination rule is strict, which work together to diffuse, clear the lung and relieve wheezing.

[Clinical Application]   This formula is the representative formula to diffuse the lung and discharge heat, with the diagnosis of essential points of fever, panting, yellow coating, rapid pulse, no matter whether sweating or not. If the patient manifests sweating and wheezing, [mostly] caused by constraint-heat in the lung, [we should]

discharge heat from the skin and body hair. In the original book, the dosage of *shí gāo* is twice as much as the dosage of *má huáng*, but based on clinical practice, the dosage of *shí gāo* can be five times as much as *má huáng* or even ten times as much. If the patients have no sweating but present wheezing, that is caused by constraint-heat in the lung with closed orifices in the skin [the lung has lost its control over the opening and closing of the pores], which requires a large quantity of *má huáng* but still less than *shí gāo*. Here *má huáng* diffuses the lung that opens a pathway for constraint-heat; *shí gāo* clears the heat and discharges the heat, which avoids the generation of pathogenic heat. The dosage of acrid cold medicines is higher than acrid warm medicines, which means it's still an acrid-cool formula essentially.

Section 3   Formulas that reinforces healthy qi and releases the exterior

These formulas are suitable for patients who are deficient but with exterior syndrome. At this point, reinforcing is for releasing the exterior not only to supplement the deficiency. Cause only with a sufficient healthy qi can the human body dispel pathogens. A deficiency of healthy qi easily leads to exterior syndrome; thus, the healthy qi must be strengthened. If we just focus on sweating, the yang qi will get hurt and yin blood consumed, even worse, the patients will have yang collapse due to profuse sweating. Therefore, one must be prudent!

The deficiencies include yang, qi, yin and blood deficiency, so releasing the exterior by reinforcing yang (tonifying qi) is different from releasing the exterior by reinforcing yin (nourishing the blood). The reinforcing yang (tonifying qi) method is designed for those who have both yang qi deficiency and externally-contracted exterior syndrome. Some commonly used medicines that warm yang and tonify qi are *rén shēn*, *fù zǐ*. They are used with the medicines that release the exterior like *má huáng*, *xì xīn* and *qiāng huó*, etc. *Bài Dú Sǎn* (Toxin-Resolving Powder, 败毒散), *Má Huáng Fù Zǐ Xì Xīn Tāng* (Ephedra, Aconite and Asarum Decoction, 麻黄附子细辛汤) are the typical formulas. The reinforcing yin (nourishing blood) method is designed for patients with insufficiency of yin blood, the commonly used medicines are *yù zhú*,

mài dōng and other exterior-releasing medicines like *cōng bái*, *dàn dòu chǐ* and *bò he*. *Jiā Jiǎn Wēi Ruí Tāng* (Solomon's Seal Variant Decoction, 加减葳蕤汤) is the typical formula.

Bài Dú Sǎn (Toxin-Resolving Powder, 败毒散，人参败毒散)
Craft of Medicines and Patterns for Children (*Xiǎo Ér Yào Zhèng Zhí Jué*, 小儿药证直诀)[11]

[Ingredient]

Chái Hú (Radix Bupleuri)　remove the sprout 1 *liang* (3 g)

Gān Cǎo (Radix et Rhizoma Glycyrrhizae)　half *liang* (1.5 g)

Jié Gěng (Radix Platycodonis)　1 *liang* (3 g)

Rén Shēn (Radix et Rhizoma Ginseng)　1 *liang* (3 g)

Chuān Xiōng (Rhizoma Chuanxiong)　1 *liang* (3 g)

Fú Líng (Poria)　remove rind　1 *liang* (3 g)

Zhǐ Ké (Fructus Aurantii)　1 *liang* (3 g)

Qián Hú (Radix Peucedani)　1 *liang* (3 g)

Qiāng Huó (Rhizoma et Radix Notopterygii)　1 *liang* (3 g)

Dú Huó (Radix Angelicae Pubescentis)　1 *liang* (3 g)

[Usage]　The original formula was ground into a coarse powder, each time the patient takes 2 *qian* with a cup of water, a little *shēng jiāng*, *bò he*, boils the mixture, filters it and then drinks it at any time. For cold syndrome, the patients should drink the hot decoction; otherwise, drink the warm decoction.

Modern usage: Add some *shēng jiāng*, *bò he*, decocted with water. The dosage should be reduced in proportion according to the original formula.

[Action]　Tonify qi, release the exterior, scatter wind and remove dampness.

[Indication]　Internal deficiency, [with] externally-contracted wind-cold-damp pathogen, aversion to cold and high fever, headache and pain in the neck, pain in the limbs, no sweat, heavy nasal sound, cough with phlegm, white and greasy coating, floating pulse but weak under pressing.

[Formula Analysis]　Deficient body constitution, with wind-cold and damp

pathogens invading the exterior. In the formula, acrid bitter and warm, *qiāng huó* and *dú huó* can dissipate the wind-cold from the exterior, remove dampness and relieve the pain, serving as chief medicines; the bitter and neutral *chái hú* scatters heat and leads the ascent of the clear. The acrid warm *chuān xiōng* dispels wind and relieves the pain. These two help *qiāng huó* and *dú huó* releases the exterior and relieve pain, serving as deputy medicines; *zhǐ qiào* and *jié gěng* respectively lead the descending and ascending of qi, loosen the chest and rectify qi. *Qián hú* and *fú líng* diffuse the lung and dissolve phlegm, acrid *shēng jiāng* and *bò he* releases the exterior. *Rén shēn* helps to strengthen the healthy qi and dispel the pathogenic qi. A strong healthy qi can dispel the pathogen out, the seven medicines serve as assistant medicines. *Gān cǎo* harmonizes the center and the actions of all medicines in a formula, rectifying the spleen, serving as the envoy medicine. In this formula, *rén shēn* strengthens the healthy qi and dispels the pathogenic qi, the cooperation between all the medicines dredges the meridians and collaterals, releases the exterior and the constrained pathogen, which is the reason that this formula is named "*Rén Shēn Bài Dú*".

[Clinical Application]

1. This formula applies to those externally contracted by wind, cold and damp due to qi deficiency. *Rén shēn* is the assistant medicine, of which the low dosage can boost qi and dispel the pathogen. If the dosage is too high, it will generate dampness, which is not conducive to removing the pathogen.

2. This formula can also be applied to treat the early stage of dysentery with wind, cold and damp exterior syndrome. Yu Jia-yan[12] thought that in the early stage of dysentery, patients had the exterior syndrome, and the pathogen invaded the interior.This formula releases the exterior pathogen. Once the qi in the exterior is fluent, the stagnation will disappear and dysentery will recovers. When the pathogen invades from the exterior, it must return by the same way it came, released from the interior to the exterior, which is called the method of hauling the boat upstream.

Má Huáng Fù Zǐ Xì Xīn Tāng (Ephedra, Aconite and Asarum Decoction, 麻黄附子细辛汤)

Treatise on Cold Damage (*Shāng Hán Lùn*, 伤寒论)

[Ingredient]

Má huáng (Herba Ephedrae)   2 *liang*, remove stem nodes (6 g)

Xì Xīn (Radix et Rhizoma Asari)   2 *liang* (3 g)

Fù Zǐ (Radix Aconiti Lateralis Praeparata)   1 *mei* [pcs], processed, peel, cut into 8 pieces (9 g)

[Usage]   Three herbs in the original formula, boil the *má huáng* first with 10 *sheng* of water. Then take 2 *sheng* away, skim off the froth, add other herbs, boil them till 3 *sheng* left, remove the precipitate and drink 1 *sheng* when it is warm, 3 times a day.

Modern Usage: Decocted with water.

[Action]   Assist yang and release the exterior.

[Indication]   People with *shaoyin* syndrome but have a fever with a deep pulse.

[Formula Analysis]   *Shaoyin* syndrome's nature is cold due to yang qi deficiency with the cprimary syndrome "thready and faint pulse but feels sleepy", and the patient should have no fever manifestation. In this situation, the presence of fever indicates that *taiyang* exterior syndrome must be combined with which should be treated by the sweating method; while the yang deficiency of *shaoyin* needs to be treated by warming. *Má huáng* can dissipate the cold of *taiyang* and induce sweating to release the exterior, *fù zǐ* can warm the *shaoyang* channel, consolidate and protect *yuan yang*. They are both chief medicines. *Xì xīn* can release the exterior of *taiyang* and dissipate the cold of *shaoyin* which can help *má huáng* induce sweating to release the exterior and help *fù zǐ* warm the channels and dissipate cold. It is the assistant medicine. With all three herbs, the wind-cold of *taiyang* can be dissipated, *yuan yang* of *shaoyin* can be consolidated and protected, which brings out the best in each other.

[Clinical Application]

1. This formula treats the root of yang deficiency and the branch of contracted cold simultaneously. The main points of syndrome differentiation are severe aversion

to cold with light fever, without sweating, deep pulse with white and moist coating.

2. The syndrome is yang deficiency and external contraction while yang deficiency is not very severe. Therefore, assisting yang and releasing the exterior can be used. If the yang qi of *shaoyin* declines with the syndromes like diarrhea with undigested food and a faint pulse that nearly stops, *Sì Nì Tāng* can be used to restore yang. If the sweating method is used erroneously, it will release the extreme cold of the limbs with yang collapse. It should be taken carefully.

Jiā Jiǎn Wēi Ruí Tāng (Solomon's Seal Variant Decoction, 加减葳蕤汤)
Revised Popular Guide to the Discussion of Cold Damage (Chóng Dìng Tōng Sú Shāng Hán Lùn, 重订通俗伤寒论)[13]

[Ingredient]

Shēng Wēi Ruí (Rhizoma Polygonati Odorati)   2–3 *qian* (6–9 g)

Shēng Cōng Bái (Bulbus Allii Fistulosi)   2–3 *mei* (2–3 slices)

Jié Gěng (Radix Platycodonis)   1–1.5 *qian* (3–4.5 g)

Dōng Bái Wēi (Radix et Rhizoma Cynanchi Atrati)   0.5–1 *qian* (1.5–3 g)

Dàn Dòu Chǐ (Semen Sojae Praeparatum)   3–4 *qian* (9–12 g)

Sū Bò He (Herba Menthae)   1–1.5 *qian* (3–4.5 g)

Zhì Gān Cǎo (Radix et Rhizoma Glycyrrhizae Praeparatacum Melle)   0.5 *qian* (1.5 g)

Hóng Zǎo (Fructus Jujubae)   2 *mei* (2 pcs)

[Usage]   In the original book, there is no record of the usage instructions.

Modern Usage: Decoct with water.

[Action]   Reinforce yin and release the exterior.

[Indication]   People who are yin deficient in the constitution and have been attacked by the exterior pathogen, manifested headache and fever, slight aversion to wind and cold, without sweating or scanty sweating, cough and dry throat, thirsty and irritable, red tongue and rapid pulse.

[Formula Analysis]   The patient with yin deficient constitution who is attacked by exogenous pathogenic factors may easily transform into a heat nature. The yin

deficient constitution lacks sufficient sources of sweat so when they are attacked by the exterior pathogen, the body fails to release the pathogen through sweating. The formula should increase fluids to reinforce the sources of sweat [body fluid]. *Shēng wēi ruí*, namely is *shēng yù zhú* which can enrich yin, moisten dryness and promote fluid production. It is a clearing and supplementing herb of which has been said, "It is good for treating febrile diseases caused by pathogenic wind and warmth with fever and spontaneous perspiration" in *The Grand Compendium of Materia Medica* (*Běn Cǎo Gāng Mù*, 本草纲目[14]), so it is the chief medicine. The deputy medicines are *cōng bái*, *dàn dòu chǐ*, *bò he* which can scatter and dissipate the exterior pathogen; the assistant medicines are *bái wēi* which can clear heat and boost yin and *jié gěng* which can relieve throat and cough; the envoy medicines are *zhì gān cǎo* and *hóng zǎo* [*dà zǎo*] which are sweet and moistening to promote fluid production and harmonize the actions of all medicines in a formula.

[Clinical Application]　　This formula is a variation of *Wēi Ruí Tāng* (Solomon's Seal Decoction, 葳蕤汤 : *wēi ruí*, *dōng bái wēi*, *má huáng*, *dú huó*, *xìng rén*, *chuān xiōng*, *gān cǎo*, *qīng mù xiāng*, *shí gāo*) in *Classical Formulas* (*Xǐao Pǐn Fāng*, 小品方[15]) which is designed for patients of yin deficient constitution with an externally contracted wind pathogen. When the exterior syndrome is not solved, medicine for enriching yin can not be used because it is easy to generate the pathogen retention inside. However, if an exterior pathogen attacks the patients with a yin deficiency constitution, then sweating not only fails to release the exterior pathogen, but also consumes fluid and yin. Therefore, the only way to satisfy both sides is to enrich yin and release the exterior at the same time.

Chapter 2

Emetic Formulas

According to the principles of legislation in *Basic Questions-The Great Treatise on Yin Yang Correspondence in phenomena* (*Sù Wèn-Yīn Yáng Yīng Xiàng Dà Lùn*, 素问·阴阳应象大论[16]): "[disease located] In the upper, vomiting should be used", every formula which consists of emetic medicines which can stimulate the upward movement and vomiting, eliminate phlegm, retained food, poison, *etc.*, that stagnated in the throat, chest, diaphragm, and the stomach cavity. It is the "vomit induction" in "eight methods" and the "diffuse to remove congestion" in "ten formula types".

This kind of formula usually consists of emetic medicines like *guā dì, bái fán*, salt, *etc.* There are typical formulas like *Guā Dì Sǎn* (Melon Stalk Powder, 瓜蒂散), *Yán Tāng Tàn Tǔ Fāng* (salt decoction of touching and vomiting formula, 盐汤探吐方) and so on.

Guā Dì Sǎn (Melon Stalk Powder, 瓜蒂散)
Treatise on Cold Damage (*Shāng Hán Lùn*, 伤寒论)

[Ingredient]

Guā Dì (Pedicellus Melo)   1 *fen*, stewed into yellow (1 g)

Chì Xiǎo Dòu (Semen Phaseoli)   1 *fen* (1 g)

[Usage]   Grind the two herbs into a powder and then mix them. Take the powder about the amount of 1 *qian bi* with *xiāng chǐ* 1 *he* and hot water 7 *he* and then boil into thin gruel, remove the precipitate and drink it warm. If the patient does not vomit, add bit by bit until vomiting.

Modern Usage: Grind and mix *guā dì* and *chì xiǎo dòu*. Every 1–2 g of the

mixture must be taken with *dàn dòu chǐ* 12 g which is made into a decoction. If the patient is in urgent need of vomiting, a clear feather or tongue depressor can be used to touch the throat to help the patient vomit after taking the medicines.

[Action] Vomit phlegm and retained food.

[Indication] People who have sputum and retained food stagnated in the chest and leads to epigastric fullness in chest, the uprushing qi result in the uncomfortable feeling in throat, or people who have reversal cold of the hands and feet, fullness in the epigastrium with vexation and hard to vomit.

[Formula Analysis] Sputum obstructs at chest or retained food stagnates in the upper third portion of the stomach cavity (*shàng wǎn*, 上脘). In *Basic Questions-The Great Treatise on Yin Yang Correspondence in phenomena* (*Sù Wèn-Yīn Yáng Yīng Xiàng Dà Lùn*, 素问·阴阳应象大论) says, "In the upper, vomiting should be used.", if the disease is located at chest, which can't be solved by sweating or purgation methods, capitalize on the trend, release the exterior pathogen from upper. *Guā dì* which is bitter-cold and can promote vomiting of retained food with little dosage, is taken as the chief medicine; *chì xiǎo dòu* which is sour and neutral can work mutually with *guā dì*, sour and bitter flavors with emetic and purgative effects, can promote the vomiting of the excess pathogen in the chest as the deputy medicine; *xiāng chǐ* which is light, floating and upward, can diffuse old pathogens in the chest and release it by moving it upward. Thus, the upper *jiao* can be unblocked, yang qi can be recovered, stagnation and hardness can vanish, and the chest can be harmonized. If the patient does not vomit after taking the decoction, "add bit-by-bit until vomiting". However, one must be careful not to impair the qi and consume the fluid.

[Clinical Application] This formula is the original type of emetic formula. *Guā dì* in the formula is *tián guā dì* which is freshly picked. The new and small one is better in comparison with the older one which will not be as effective. If there is not *tián guā dì*, *sī guā dì* can be used.

Yán Tāng Tàn Tǔ Fāng (salt decoction of touching and vomiting formula, 盐汤探吐方)

Essentials from the Golden Cabinet (*Jīn Guì Yào Lüè*, 金匮要略[17])

[Ingredient]

Salt   1 *sheng*

Water   3 *sheng* (appropriate amount)

[Usage]   Boil salt until it melts. Drink it three times, stop taking it when the patient vomits out.

Modern Usage: Boil salt with water into a saturated salt solution. After drinking about 200 ml, use a clear feather or fingers to touch the throat to stimulate vomiting, and stop after vomiting all the retained food. If the patient does not vomit after taking medicine, more hot salt soup is needed for vomiting.

[Action]   Vomit retained food.

[Indication]   Retained food makes the patient feel stiffness, fullness and pain in the abdomen. Or the patient suffers from dry cholera and prefers to vomit or defecate, but fails to perform, combined with colicky pain, irritability and fullness.

[Formula Analysis]   Improper diet causes food retention in the stomach cavity and obstructs the qi movement. The *Basic Questions-Comprehensive Discourse on the Essentials of the Most Reliable* (*Sù Wèn-Zhì Zhēn Yào Dà Lùn*, 素问·至真要大论) says, "Salty flavor pertains to Yin because it induces vomiting and purgation." This formula uses salt decoction to promote vomiting thanks to the extreme taste. *Shen Nong's Classic of the Materia Medica* (*Shén Nóng Běn Cǎo Jīng*, 神农本草经) has the record of "salt can make one vomit". But the power of salt decoction to vomit is weak, so we always prefer to use a feather, fingers, or a tongue depressor to help move the retained food upward and remove the obstruction, and then all the syndromes can be healed successfully.

[Clinical Application]   Properties of herbs in this description are gentle, convenient to use, and have a rapid effect. It is a commonly-used emetic formula.

Chapter 3

Purgative Formulas

According to the principle that "pathogen in the lower requiring dredging; abdominal fullness should be treated by elimination" and "when there is excess, treat it with dissipation and drainage.", in *Basic Questions-The Great Treatise on Yin Yang Correspondence in phenomena* (*Sù Wèn-Yīn Yáng Yīng Xiàng Dà Lùn*, 素问·阴阳应象大论), purgative formulas refer to those that are mainly composed of purgatives with therapeutic effects of relieving constipation, eliminating gastrointestinal stagnation, purging away excess heat, evacuating cold retention, and eliminating retained fluid, which is used in the treatment of interior syndrome of excess type. The purgative formula is also called a prescription of attacking the interior that belongs to the "purgative method" in "eight methods".

Section 1   Purgatives formulas of cold nature

Purgative formulas of cold nature (cold purgation formula) are applied in the treatment of excess syndrome of interior heat stagnation. Symptoms like constipation, distending abdominal pain, tidal fever, yellowish coating, excess pulse, *etc.* Formulas of cold purgation are aimed at purging stagnation and eliminating pathogenic heat and mainly consist of purgative herbs with cold nature such as *dà huáng*, *máng xiāo*, *lú huì*. Suppose dry stool, stained food and excess heat accumulate in the stomach and intestines which causes the blockage of *fu* qi, the formula can combine medicines with the efficacy of moving *qi* like *hòu pò*, *zhǐ shí*, which can eliminate retained food and evacuate stagnated heat. The representative formula is *Dà Chéng Qì Tāng* (Major

Purgative Decoction, 大承气汤). If dampness heat stagnates in the intestines and develops into intestinal abscesses, the formula can be combined with herbs that reduce dampness and dissipate stasis like *yì yǐ rén*, *dōng guā zǐ*, *táo rén*, *mǔ dān pí*, *etc*. The representative formula is *Dà huáng Mǔ Dān Tāng* (Decoction of Rhubarb Root and Moutan Bark, 大黄牡丹汤). If patients have gastrointestinal dry heat, and exuberance of heart and liver fire, the formula can be combined with *zhū shā* to calm the heart and clear away fire. The representative formula is *Gēng Yī Wán*.

Dà Chéng Qì Tāng (Major Purgative Decoction, 大承气汤)
Treatise on Cold Damage (*Shāng Hán Lùn*, 伤寒论)

[Ingredient]

Dà Huáng (Radix et Rhizoma Rhei) 4 *liang* (12 g)

Hòu Pò (Cortex Magnoliae Officinalis) rough skin removed, fired with ginger juice half *jin* (15 g)

Zhǐ Shí (Fructus Aurantii Immaturus) 5 *mei*, fluid-fried (12 g)

Máng Xiāo (Natrii Sulfas) 3 *he* (9 g)

[Usage] Add 1 *dou* water to decoct the above herbs. Firstly, decoct *hòu pò* and *zhǐ shí* till 5 *sheng*, then abandon the dregs. Secondly, add *dà huáng* and stew till 2 *sheng*, then abandon the dregs. Thirdly, add *máng xiāo*, and then boil with mild fire when it bubbles up once or twice. Divide it into several dosages and take it when it is warm. Stop taking when the decoction works.

Modern Usage: First boil *hòu pò* and *zhǐ shí*, and then add *dà huáng* and *máng xiāo*.

[Action] Drastic purgation for eliminating [accumulated] heat.

[Indication]

1. This recipe is used to treat excessive heat syndrome of *yangming fu* visceral syndrome, manifested as no aversion to cold while aversion to heat, late afternoon tidal fever, delirious speech and unconsciousness, profuse flatulence, constipation and continuous sweating in the hands and feet, abdominal fullness pain and stuffiness, blurred vision and uneven movement of the eyeballs, yellowish fur, prickly tongue

with dry yellowish coating or dry blackish coating with fissures, deep and excessive pulse.

2. Heat retention but with watery discharge, which has a sour and filthy smell, peri-navel pain, lumps felt during the press, dry mouth and throat, slippery and rapid pulse.

3. Interior excess heat of *yangming* bowel syndrome includes heat syncope, convulsive disease, and delirium.

[Formula Analysis]   The indication of this formula is "*pi*, fullness, dryness, excess". "*pi*" means chest or abdominal mass causing stuffiness and stagnation. The patient feels *pi* (*pǐ* 痞) in the abdomen due to the *qi* accumulated in the stomach and intestines with a disorder of *qi* movement in ascending and descending. "fullness" (*mǎn* 满) is visible distention that is hard and painful to palpation. This is due to the retained food stagnating in the bowels that obstruct the *qi* movement. "dryness" (*zào* 燥) refers to the dry stool that accumulates in the intestines and causes parts of the abdomen to become tense and firm. The stool in the bowels is dry and hard. "excess" (*shí* 实) refers to the heat that accumulates which causes constipation and abdominal fullness and pain. Some fluid flows around the clogged stools and manifests as watery green diarrhea with a sticky odor while the abdominal fullness will not be relieved. *Dà huáng*, which is bitter and cold, serves as the chief medicine to eliminate heat and move stools in the gastrointestinal tract to relieve constipation. *Máng xiāo*, which is salty and cold, possesses the effect of draining heat, moistening dryness and softening masses, and is used as a deputy medicine to reinforce the effect of the chief medicine, which is effective for purging heat accumulation.

Stagnation accumulates and obstructs the interior, which causes *qi* stagnation and abnormality of *qi* movement. *Zhī shí* and *hòu pò* are the assistant medicines for dispersing *pi* and relieving fullness, which are capable of promoting the flow of *qi* and helping the chief and deputy medicines with purging accumulated heat. These four medicines together generate a drastic efficacy in purging heat accumulation. The normal stomach *fu*-organ *qi* direction is downward or descending. This formula has a drastic effect of purgation for eliminating accumulated heat, which follows the normal

descending flow of the stomach *qi*, relieving the stagnation and blockage. That is the reason for the name "purgative decoction".

[Clinical Application] The patient can take this formula only if he/she has four syndromes of "*pi*, fullness, dryness, excess". The misapplication of this formula can impair interior *qi*, which easily causes cold apoplexy, thoracic accumulation, *pi* qi.

Dà huáng Mǔ Dān Tāng (Decoction of Rhubarb Root and Moutan Bark, 大黄牡丹汤)
Essentials from the Golden Cabinet (*Jīn Guì Yào Lüè*, 金匮要略)

[Ingredient]

Dà Huáng (Radix et Rhizoma Rhei)   4 *liang* (12 g)

Mǔ Dān Pí (Cortex Moutan)   1 *liang* (9 g)

Táo Rén (Semen Persicae)   50 *mei* (9 g)

Dōng Guā Zǐ (Semen Benincasae)   half *sheng* (15 g)

Máng Xiāo (Natrii Sulfas)   3 *he* (9 g)

[Usage]   Add 1 *dou* water to decoct the above herbs. Firstly, decoct the first four ingredients in water till 1 *sheng*, and then remove the dregs from the decoction. Secondly, dissolve *máng xiāo* in it and boil. The decoction is to be taken separately.

Modern Usages: Decoct the first four ingredients in water, and then dissolve *máng xiāo* in it.

[Action]   Purge away heat and remove blood stasis, disperse pathogenic accumulation and subdue abscess.

[Indication]   This formula is indicated for intestinal abscess in the early stage, marked by pain and tenderness in the right lower abdomen, even with local swelling and mass, normal urination, but constant fever, spontaneous sweating with aversion to cold, or limitation of the right foot to stretch, thin yellowish and greasy coating, slow, tight and powerful pulse.

[Formula Analysis]   Intestinal abscess refers to a type of disease in which there is swelling and abscess in the intestines and causing right lower abdominal

pain. *Dà huáng*, which is bitter and cold, purges away intense heat and stagnation, removing toxins and heat stasis from the intestines. *Dà huáng* is described as "purge away the blood stasis...remove pathogens in the stomach and intestines, get rid of the stale and bring forth the fresh" in *Shen Nong's Classic of the Materia Medica* (*Shén Nóng Běn Cǎo Jīng*, 神农本草经) [as know as *Běn Jīng*]. *Mǔ dān*, pungent, bitter and slightly cold, is described as "relieve hard concretions and blood stasis in stomach and intestines" in *Běn Jīng*, and functions as clearing away heat, cooling the blood and dissipating stasis. The first two herbs both act as chief medicines. *Máng xiāo*, which is salty, bitter and very cold, possesses the efficacy of draining heat and stagnation, softening hardness and dissipating masses. *Máng xiāo* helps *dà huáng* with removing pathogens in the stomach and intestines, getting rid of the stale and bringing forth the fresh. *Táo rén*, which is neutral, bitter and sweet, possesses the functions of breaking up blood, moistening the intestines to promote defecation, and helps *mǔ dān* with the efficacy of invigorating blood and dissipating stasis. *Máng xiāo* and *táo rén* both serve as deputy medicines. *Dōng guā zǐ*, which is sweet and cold, possesses the efficacy of expelling pus and dissipating masses. It is the necessary drug for treating internal abscesses and acts as an assistant medicine. *The Grand Compendium of Materia Medica* (*Běn Cǎo Gāng Mù*, 本草纲目) records it with the function of 'treating intestinal abscess'. The combination of the above herbs will eliminate damp-heat and relieve stasis, freeing the heat accumulation and dissipateing abscesses spontaneously, smoothing the blood flow and relieving pain spontaneously. It agrees with the saying "pathogen in the lower requiries dredging" in *Basic Questions-The Great Treatise on Yin Yang Correspondence in phenomena* (*Sù Wèn-Yīn Yáng Yīng Xiàng Dà Lùn*, 素问·阴阳应象大论).

[Clinical Application] Intestinal abscess is divided into the stagnation of damp-heat and stagnation of damp-cold. This formula can only treat damp-heat stagnation.

Gēng Yī Wán (Defecation Pill, 更衣丸)

Medicine Notes of Xian Xing Zhai (*Xiān Xǐng Zhāi Yī Xué Guǎng Bǐ Jì*, 先醒斋医学广笔记)[18]

[Ingredient]

Zhū Shā (Cinnabaris)   grind into a fine powder like flour, 5 *qian* (15 g)

Lú Huì (Aloe)   grind into a fine powder, 7 *qian* (21 g)

[Usage]   Drop a few drops of yellow rice wine in the above herbs and knead into pills. Take 1 *qian* and 2 cents each dosage, and swallow with wine. Bowel movement will be smooth in the evening if taken in the morning, while it will be smooth the following day if taken in the evening the night before. It is better to collect and process the herbs on sunny days.

Modern Usages: Knead the above herbs into pills with yellow wine, and swallow it with warm boiled water, 4.5–6 g each time.

[Action]   Purge fire to promote constipation.

[Indication]   Heat accumulation in intestines and stomach manifested as constipation, vexation and irritability, restless sleep at night.

[Formula Analysis]   The large intestine has the functions of conducting and transmitting. If dry heat is located in the intestines and the stomach, it will consume the body fluids and it will cause dry stool and constipation. Vexation and irritability, restless sleep at night are indicate heart-liver fire hyperactivity. *Lú huì*, bitter and cold, acts as the chief medicine. It is taken in larger dosages and enters the liver, stomach, and large intestine channels to reduce fire, relieve constipation, clear away heat and cool the liver. *Zhū shā*, which is sweet and cold, acts as the deputy medicine. It possesses the efficacy of purging pathogenic heat in the heart channel, as well as a descending function due to its heavy nature. Because *lú huì* has a bad and filthy smell, a bit of wine is applied to dispel filth and harmonize the stomach, which acts as an assistant and envoy medicine. The combination of the above herbs is effective in draining fire and promoting constipation.

[Clinical Application]   This formula treats dry accumulation in the intestines

and stomach with constipation. When constipation is due to vigorous heart-liver fire, the moisten medicine like *rén* (seed) is unsuitable.

Section 2   Purgative formulas of warm nature

The purgative formula of warm nature is applied for the disease of cold stagnation in *zang-fu*, with warmth used to dissipate coldness and purge to dissipate accumulations. Cold accumulation is caused by the constitution of internal cold with *yang* deficiency, as well as accumulation and stagnation of food. The manifestation includes a white glossy coating, or thick greasy coating at the root of the tongue. The purgative formulas of warm nature are usually made up of *dà huáng*, *bā dòu* in combination with herbs capable of warming the interior like *fù zǐ*, *gān jiāng*, *zhì gān cǎo, etc*. Medicines with bitterness in taste and cold in nature are combined with large dosages of medicines that are warm, to not only restrict the nature of bitter and cold, but also increase the efficacy of warm purgation. The representative formula is *Wēn Pí Tāng* (Spleen-Warming Decoction, 温脾汤). As for the abrupt diseases with an exuberance of pathogen, cold stagnation with food accumulation, stagnation and jamming of *qi* movement, it should be purged drastically, like *Sān Wù Bèi Jí Wán* (Three Substances Emergency Pill, 三物备急丸).

Wēn Pí Tāng (Spleen-Warming Decoction, 温脾汤)
Valuable Prescriptions of Emergency (*Bèi Jí Qiān Jīn Fāng,* 备急千金方)

[Ingredient]

Dà Huáng (Radix et Rhizoma Rhei)   4 *liang* (12 g)

Fù Zī (Radix Aconiti Lateralis Praeparata)   1 large piece (9 pcs)

Gān Jiāng (Rhizoma Zingiberis)   2 *liang* (6 g)

Rén Shēn (Radix Et Rhizoma Ginseng)   2 *liang* (6 g)

Gān Cǎo (Radix et Rhizoma Glycyrrhizae)   2 *liang* (6 g)

[Usage]   Add 8 *dou* water to boil the above herbs after cutting them into pieces. Until two and a half liquid is left and take it separately three times. Add *dà*

huáng at the end.

Modern Usage: Boil the medicines in water for oral application, *dà huáng* added later.

[Action]　Warm and invigorate spleen-*yang*, eliminate cold accumulation.

[Indication]　Cold accumulation with constipation, protracted diarrhea with pus and blood, abdominal pain, cold limbs, wiry and deep pulse.

[Formula Analysis]　Deficiency of spleen-yang causes interior accumulation and stagnation. If we warm and invigorate only the spleen yang, stagnation will not be eliminated. If we purge hastily, the yang of middle *jiao* will be impaired. That is why warming and invigorating spleen-yang should be combined with eliminating cold and accumulation. The first two herbs achieve those functions as chief medicines, with *dà huáng* relaxing the bowels to eliminate stagnation and *fù zǐ* strengthening spleen-yang to dissipate coagulated cold. *Gān jiāng*, *rén shēn*, and *gān cǎo* act as assistant medicines, which help *fù zǐ* with warming and invigorating spleen-*yang*. *Gān cǎo* also serves as an envoy medicine to mediate the properties of other herbs. The above medicines are combined to make a formula of purgation with warming the spleen.

[Clinical Application]　The formula is used to treat the syndrome of cold accumulation due to spleen-yang deficiency, manifested with constipation or protracted diarrhea with pus and blood. If the abdominal pain is severe, apply *ròu guì*, *hòu pò*, and *mù xiāng* to reinforce the function of warming and moving qi to relieve pain. If the patient also vomits, apply prepared *bàn xià*, *shā rén* to harmonize the stomach and direct counterflow downward. If the stagnation and accumulation are slight, the dosage of *dà huáng* can be reduced.

Sān Wù Bèi Jí Wán (Three Substances Emergency Pill, 三物备急丸)
Essentials from the Golden Cabinet (*Jīn Guì Yào Lüè*, 金匮要略)

[Ingredient]

Dà Huáng (Radix et Rhizoma Rhei)　1 *liang* (3 g)

Gān Jiāng (Rhizoma Zingiberis)　1 *liang* (3 g)

Bā Dòu (Fructus Crotonis)　1 *liang*, skin and core removed, boil, grind as

processed as powder (3 g)

[Usage]　The above medicines need to be refined before using. Grind *dà huáng* and *gān jiāng* into a powder, and mix *bā dòu* [powder] with the two former herbs, pestle repeatedly [for a thousand times], and use as a powder or honey pill. Keep it in a sealed container. Take three or four pills with warm water or wine. If the patient cannot swallow, hold his head upward and pour it down the throat. Within a moment, the patient will be relieved. If not, apply three more pills; when the sound in the abdomen are heard and the patient gets vomiting with diarrhea, it will be relieved and cured soon. If the patient cannot swallow down, the doctor must pry the mouth and pour it in.

Modern Usage: Grind the above herbs into powder, take 0.3–1.5 g each time with warm boiled water. If the patient has the inability to swallow, it can be administered by nasal feeding.

[Action]　Expele and eliminate cold accumulation.

[Indication]　Cold coagulated with food stagnation, abrupt distending pain in the heart and abdomen, stabbing pain, shortness of breath with an inability to eat, sudden fainting.

[Formula Analysis]　Coagulated cold and food stagnation obstruct the intestines and stomach, causing the *qi* movement blockage. *Bā dòu*, which is pungent and hot, severely toxic, acts as the chief medicine, and it enters the stomach and large intestine channels to purge drastically and eliminateing accumulation. *Gān jiāng*, which is pungent and hot, acts as a deputy medicine, and it possesses the functions of warming the middle and dissipating accumulation to help *bā dòu* with expelling coldness. *Dà huáng*, which is bitter and cold, acts as an assistant and envoy medicine with the functions of clearing up bowels to eliminate stagnation, getting rid of the stale and bringing forth the fresh, as well as restricting the pungent hot toxicity of *bā dòu*. The combination of the above herbs makes a powerful and efficient formula, which is prepared and used for the syndrome of abrupt acute cold excess. That is the reason for its name, 'Three Substances Emergency Pill'.

[Clinical Application]　This formula is used for eating or drinking disorder.

Food stagnation in the intestines and the stomach causes the disorder of upper *jiao*, an unsmooth of the lower-third portion of the stomach cavity (*xià wǎn*, 下脘). When abrupt acute cold excess diseases break out, it is necessary to take to possess efficacy, or the patient can't be saved.

Section 3　Purgative formulas for moistening

Moisten purgation formulas, with the function of relaxing the bowels to relieve constipation, is used for constipation due to a deficient constitution for its mild laxative efficacy. If the constipation is caused by pathogenic heat impairing the body fluids, the exuberance of fire, or dryness of the intestines and stomach, the treatment should be a combination of moistening the dryness and draining heat. The representative formula like *Má Zǐ Rén Wán* (Cannabis Fruit Pill, 麻子仁丸) is composed of moistening herbs like *má zǐ rén, xìng rén, sháo yào* and purgative herbs like *dà huáng*. If the patient has a fluid impairment and intestinal dryness without fire, the dominant formula should be *Wǔ Rén Wán* (Five Seed Pill, 五仁丸).

Má Zǐ Rén Wán /Pí Yuē Má Rén Wán (Cannabis Fruit Pill, 麻子仁丸, 脾约麻仁丸)
Treatise on Cold Damage (Shāng Hán Lùn, 伤寒论)

[Ingredient]

Má Zǐ Rén (Fructus Cannabis)　2 *sheng* (500 g)

Sháo Yào (Radix Paeoniae)　half *jin* (250 g)

Zhǐ Shí (Fructus Aurantii Immaturus)　half *jin*, fluid-fried (250 g)

Dà Huáng (Radix et Rhizoma Rhei)　1 *jin*, skin removed (500 g)

Hòu Pò (Cortex Magnoliae Officinalis)　1 *chi*, fired with ginger juice, skin removed (250 g)

Xìng Rén (Semen Armeniacae Amarum)　1 *sheng*, skin and sprout removed, boil but not boil the lipid out (250 g)

[Usage]　Grind the above herbs into a fine powder and then make them into

pills as large as *wú tóng zǐ* (Semen Firmianae) by mixing them with honey, take 10 pills with water, three times daily. Increase the dosage gradually. Stop taking the pills when the patient gets better.

Modern Usage: Grind the above herbs into a fine powder, and then make them into pills by mixing them with honey, take 9 g with warm boiled water, once or twice daily.

[Action]　Moisten the intestine, relieve constipation and clears away heat with mild purgation.

[Indication]　Gastrointestinal dryness and heat, deficiency of body fluid, constipation, frequent urination.

[Formula Analysis]　The syndrome is spleen constipation due to gastrointestinal dryness-heat. *Má zǐ rén*, mild and sweet in nature, is used in the largest dosages and acts as the chief medicine that moistens the large intestine to relieve constipation. It is said, "enter the foot *taiyin* spleen channel, the hand *taiyang* large intestine channel...*Nèi Jīng* says, when there is dryness, treat it by moistening, so Zhang Zhong-jing uses *má rén* to moisten dryness of *taiyin* and relax intestines" in *Decoction and Material Medica* (*Tāng Yè Běn Cǎo*, 汤液本草). *Xìng rén* descends *qi* and relaxes bowels, and *sháo yào* nourishes *yin*. The above two are deputy medicines. *Zhǐ shí* and *hòu pò* promote the flow of *qi* and dissolve masses, *dà huáng* clears away heat and promotes defecation, serving as assistant medicines. Honey is meant to strengthen further the effect of moistening dryness and relaxing the bowels. The above herbs made into pills have the efficacy of moistening intestines to relieve constipation and clearing away heat with mild purgation.

[Clinical Application]　This formula is used to treat spleen confinement syndrome. The point of the syndrome differentiation is frequent urination, difficulty in defecation, yellowish coating. It is composed of moistening and purgative herbs, moistening but not cloying, purgative but not drastic. The usage of formula is only takeing ten pills as big as *wú tóng zǐ*. Increase the dosage gradually. Stop taking the medicine of mild purgation when the patient gets better. The formula is for mild purgation.

Section 4　Formulas that expels water retention

Formulas that eliminate retained water are used for patients with a strong constitution to treat water retention in the chest and abdomen and edema. It is capable of expelling stagnated water in the body through defecation and urination to eliminate retained fluids and edema. The formula for eliminating fluid retention is only used to treat those with the excessive syndrome but without deficiency in healthy qi. According to the method of treating the branch in urgent conditions, there is a saying, "diseases causing the center fullness, and difficulty in urination and defecation, treat the branch" in *Basic Questions-Discourse on Tip and Root and on the Transmission of Disease* (*Sù Wèn-Biāo Běn Bìng Chuán Lùn*, 素问·标本病传论). So purgation with eliminating fluids cannot be used for the long term or overdose, or it will purge hut impair healthy qi, expel water hut damage yin. This sort of formula usually has toxicity with drastic purgation, and is mostly composed of the herbs like *yuán huā*, *gān suì*, *dà jǐ*, *qiān niú zǐ*, etc. The representative formulas are *Shí Zǎo Tāng* (Ten Jujubes Decoction, 十枣汤), *Zhōu Chē Wán* (Vessel and Vehicle Pill), etc.

Shí Zǎo Tāng (Ten Jujubes Decoction, 十枣汤)
Treatise on Cold Damage (*Shāng Hán Lùn*, 伤寒论)

[Ingredient]

Yuán Huā (Flos Genkwa)

Gān Suí (Radix Kansui)

Dà Jǐ (Radix Knoxiae)

equal in dosage

Dà Zǎo (Fructus Jujubae)　10 pieces

[Usage]　First, take the first three medicines in equal dosages, then grind them into a powder. Secondly, boil 10 grains of large *dà zǎo* with one and a half *sheng* water and take 8 *he* (800 ml), mix them with powder after abandoning sediments. Take it early in the morning before a meal with warm boiled water, 1 coin if the patient has a strong constitution, while taking half *qian* if the patient is weak and

tabid. Let the patient take half more coin the next day if the disease is not cured after purgation. After the purgation, let the patient take porridge to harmonize the stomach.

Modern Usage: Grind the first three medicines into powder with equal dosage, or put them into a capsule. Take the powder 1.5–3 g with the decoction of 10 grains of *dà zǎo* early in the morning before a meal, once daily.

[Action]　Expel water by purgation.

[Indication]

1. Pleural rheum, thoracic retention of fluid, causing pain in the chest and rib-side when coughing, epigastric *pǐ* (stiffness and fullness), nausea and shortness of breath, headache, dizziness, or persistent pulling pain in chest and back, glossy coating, deep wiry pulse.

2. Edema and abdominal fullness, which belongs to the excessive syndrome.

[Formula Analysis]　The rib-sides are the ways for ascending and descending yin and yang, qi. Water retention in rib-side obstructs the channels, causing disorder of ascending and descending, resulting in pain in the chest and rib-side when coughing with sputum and phlegm, this is pleural rheum. This formula refers to purgation with water expelling drastically. *Yuán huā*, which is pungent, warm and toxic, is capable of removing fluid and phlegm from the chest and rib-sides. It acts as chief medicine, and is described as "treat water fluid phlegm retention, and rib-side pain" in *The Grand Compendium of Materia Medica* (*Běn Cǎo Gāng Mù*, 本草纲目). *Gān suí*, which is bitter cold and toxic, is good at eliminating the retention of fluid and dampness from channels. *Dà jǐ*, which is bitter, cold and toxic, is good at eliminating the retention of fluid and dampness from the six *fu* organs. The above two herbs act as assistant medicines. According to the saying in *Běn Cǎo Gāng Mù*, "*yuán huā, dà jǐ, gān suí* can expel water and drain dampness through the shelter of water and fluid. It will be efficient if used mildly, while it will cause desertion of original *qi* if used in too big dosage." The decoction of *dà zǎo*, reinforcing healthy *qi* and boosting *qi*, banks up the earth to control water. Therefore, it is meant to reduce the toxic and drastic properties of the herbs so that the formula can achieve the purgative result without affecting the healthy *qi*. It functions as an envoy medicine. *Discussion of Medical Prescription*

(*Yī Fāng Lùn*, 医方论) [19]says, "Zhang Zhong-jing named the formula Ten Jujubes Decoction because of the importance of *dà zǎo* to reinforce the spleen and stomach to achieve the effect of restriction and controlling". The name of the formula is meaningful.

[Clinical Application] *Essential Teachings of [Zhu] Dan Xi (Dān Xī Xīn Fǎ,* 丹溪心法) [20] suggests processing this formula with pounded boiled meat of *dà zǎo* into pills, and the formula is named *shí zǎo wán*. This formula treats fluid retention, edema of four limbs, the abnormal rising of qi, panting and dyspnea, difficulty in urination and defecation. It will be more convenient if it changes into pills. The formula states "treat it with drastic purgation; promote the movement with mild effect".

Zhōu Chē Wán (Vessel and Vehicle Pill, 舟车丸)
Indispensable Tools for Pattern Treatment (Zhèng Zhì Zhǔn Shéng, 证治准绳) [21]
quota from Liu He-jian [22]

[Ingredient]

Gān Suí (Radix Kansui) 1 *liang* dry-fried with vinegar (30 g)

Yuán Huā (Flos Genkwa) 1 *liang* dry-fried with vinegar (30 g)

Dà Jǐ (Radix Knoxiae) 1 *liang* dry-fried with vinegar (30 g)

Dà Huáng (Radix et Rhizoma Rhei) 2 *liang* (60 g)

Hēi Qiān Niú (Semen Pharbitidis) Grind into powder, 4 *liang* (120 g)

Qīng Pí (Pericarpium Citri Reticulatae Viride) half *liang* (15 g)

Chén Pí (Pericarpium Citri Reticulatae) half *liang* (15 g)

Mù Xiāng (Radix Aucklandiae) half *liang* (15 g)

Bīng Láng (Semen Arecae) half *liang* (15 g)

Qīng Fěn (Calomelas) 1 *qian* (3 g)

[Usage] Grind the above herbs into powder, mix with water and knead into pills. Take five pills as the first dosage before a meal, three times daily. Increase the dosage gradually until urination and defecation are promoted. Take the pills until the syndromes are relieved.

Modern Usage: Grind the above herbs into powder, mix with water and knead into pills. Take 3–6 g with warm boiled water every morning before a meal, once daily.

[Action]　Expell water and move qi.

[Indication]　Edema and water fullness, excess in both body fluids and qi, thirst with the coarse breath, distending and hardness in the abdomen, difficulty in defecation and urination, deep, rapid and powerful pulse.

[Formula Analysis]　Water-dampness stagnation transforms into heat, obstructing the abdomen and channels, causing gastrointestinal qi movement obstruction. *Hēi qiān niú*, which is bitter cold and toxic, acts as chief medicine in large dosage, promoting defecation and urination as well as expelling water and dissipating edema. *Dà huáng* relaxes the bowels to promote purgation. *Gān suí, dà jǐ, yuán huā* eliminate water and dissipate edema. The above four act as deputy medicines. Turbid water retention results in the disorder of qi movement in ascending and descending. Therefore, *qing pí* breaks the qi stagnation and dissipates accumulation, *chén pí* rectifies qi and dry dampness, *mù xiāng* and *bīng láng* smooth the flow of qi in *sanjiao* to promote water transportation. *Qing fěn* (also called *shui yin fen*, powder of mercury, 轻粉) in little quantity, pungent, cold and extremely toxic, is good at wandering but not staying, so it can expel water to promote defecation. The above five herbs act as assistant medicines. All the herbs function together to purge drastically and expel water, as well as break qi stagnation. It will purge the water congestion and heat accumulation through defecation and urination, like a boat floating downstream in a river, or a car driving downhill. Going down with the trend, that is why the formula is called "Vessel and Vehicle".

[Clinical Application]　Because of the extreme purgative function, this formula is used for excess in yang edema, body and qi. It is also called "*Jìng Fǔ Wán*". This formula is usually used to treat liver cirrhosis with ascites; excess in both pulse and syndrome, healthy qi is still supportive. If there is an exuberance of edema with a weak constitution, this formula is banned. Besides, it is forbidden to be used with *gān cǎo*, and is also contraindicated during pregnancy.

Section 5　Formulas that simultaneously attacks and supplement

Formulas for treatment with both attacking and supplementing are applied to treat excess interior accumulation with healthy qi deficiency. Because the excessive pathogenic qi coexists with deficient healthy qi, so, supplementing healthy qi will cause the congestion of excess pathogenic qi to become more severe. Thus, purgation associated with reinforcement can dispel pathogens and reinforce healthy qi, which is the best choice. At the same time, the body with excessive pathogenic accumulation and deficiency of healthy qi usually gets consumption of qi or impairment of yin due to the qi deficiency, and it not capable of expelling the pathogen as well as relieving dry stool. The body may be at risk of healthy qi desertion even though the excess pathogen is dissipated. Therefore, combing purgation and supplementation is the right way to treat such a condition. The commonly used purgative herbs in this condition are *dà huáng, máng xiāo*, and the supplementing herbs are *rén shēn, dāng guī, dì huáng, xuán shēn, etc.* The representative formulas are *Huáng Lóng Tāng* (Yellow Dragon Decoction, 黄龙汤) and *Zēng Yè Chéng Qì Tāng* (Humor-Increasing and Qi-Guiding Decoction, 增液承气汤).

Huáng Lóng Tāng (Yellow Dragon Decoction, 黄龙汤)
Six Books on Febrile Diseases (Shāng Hán Liù Shū, 伤寒六书)[23]

[Ingredient]

Dà Huáng (Radix et Rhizoma Rhei)　(9 g)

Máng Xiāo (Natrii Sulfas)　(9 g)

Zhǐ Shí (Fructus Aurantii Immaturus)　(6 g)

Hòu Pò (Cortex Magnoliae Officinalis)　(6 g)

Gān Cǎo (Radix et Rhizoma Glycyrrhizae)　(3 g)

Rén Shēn (Radix et Rhizoma Ginseng)　(6 g)

Dāng Guī (Radix Angelicae Sinensis)　(9 g)

[The original book did not record the dosage]

[Usage] Add 2 *zhan*① water to decoct the above herbs (except *máng xiāo*) with *shēng jiāng* (3 pieces), *dà zǎo* (2 grains). Decoct it, and then add 1 pugil of *jié gěng*, boiled for oral application.

Modern Usage: Decoct the above herbs with *jié gěng* (3 g), *shēng jiāng* (3 pieces), *dà zǎo* (2 grains) in water for oral application.

[Action] Purge and reinforce healthy qi.

[Indication] The syndrome with excessive interior heat and qi and blood deficiency; or the heat disease but applied with unsuitable purging method which leads to epigastric stuffiness and pain, feverish body with thirst, incoherent speech, watery diarrhea; or qi and blood deficiency combined with *yangming* bowel syndrome; or the erroneous treatment caused deficiency but still with [fu] excess remaining, manifested with weak breathing and mental fatigue, constipation, abdominal fullness, stuffiness and pain, or even picking at bedclothes, unconscious and reversal counterflow cold of the four limbs, parched yellowish or dark tongue coating, deficient pulse.

[Formula Analysis] This formula is used to treat the syndrome of heat retention with watery discharge that coexists with qi and blood deficiency. The situation of *yangming* bowel syndrome with depletion of qi and blood, or unfair treatment causing the deficiency and excess in the bowel, is hard to treat without tonifying healthy qi deficiency to overcome the pathogen. This formula refers to the *Dà Chéng Qì Tāng* (Major Purgative Decoction) and combines *rén shēn, dāng guī, gān cǎo, jié gěng, shēng jiāng, dà zǎo*. *Dà huáng, máng xiāo, zhǐ shí, hòu pò* are combined for the purgative function to drain heat, which relaxes the bowels and eliminates excess heat stagnation in the intestines and stomach. *Rén shēn* and *dāng guī* function as supplementation of qi and blood to reinforce healthy qi and expel pathogens, which protect the healthy qi from the purgative herbs. The above herbs are the central part of the formula. *Jié gěng* in little quantity acts as assistant medicine. It is meant to disperse the stagnated lung-*qi* and eliminate accumulation from the intestines and stomach, which helps to ascend before descending. *Gān cǎo, shēng jiāng* and *dà zǎo* are meant

①　zhan, [original meaning] small cup, the capacity is zooml.

to reinforce the stomach qi and harmonize the actions of all medicines in the formula. The above herbs compose the formula of purging and supplementing.

[Clinical Application] This formula is used to treat *yangming* bowel syndrome coexists with a deficiency of qi and blood. The purgative function is necessary to treat the excess, while supplementation is necessary to reinforce the deficiency. Therefore, this formula is appropriate.

Zēng Yè Chéng Qì Tāng (Purgative Decoction for Increasing Fluid, 增液承气汤) *Systematic Differentiation of Warm Diseases* (*Wēn Bìng Tiáo Biàn*, 温病条辨)

[Ingredient]

Xuán Shēn (Radix Scrophulariae)   1 *liang* (30 g)

Mài Dōng (Radix Ophiopogonis)   core not removed, 8 *qian* (24 g)

Shēng Dì Huáng (Radix Rehmanniae)   8 *qian* (24 g)

Dà Huáng (Radix et Rhizoma Rhei)   3 *qian* (9 g)

Máng Xiāo (Natrii Sulfas)   1 *qian* and 5 cents (4.5 g)

[Usage] Adopt eight bottles of water to decoct the above herbs, and boil it until three bottles volume left. Take one bottle first, If the purgative effect has not been achieved, take the rest again.

Modern Usage: Boil the above herbs with water, and take it in three times. Do not take the leftover when the purgative effect occurs.

[Action] Nourish yin, nourish fluid, purge heat and induce defecation.

[Indication] *Yangming* warm disease, heat accumulation and yin deficiency, dry stool and constipation.

[Formula Analysis] Warm pathogens impair and consume body fluids. The syndrome emerges when the accumulated *yangming* heat consumes body fluids and causes it to fail to moisten the intestines, aggravateing the fluid consumption. *Xuán shēn*, *shēng dì huáng*, *mài dōng*, in large dosage, being sweet, cool, and moistening, function as nourishing yin for the production of body fluids, and moistening the intestines to promote defecation. *Dà huáng*, *máng xiāo*, function to soften and moisten hard masses, as well as draining and purging heat in combination with the first three

herbs to achieve a purgative effect and supplementation. This formula is meant to supplement yin fluids, purge heat accumulation, expel pathogens and reinforce healthy qi. The name "*Zēng Yè Chéng Qì*" comes from the formula combined by *Zēng Yè Tāng* (Humor-Increasing Decoction) and *Tiáo Wèi Chéng Qì Tāng* (Stomach-Regulating and Purgative Decoction) excluding *gān cǎo*.

[Clinical Application]   This formula is used to treat *yangming* warm disease, syndrome of dry heat accumulation and fluid depletion. The syndrome of yin deficiency and heat accumulation manifesting with dry stool and protracted hemorrhoids is also appropriate for this formula.

Chapter 4

Harmonizing Formulas

~~

All the formulas that eliminate the disease by means of harmonization and regulation are collectively referred to as harmonizing formulas. The harmonizing formulas are often used to treat *shaoyang* syndrome and liver-spleen or stomach-intestine disharmony. They have the functions of harmonizing *shaoyang*, harmonizing liver-spleen, harmonizing intestine-stomach. It belongs to the "*harmonization*" in the "eight methods".

Section 1   Formulas that harmonizes *shaoyang*

Harmonizing *shaoyang* formulas are suitable for sitution where a pathogen dwells in the foot *shaoyang* gallbladder channel. Symptoms include alternating chills and fever, fullness and discomfort in the chest and rib-side, vexation and frequent vomiting, lack of desire to eat or drink, bitter taste in the mouth, dry pharynx, dizzy vision and so on. *Shaoyang* is located in the half-exterior half-interior, which is the pivot of yang channels. The pathogen can be solved by venting the exterior through the *taiyang* channel, or it can invade the *yangming* channel and *taiyin* channel inward, leading to excess-heat syndrome or deficiency-cold syndrome. This disease is neither in the exterior nor in the interior, so sweat promotion, vomit induction and purgation are forbidden while harmonization is the only choice. For this method, *chái hú*, *huáng qí, bàn xià,* and *qīng hāo* are commonly used as the main parts in formulas, such as *Xiǎo Chái Hú Tāng* (Minor Bupleurum Decoction, 小柴胡汤), *Dà Chái Hú Tāng* (*Major Bupleurum Decoction*, 大柴胡汤), *Hāo Qín Qīng Dǎn Tāng* (*Sweet Wormwood and Scutellaria Gallbladder-Clearing Decoction*, 蒿芩清胆汤), and so on.

Xiǎo Chái Hú Tāng (Minor Bupleurum Decoction, 小柴胡汤)
Treatise on Cold Damage (*Shāng Hán Lùn*, 伤寒论)

[Ingredient]

Chái Hú (Radix Bupleuri)   half *jin* (12 g),

Huáng Qín (Radix Scutellariae)   3 *liang* (9 g)

Rén Shēn (Radix et Rhizoma Ginseng)   3 *liang* (9 g)

Gān Cǎo (Radix et Rhizoma Glycyrrhizae)   3 *liang*, liquid-fried (6 g)

Bàn Xià (Rhizoma Pinelliae)   half *sheng*, washed (9 g)

Shēng Jiāng (Rhizoma Zingiberis Recens)   3 *liang*, cut (9 g)

Dà Zǎo (Fructus Jujubae)   12 *mei*, split (4 pcs)

[Usage]   The original formula includes seven herbs. Adopt 1 *dou* 2 *sheng* water to boil the formula till 6 *sheng* is left. Discard the dregs. Continue to boil the liquid till 3 *sheng* is left. Take the decoction when it is warm 3 times a day.

Modern Usage: Decoct with water.

[Action]   Harmonize *shaoyang*.

[Indication]

1. *Shaoyang* syndrome, with symptoms of alternating chills and fever, fullness and discomfort in the chest and rib-side, no desire to eat or drink, vexation and frequent vomiting, bitter taste in the mouth, dried pharynx, dizzy vision, white and thin coating, wiry pulse.

2. Women get attacked by wind, which penetrates the blood chamber where it binds the blood, leading to irregular menstruation [sometimes stopped], alternating fever and chills. As well as malaria, jaundice and other miscellaneous diseases which have *shaoyang* syndrome.

[Formula Analysis]   This formula is the main formula for harmonizing *shaoyang*. In this formula, *chái hú* is bitter and neutral, which can enter the liver and gallbladder channel. It can vent the *shaoyang* pathogen outwards, solve the constraint and stagnation of the qi mechanism, so act as the chief medicine; the deputy medicine, *huáng qín* is bitter and cold, which helps *chái hú* to clear away the pathogenic heat of *shaoyang*. *Chái hú* is ascending while *huáng qín* is descending, which avoids the

harm of raising yang but consuming yin. Stomach qi failed to descend because of gallbladder qi invading the stomach, so *bàn xià* and *shēng jiāng* are used to harmoniz the stomach, direct counterflow downward, eliminate fluid retention and stop vomiting. *Rén shēn* and *dà zǎo* can reinforce healthy qi. If healthy qi is vigorous, then pathogen has no chance of inward development and can be resolved directly from the outside; envoy medicine *zhì gān cǎo* can assist *rén shēn* and *dà zǎo* to strengthen healthy qi, and can also harmonize the actions of all medicines in a formula. This formula's legislation mainly focuses on harmonizing *shaoyang*. Ke Qin[24] regards it as "the formula of *shaoyang* pivot and the general formula of harmonizing the exterior and interior", so it ranks first among all the harmonizing formulas.

[Clinical Application]　This formula is designed for *shaoyang* syndrome. The key points of syndrome differentiation are "alternating chills and fever, fullness and discomfort in the chest and rib-side, lack of desire to eat or drink, vexation and frequent vomiting". As long as we grasp one of the main symptoms, we can use *Xiǎo Chái Hú Tāng* directly without waiting for other symptoms all manifested. In addition, to treat the *shaoyang* cold damage syndrome, for other miscellaneous diseases such as heat entering wowen's blood chamber (uterus), postpartum depression and dizziness, malaria, jaundice, all of these we can apply the formula if we see the above main symptoms.

Dà Chái Hú Tāng (Major Bupleurum Decoction, 大柴胡汤)
Treatise on Cold Damage (*Shāng Hán Lùn*, 伤寒论)

[Ingredient]

Chái Hú (Radix Bupleuri)　half *jin* (12 g)

Huáng Qín (Radix Scutellariae)　3 *liang* (9 g)

Sháo Yào (Radix Paeoniae)　3 *liang* (9 g)

Bàn Xià (Rhizoma Pinelliae)　half *sheng*, washed (9 g)

Shēng Jiāng (Rhizoma Zingiberis Recens)　3 *liang*, cut (9 g)

Zhǐ Shí (Fructus Aurantii Immaturus)　4 pcs, liquid-fried (9 g)

Dà Zǎo (Fructus Jujubae)　12 *mei*, split (4 *mei* [pcs])

Dà Huáng (Radix Et Rhizoma Rhei) 2 *liang* (6 g)

[Usage] The original formula includes eight herbs. Adopt 1 *dou* 2 *sheng* water to boiling the formula till 6 *sheng* is left. Dischard the dregs. Continue to boil the liquid till 3 *sheng* is left. Take the decoction when it is warm 3 times a day.

Modern Usage: Decocted by water.

[Action] Harmonize *shaoyang*, discharge accumulation heat internally.

[Indication] Overlap of diseases of *shaoyang* and *yangming*, alternating chills and fever, fullness and discomfort in the chest and rib-side, persistent vomiting, depression and slight vexation, epigastric *pǐ* and hardness or epigastric fullness and pain, constipation or diarrhea, yellow tongue coating, wiry rapid and powerful pulse.

[Formula Analysis] This disease is caused by unresolved *shaoyang* syndrome affecting *yangming* which products head bind, so it is called overlap of diseases of *shaoyang* and *yangming*. This formula is to remove *rén shēn* and *gān cǎo* from *Xiǎo Chái Hú Tāng* then add *dà huáng*, *zhǐ shí*, *sháo yào*. In this formula, *chái hú* and *huáng qín* harmonize *shaoyang*, for treating alternating chills and fever, fullness and discomfort in the chest and rib-side. They are the chief medicines. Deputy medicines *dà huáng* and *zhǐ shí* discharge heat bind internally, for treating epigastric *pǐ* and hardness or epigastric fullness and pain, depression and slight vexation, constipation or diarrhea, yellow coating, wiry rapid and powerful pulse. *Sháo yào* can harmonize interior and have a good mastery of relieving abdominal pain. It can help *chái hú* and *huáng qín* to clear liver and gallbladder. *Bàn xià* harmonizes the stomach and direct counterflow downward for solving persistent vomiting. Attach importance to use ginger, because it can not only help *bàn xià* to harmonize the stomach and stop vomiting, but also help *dà zǎo* to harmonize *ying-wei* and transport fluids. They are envoy medicines. In a word, it is the formula that is designed for treating the overlap of diseases of *shaoyang* and *yangming*. It is the combination of *harmonization* and *purgation*. Compared with *Xiǎo Chái Hú Tāng* which specializes in harmonizing *shaoyang*, this formula is more powerful, so it is entitled "*Dà Chái Hú Tāng*".

[Clinical Application] This formula is designed for treating the overlap of diseases of *shaoyang* and *yangming*. *Shaoyang* syndrome should have prohibited

to use the purgative method, however, if only the harmonization method is used, interior excess can not be removed, but if only purge heat bind, then the syndrome of *shaoyang* can't be solved. Therefore, this formula is used to solve the *shaoyang* exterior and purge heat bind interior. Wang Ang[25] says, "This formula fuses *Xiǎo Chái Hú Tāng* and *Xiǎo Chéng Qì Tāng* into one formula by adding or subtracting herbs. *Shaoyang* can't use purgation method, but it should use the purgation for *shaoyang* accompanied by *yangming* bowel syndrome." This does not violate the principle of *shaoyang* purgation prohibition, and can cure this syndrome with only one formula. It is indeed a way to kill two birds with one stone.

Hāo Qín Qīng Dǎn Tāng (Sweet Wormwood and Scutellaria Gallbladder-Clearing Decoction, 蒿芩清胆汤)
Revised Guide to the Discussion of Cold Damage (*Tōng Su Shāng Hán Lùn*, 通俗伤寒论)[26]

[Ingredient]

Qīng Hāo Burgeen (Herba Artemisiae Annuae Burgeen)　0.5 to 2 *qian* (4.5 to 6 g)

Zhú Rú (Caulis Bambusae In Taenia)　3 *qian* (9 g)

Xiān Bàn Xià Impregnated　(4.5 g)

Chì Fú Líng (Poria Rubra)　3 *qian* (9 g)

Qing Huáng Qín (Green Radix Scutellariae)　0.5 to 3 *qian* (4.5 to 9 g)

Sheng Zhǐ Qiào (Fructus Aurantii)　0.5 *qian* (4.5 g)

Chén Pí (Pericarpium Citri Reticulatae)　0.5 *qian* (4.5 g)

Bì Yù Sǎn (Jasper Jade Powder) Packeted　3 *qian* (9 g)

[Usage]　The usage is not mentioned in the original formula.

Modern Usage：Decocted with water.

[Action]　Clear gallbladder and drain dampness, harmonize the stomach and dissolve phlegm.

[Indication]　Dampness trapping and heat constraint, alternating light chills and severe fevers similar to malaria, mild cold but more heat, bitter taste in the mouth,

diaphragm oppression, bitterness and acid regurgitation, or yellow and sticky drool vomiting, even belching and hiccup, distending pain in the chest and rib-side, short and dark urine, red tongue, white greasy coating mixing with other colors, a rapid pulse which the left is glossy and the right is wiry.

[Formula Analysis] The syndrome of this formula is caused by the dampness trapping and heat constraint that blocked in the *shaoyang* gallbladder channel and the *sanjiao* channel. In this formula, *qīng hāo* is bitter-cold and aromatic, it can vent *shaoyang* pathogenic heat; *huáng qín* is also bitter-cold, which is good at clearing gallbladder heat as well as drying dampness, these two herbs are chief medicines; *zhú rú*, *zhǐ qiào*, *bàn xià* and *chén pí*, the deputy medicines, can clear heat and harmonize the stomach, dissolve phlegm and direct counterflow downward; clearing heat and draining dampness, *chì fú líng*, *bì yù sǎn* lead pathogen eliminated with urination, at the same time, they harmonize the center. They are assistant and envoy medicines. All the above herbs together can play a role in clearing the gallbladder, draining dampness, harmonizing the stomach and dissolving phlegm.

[Clinical Application] This formula clears the gallbladder, drains dampness, harmonizes the stomach and dissolves phlegm. It is mainly applicable to treat damp-heat constraints in the *shaoyang* gallbladder and *sanjiao* channels. For solving excessive vomiting, we can add *huáng lián* and *sū yè* to clear heat and arrest vomiting; if dampness is severe, *huò xiāng*, *yì yǐ rén*, *bái kòu rén*, *hòu pò* can be added for removing damp-turbidity; inhibited urination can be solved with *chē qián zǐ*, *zé xiè*, *tōng cǎo* to treat dampness and promote urination.

Section 2   Formulas that harmonizes liver-spleen

Harmonizing liver-spleen formula is suitable for emotional depression, liver-spleen disorders, in which we would see a lack of warmth in the extremities, distending pain in the epigastric abdomen and chest and rib-side, mental weariness, poor appetite, menstrual irregularities, abdominal pain, diarrhea, *etc.* The liver stores the blood and governs the free flow of qi, it prefers free activity, and it depots the

ministerial fire. If the emotion is depressed, the qi flow will be disordered. Constrained for a long time, it transforms into a fire then it must consume yin-blood. On the contrary, blood deficiency can't nourish the liver, liver qi can't be smooth. Hence, liver constraint is enough to cause blood deficiency; blood deficiency can also lead to liver constraint. Liver disease can spread to the spleen, which is called wood restrict earth; the spleen and stomach are the sources of qi and blood production, insufficient due to spleen deficiency can also lead to liver blood deficiency, the liver loses its softness and gracefulness, which also leads to liver constraint, which is called earth deficiency and wood constraint. Because of the close relationship between the liver and the spleen, it is a common clinical treatment to harmonize the liver and spleen. We commonly use herbs that can soothe the liver and fortify the spleen such as *chái hú*, *sháo yào*, *bái zhú* and *gān căo*. They are the main components of formulas. The representative formulas include *Sì Nì Săn* (Frigid Extremities Powder, 四逆散), *Xiāo Yáo Săn* (Free Wanderer Powder, 逍遥散), *Tòng Xiè Yào Fāng* (Important Formula for Painful Diarrhea, 痛泻要方) *etc.*

Sì Nì Săn (Frigid Extremities Powder, 四逆散)
Treatise on Cold Damage (*Shāng Hán Lùn*, 伤寒论)

[Ingredient]

Gān Căo (Radix Et Rhizoma Glycyrrhizae)   liquid-fried

Zhǐ Shí (Fructus Aurantii Immaturus)   broken, water stained, dried

Chái Hú (Radix Bupleuri)

Sháo Yào (Radix Paeoniae)

(equal division) (6 g)

[Usage]   The original formula includes four herbs, each 10 *fen*, smash and sieved, water blending, swallow a small tablespoon [方寸匕 *fāng cùn bǐ*] of powder three times a day.

Modern Usage: Decocted by water.

[Action]   Vent pathogen and dissipate constrained heat, soothe the liver and rectify the spleen.

[Indication]   Yang qi internal constraint, reversal counterflow cold of the four limbs (cold distal extremities with cold moving proximally; *sì zhī jué nì*), or epigastric pain, or diarrhea with rectal heaviness, wiry pulse.

[Formula Analysis]   There are two types of counterflow cold of the four limbs syndrome: cold and heat, this formula is designed for treating heat type: heat syncope, which is caused by the binding constraint of liver qi, [it blocks]the diffusion and flowing of qi, yang qi is constrained and fails to reach the extremities. In this formula, soothing the liver and resolving constraint, *chái hú*, as the chief medicine, can vent constrained heat. The deputy medicine *sháo yào* nourishes the blood, softens the liver, harmonizes *ying* and relieves pain. *Chái hú* accompanis with *sháo yào*, dispersing but astringing, and there is no disadvantage of excessive dispersion and exhaustion of liver-*yin*; *zhǐ shí* is the assistant medicine, loosen the center and direct qi downward; the envoy medicine *gān cǎo* harmonizes the actions of all medicines in a formula. Moreover, *chái hú* and *zhǐ shí* are used together, one ascending and one descending, strengthening the effect of soothing the liver and rectifying qi; *sháo yào* and *gān cǎo* are used together, which can harmonize liver-spleen, relieve urgency and pain. The above herbs are combined. They can play the effect of venting constrained heat, soothing the liver and rectifying the spleen. The original formula is used as a powder to treat "counterflow cold of the four limbs (cold distal extremities with cold moving proximally past elbows and knees; *sì zhī nì lěng*)", so the formula is named "*Sì Nì Sǎn*".

[Clinical Application]   This formula is mild for soothing the liver and rectifying the spleen. Clinically, it can treat the lack of warmth in the extremities caused by liver constraint, epigastric or lateral thorax pain and diarrhea with a rectal heaviness caused by liver-spleen disharmony.

Xiāo Yáo Sǎn (Free Wanderer Powder, 逍遥散)
Formulary of the Pharmacy Service for Benefiting the People in the Taiping Era
(*Tài Píng Huì Mín Hé Jì Jú Fāng*, 太平惠民和剂局方)

[Ingredient]

Chái Hú (Radix Bupleuri)   remove plantlet (30 g)

Dāng Guī (Radix Angelicae Sinensis)   remove plantlet, file, light (30 g)

Dry-Fried Sháo Yào (Radix Paeoniae)   white (30 g)

Bái Zhú (Rhizoma Atractylodis Macrocephalae)   (30 g)

Fú Líng (Poria)   1 *liang* of peeled and white ones (30 g)

Gān Cǎo (Radix Et Rhizoma Glycyrrhizae)   light liquid-fried to red, 0.5 *liang* (15 g)

[Usage]   The original formula is crude powder. Each takes 1 *qian*, needs a large glass of water, add a piece of burned *shēng jiāng* cut, a little *bò he*, decocted together until seven-tenths left. Abandon the dregs, take in when it is hot without time limits.

Modern Usage: All herbs are made into powder. Take 6–9 g each time, add a little *shēng jiāng* and *bò he* together to cook the soup, and take it three times a day. It can also be used as a decoction and be taken in after boiled. The dosage should be increased or reduced according to the original proportion. There are also [processed into] pills, 6–9 g each time, twice a day.

[Action]   Soothe the liver and resolve constraints, nourish the blood, and fortify the spleen.

[Indication]   liver constraint and blood deficiency, rib-side pain, headache, dizzy vision, dry mouth and throat, mental weariness and poor appetite, alternating chills and fever, or menstrual irregularities, breast distension, wiry and deficient pulse.

[Formula Analysis]   This is a syndrome of stagnation of liver constraint and blood deficiency. *Dāng guī* in this formula is sweet, acrid, bitter, and warm, supplementing the blood and harmonizing the blood, its fragrance can enter the spleen, which relaxes the spleen qi, *bái sháo*, sour, bitter, and a little cold. It can nourish

the blood, soften the liver, accumulate yin and benefit the spleen. *Dāng guī* and *bái sháo* are used together to harmonize the blood and liver, [with] plentiful blood will soften the liver, they are chief medicines; wood excess lead to earth weakness, liver disease is easy to spread to the spleen, so deputy medicines *bái zhú*, *fú líng* and *gān cǎo* are used to fortify the spleen and boost qi, strengthen the earth to resist wood's restriction; *chái hú* soothes the liver and resolves constraint so that the liver can be free, a little *bò he* can vent constrained heat of liver channel, disperse constrained qi, *wèi jiāng* warms the stomach and harmonizes the center, it can also resolve constraint with its dispersing acrid. They are assistant and envoy medicines. The combination of the above herbs is in line with the tenets of *Basic Questions-Discourse on How the QI in the Depots Follow the Pattern of the Seasons* (*Sù Wèn-Zāng Qì Fǎ Shí Lùn*, 素问·藏气法时论), "When the liver [tenders to] suffer from rapid flow of qi, quickly consume sweet [flavor] to alleviate it.", "When the spleen needs to be moderated, requires the immediate use of sweet[flavor] to moderate.", "When the liver needs to be dissipated, immediate use of pungent [flavor] to dissipate it", ensure the blood deficiency to gets nourished, spleen deficiency gets solved, liver constraint gets eased, then all symptoms recover naturally, qi and blood regulating smoothly, so the formula is named "*Xiāo Yáo Sǎn*".

[Clinical Application]

1. This formula is an important prescription to harmonize liver-spleen, the liver storing blood and the spleen controlling blood, they are in close relationship with menstruation, so it is also one of the commonly used formulas for menstruation regulation. Anyone with liver qi deficiency and spleen weakness can be treated with this formula.

2. Liver constraint is mostly caused by an emotional disorder. When we treat constraint syndrome, we should encourage patients to be optimistic. Otherwise, the formula means "free and unfettered", while people are not really "free".

***Bái Zhú Sháo Yào Săn (Tòng Xiè Yào Fāng,* Important Formula for Painful Diarrhea, 白术芍药散，痛泻要方)**

***Collected Treatises of [Zhang] Jing-yue (Jǐng Yuè Quán Shū,* 景岳全书)**[27]

Quote From (*Liu Cao-chuang Formula,* 刘草窗方)[28]

[Ingredient]

Bái Zhú (Rhizoma Atractylodis Macrocephalae)   dry-fried, 3 *liang* (9 g)

Sháo Yào (Radix Paeoniae)   dry-fried, 2 *liang* (6 g)

Fáng Fēng (Radix Saposhnikoviae)   1 *liang* (3 g)

Chén Pí (Pericarpium Citri Reticulatae)   fried, 1.5 *liang* (4.5 g)

[Usage]   The original formula filed is divided into 8 *tie*, decocted by water or made pills.

Modern Usage: Make decoction. Take in after it is decocted by water, and the dosage should be reduced according to the original proportion.

[Action]   Suppress the liver and supporting the spleen.

[Indication]   Wood restricting the earth, borborygmus and abdominal pain, diarrhea, diarrhea must be with abdominal pain, thin white tongue coating, irregular *guan* pulse in both hands: left wiry and right moderate.

[Formula Analysis]   This syndrome is caused by wood restricting the earth, causing liver and spleen disharmony and spleen dysfunction. In the formula, *bái zhú* is used to fortify the spleen, harmonize the center and remove dampness, *bái sháo* suppresses the liver and relieves urgency and pain. They are chief medicines; *chén pí* rectifies qi and harmonizes the center, *fáng fēng* has the property of ascending and dispersing, acrid can disperse liver constraint, and fragrance can smooth spleen qi. They are assistant medicines. The formula is only four herbs, it combines soothing with supplementation, suppresses the liver and supports the spleen, regulates the qi mechanism. In this way, pain and diarrhea [all] disappear naturally.

[Clinical Application]   This formula is commonly used for treating liver-restricting spleen, abdominal pain, and diarrhea. The syndrome of pain and diarrhea is often seen in patients with liver constraints and a short temper, and it is always stirred by emotion. Apart from painful diarrhea, appetite loss, abdominal distension and

incomplete digestion of food in stool can be seen in this syndrome. So it can easily be misdiagnosed as diarrhea due to indigestion. However, abdominal pain caused by diarrhea due to indigestion can be relieved by diarrhea and defecation. [but in here] Although the painful diarrhea is slightly relieved after diarrhea, abdominal pain and diarrhea remain, for a short time, whose symptoms do not relieve, but repeats attacks. This is a point of differentiation.

Section 3　Formulas that harmonizes intestine-stomach

Harmonizing intestine-stomach formulas are suitable for treating pathogens in the intestines and stomach, abnormal ascending and descending, cold-heat complex, appearing epigastric *pǐ*, vomiting, borborygmus, diarrhea, abdominal pain and other syndromes. This is purely a case of weakness of center qi, cold-heat complex; therefore, it is necessary to treat with acrid and bitter medicines to promote descent to harmonize the intestines and stomach. The combination of medicines in this formula is characterized by acrid-hot and bitter-cold herbs, enriching-nourishing herbs and warming-clearing herbs. The main herbs are *bàn xià, huáng qín, gān jiāng, huáng lián, rén shēn, gān cǎo etc.* Representative formulas includes: *Bàn Xià Xiè Xīn Tāng* (Pinellia Heart-Draining Decoction, 半夏泻心汤) and *Huáng Lián Tāng* (Coptis Decoction, 黄连汤).

Bàn Xià Xiè Xīn Tang (Pinellia Heart-Draining Decoction, 半夏泻心汤)
Treatise on Cold Damage (Shāng Hán Lùn, 伤寒论)

[Ingredient]

Bàn Xià (Rhizoma Pinelliae)　half *sheng*, washed (12 g)

Huáng Qín (Radix Scutellariae)　3 *liang* (9 g)

Gān Jiāng (Rhizoma Zingiberis)　3 *liang* (9 g)

Rén Shēn (Radix Et Rhizoma Ginseng)　3 *liang* (9 g)

Huáng Lián (Rhizoma Coptidis)　1 *liang* (3 g)

Dà Zǎo (Fructus Jujubae)　12 pcs, split (4 *mei*)

Gān Cǎo (Radix Et Rhizoma Glycyrrhizae)   3 *liang*, liquid-fried (6 g)

[Usage]   The original formula includes seven herbs. Adopt 1*dou* water to boil the formula till 6 *sheng* is left. Abandon the dregs. Continue to boil the formula till 3 *sheng* is left. Take the decoction 1*sheng* when it is warm, 3 times a day.

Modern Usage: Decocted by water.

[Action]   Harmonize the stomach and direct counterflow downward, remove masses and dissipate *pǐ*.

[Indication]   Stomach qi disharmony, epigastric *pǐ*, vomiting, borborygmus and diarrhea, greasy and light yellow coating.

[Formula Analysis]   *Pǐ*, it means cold-heat obstructing in the center with blockage and stuffiness, and the upper and lower cannot communicate with each other. It belongs to the disease of the spleen and stomach. In the formula, acrid-warm *bàn xià* is used to disperse *pǐ* and masses, direct counterflow downward and arrest nausea, fullness, and vomiting, so it is the chief medicine; deputy medicine *gān jiāng* is acrid-warm and can be used to disperse cold, *huáng lián* and *huáng qín* discharge heat with bitter-cold. Bitterness and acrid taste using together, the combination of *bàn xià*, *huáng qín*, *gān jiāng*, *and huáng lián* can unblock and purge pathogens, which are enough to remove masses and dissipate *pǐ*; assistant with *rén shēn* and *dà zǎo* to boost qi with sweet-warm to supplement deficiency; envoy medicine *gān cǎo* can supplement the stomach qi and harmonize the actions of all medicines in a formula. The formula combines cold and heat to harmonize yin-yang, uses bitter and acrid tastes together to regulate ascend and descend, uses supplementation and drainage together to regulate deficiency and excess. To make the middle *jiao* harmonious, ascend and descend recovered, all the syndromes such as epigastric *pǐ*, fullness, vomiting, diarrhea healed. This formula takes *bàn xià* as the chief medicine, has the effect of eliminating epigastric *pǐ* and fullness. Therefore, it is called *Bàn Xià Xiè Xīn Tang*.

[Clinical Application]   The formula is designed initially for treating the damage of middle qi which is caused by inappropriate purgative method, [leads to] disharmony of the stomach, cold-heat complex, epigastric *pǐ* and fullness. Later

generations use it with a wide range, not only treating the *pǐ* which is caused by misusing purgative method in cold damage syndrome, but also treating the cold-heat obstructing in the center which is not caused by misusing purgative method, besides that, the *pǐ* caused by the spleen and stomach weakness, damp-heat stagnation, abnormal ascent and descent,etc, can all be applied with the modified formula. The effect is remarkable.

Huáng Lián Tāng (Coptis Decoction, 黄连汤)
Treatise on Cold Damage (*Shāng Hán Lùn*, 伤寒论)

[Ingredient]

Huáng Lián (Rhizoma Coptidis)   3 *liang* (9 g)

Liquid-Fried Gān Cǎo (Radix Et Rhizoma Glycyrrhizae)   3 *liang* (9 g)

Liquid-Fried Gān Jiāng (Rhizoma Zingiberis)   3 *liang* (9 g)

Guì Zhī (Ramulus Cinnamomi)   3 *liang* (9 g)

Rén Shēn (Radix Et Rhizoma Ginseng)   2 *liang* (6 g)

Bàn Xià (Rhizoma Pinelliae)   half *sheng*, washed (9 g)

Dà Zǎo (Fructus Jujubae)   12 pcs, split (4 *mei*)

[Usage]   The original formula includes seven herbs. Adopt 1dou water to boil the formula till 6 *sheng* is left. Abandon the dregs. Take the decoction 1 *sheng* when it is warm 3 times during the daytime, 2 times at night.

Modern Usage: Decocted by water.

[Action]   Regulate cold and heat, harmonize the stomach, direct counterflow downward.

[Indication]   Heat in the chest, pathogens in the stomach, abdomen pain and desire for vomiting.

[Formula Analysis]   This formula applies to the syndrome of stomach-intestine ascend-descend disorders, cold-heat complex. There is heat in the chest, so chief medicine: *huáng lián* clears heat with bitter-cold; pathogenic-qi in the stomach, so use deputy medicines *gān jiāng* and *guì zhi to* disperse cold with acrid-warm. A combination of cold and heat [nature] herbs can harmonize the cold and heat in the

body; assistant with *bàn xià* to harmonize the stomach, direct counterflow downward and arrest vomiting, *rén shēn* and *dà zǎo* are used to boost qi, harmmies center, and relieve urgency and pain; envoy medicine *gān cǎo*, it can relieve urgency, stop pain and harmonize the actions of all medicines. This formula uses cold and warm together, bitter and acrid tastes together, to make the cold dispersed, heat eliminated, upper and lower harmonious, ascend and descend recovered, and all the syndromes healed.

[Clinical Application] This formula applies to the syndrome of stomach-intestine ascend-descend disorders, cold-heat complex. The main points of pattern differentiation include cold abdominal pain, desire to vomit, water-glossy tongue and thin yellow coating.

Chapter 5

Warming Interior Formulas

According to the principles: "when there is cold, treat it with heat", "when there is cool, treat it with warm", "when cold pathogenic factors accumulated internally, treat it with sweet and warm", "when cold pathogenic factors are excessive, relieve it with pungent and heat" from *Basic Questions-Comprehensive Discourse on the Essentials of the Most Reliable* (*Sù Wèn-Zhì Zhēn Yào Dà Lùn*, 素问·至真要大论), the formula consists of warm-heat medicine, which could warm the center and dispel cold, restore yang to rescue from counter flow and treat interior cold disease, can be called formulas for warming the interior generally. It is "warming method" from "the eight methods".

Section 1   Formulas that warms the center and dispels cold

Formulas for warming the center and dispelling cold are to treat middle *jiao* and deficiency-cold of the spleen and stomach disease. The spleen and stomach ascribe to earth, located at middle *jiao*, the stomach governs intake, the spleen governs transportation and transformation, the stomach governs descent of the turbid, the spleen governs ascent of the clear. If yang qi of spleen-stomach in middle *jiao* is deficient and declined, transportation and transformation will be in failure, ascending and descending will be in disorder, which will cause yin cold to grow from inside, presenting with fatigue limbs and body, four limbs being not warm, distention and fullness feeling in the stomach duct and abdomen, abdominal cold pain, poor appetite, bland taste in the mouth and no dryness, vomiting diarrhea, acid swallowing and

drool vomiting, pale tongue, white and moist coating, deep and thready pulse or a slow and moderate pulse and other symptoms. Warming the center and dispelling cold medicines are usually used, such as formula consisting of *gān jiāng, wú zhū yú, shǔ jiāo, shēng jiāng* and so on, combined with medicines of fortifying the spleen and supplementing qi, such as *rén shēn, yí táng, bái zhú, zhì gān cǎo etc. Lǐ Zhōng Wán* (Center-Regulating Pill, 理中丸), *Wú Zhū Yú Tāng* (Evodia Decoction, 吴茱萸汤), *Xiǎo Jiàn Zhōng Tāng* (Minor Center-Fortifying Decoction, 小建中汤), *Dà Jiàn Zhōng Tān* (Major Center-Fortifying Decoction, 大建中汤) and others are representative.

Lǐ Zhōng Wán (Center-Regulating Pill, 理中丸)
Treatise on Cold Damage (Shāng Hán Lùn, 伤寒论)

[Ingredient]

Rén Shēn (Radix Et Rhizoma Ginseng)   3 *liang* (9 g)

Gān Jiāng (Rhizoma Zingiberis)   3 *liang* (9 g)

Zhì Gān Cǎo (Radix Et Rhizoma Glycyrrhizae Praeparata Cum Melle)   3 *liang* (9 g)

Bái Zhú (Rhizoma Atractylodis Macrocephalae)   3 *liang* (9 g)

[Usage]   Pound and sieve, mix them into pills as big as yolk. Fuse with boiled water many times into a pill and grind it. Take it warm three or four times in the daytime and two times at night. If there has no heat feeling in the abdomen, increase to three or four pills, but the pill is not as good as a decoction. Bisect four flavors, adopt 8 *sheng* water, boil till 3 *sheng* left, remove the residue, take 1 *sheng* in warm 3 times a day.

Modern usage: Pill, 6 to 9 g per time, 2 to 3 times per day, take in with warm water. Alternatirely take it as a decoction, decocted by water, the dosage can be changed according to the original proportion.

[Action]   Warm the center and dispell cold, supplement qi and fortify the spleen.

[Indication]

1. Deficiency-cold of the spleen and stomach syndrome, manifested with diarrhea and no thirst, abdominal fullness, vomiting, abdominal pain, retention of dietary, white and glossy tongue coating, moderate and weak pulse, or deep pulse, or slow and feeble pulse. Futhermore cholera belongs to the spleen-stomach deficiency-cold syndrome.

2. Yang deficiency and loss of blood.

3. Patients with deficiency-cold middle *jiao* manifested with frequent spitting phlegm-drool or kids with chronic infantile convulsion.

[Formula Analysis]　The yang deficiency of the spleen and stomach [leads to] cold, transportation and transformation will be in failure, ascending and descending will be in disorder. Deficiency-cold of middle *jiao*, cold and pathogenic will not be eliminated without warming, healthy qi will not recover when without nourishing. In the formula, *gān jiāng*, the chief medicine, is very pungent and heat, warms the center and dispels cold, *Miscellaneous Records of Famous Physicians* (*Míng Yī Bié Lù*, 名医别录)[29] says it as "treat cold and abdominal pain, counteract aversions, cholera and full abdomen", *Pouch of Pearls* (*Zhēn Zhū Náng*, 珍珠囊)[30]says it as "dispel deep and long-term cold of viscera and bowels"; *rén shēn*, the deputy madicinal, that is sweet, bitter and mildly warm, supplements qi and fortifies the spleen, and has the function of warming the center, *Míng Yī Bié Lù* says it as "treat the cold center of the stomach and intestines"; deficiency-cold and damp in the spleen can not be dispelled, so take *bái zhú* as assistant medicine to supplement the spleen qi and dry the damp spleen, *Zhēn Zhū Náng* says it as "eliminate the dampness and boost qi, supplement the center and yang"; *zhì gān cǎo* is as envoy medicine, nourishes the earth and warms the center, conciliates all medicines. The combination of these four medicines together can achieve the function of warming, supplementing, drying and harmonizing. It is a decoction that warms the center and dispels cold, supplements qi and fortifies the spleen. This formula is used to treat deficiency cold of middle *jiao*, so call it as "rectify the center". *Basic Questions-Comprehensive Discourse on the Essentials of the Most Reliable* (*Sù Wèn-Zhì Zhēn Yào Dà Lùn*, 素问·至真要大论) says, "restrict cold and

pathogenic, relieve it with sweet and heat, assist it with sweet and bitter", so they are. The original formula can be administered as a decoction or pill, depending on the degree of the syndrome. After taking the medicine, hot porridge is allowed to help the medicine warm and nourish the center qi.

[Clinical Application] The formula is mainly used in deficiency-cold of middle *jiao*, causing vomiting, diarrhea, abdominal pain and other syndromes. The pill is the mild regulating form, which is suitable for patients with mild syndromes; if the condition is urgent, transform the pill into a decoction to make it absorbed fast. After taking the decoction, the heat feeling around the abdomen will be an efficacious sign.

Wú Zhū Yú Tāng (Evodia Decoction, 吴茱萸汤)
Treatise on Cold Damage (*Shāng Hán Lùn*, 伤寒论)

[Ingredient]

Wú Zhū Yú (Fructus Evodiae)   1 *sheng*, washed (9 g)

Rén Shēn (Radix Et Rhizoma Ginseng)   3 *liang* (9 g)

Shēng Jiāng (Rhizoma Zingiberis Recens)   6 *liang*, cut (18 g)

Dà Zǎo (Fructus Jujubae)   12 grains, split (4 mei)

[Usage]   Adopt 7 *sheng* water to boil the above herbs till 1 *sheng* is left, remove the residue, take the decoction 3 times a day for 7 days when it is warm.

Modern Usage: Decocted by water.

[Action]   Warm the center and supplement deficiency, direct counterflow downward and arresting vomit.

[Indication]

1. Patients with deficiency-cold of stomach, frequent nausea, vomiting feeling after eating, gastric cavity pain, epigastric upset of acid swallowing, white and glossy coating, wiry and slow pulse.

2. *Jueyin* head pain, belching, vomiting drool.

3. Promoting vomiting, cold in hands and feet, vexing and agitating with a desire to die.

[Formula Analysis] Excessive yin cold in the inside, stomach qi fails to descend [but with] ascending counterflow of turbid yin. In this formula, *wú zhū yú*, the chief medicine, that is acrid, bitter and very heat, warms the center and dissipates cold, directs counterflow downward. *Shen Nong's Classic of the Materia Medica* (*Shén Nóng Běn Cǎo Jīng*, 神农本草经) says it as "warms the center, lowers qi and relieves pain mainly"; take *shēng jiāng* as deputy medicine especially to help chief medicine warm the center and dissipate cold, ascend counterflow and arrest vomiting; *rén shēn*, the assistant medicine, is sweet, bitter and mild warm, supplements deficiency and weakness, and boosts stomach qi; *dà zǎo* is sweet and warm, sweet can supplement the center, warm can boost qi, and can conciliate each medicine, used as envoy medicine. Combine them into the decoction for warming the center and supplementing deficiency, directing counterflow downward and arresting vomiting.

[Clinical Application] The formula uses acrid, bitter, sweet and warm medicines together, has the functions of warming the center and supplementing deficiency, directing counterflow downward. Clinics take the following symptoms as the main differentiation points: vomiting drool, tongue body not red, white and glossy tongue coating, wiry and slow pulse.

Xiǎo Jiàn Zhōng Tāng (**Minor Center-Fortifying Decoction**, 小建中汤)
Treatise on Cold Damage (*Shāng Hán Lùn*, 伤寒论)

[Ingredient]
Guì Zhī (Ramulus Cinnamomi)   skin removed (9 g)
Sháo Yào (Peony Root)   6 *liang* (18 g)
Gān Cǎo (Radix Et Rhizoma Glycyrrhizae)   2 *liang*, honey fired (6 g)
Shēng Jiāng (Rhizoma Zingiberis Recens)   3 *liang*, cut (9 g)
Dà Zǎo (Fructus Jujubae)   12 grains, split
Jiāo Yí (barley-sugar)   1 *sheng* (30 g)

[Usage] Adopt 7 *sheng* water to boil till 3 *sheng* is left, then remove the residue, put *jiāo yí* in it, melt it with mild fire, take the decoction 1 *sheng* in warm for 3 times a day.

Modern Usage: Decocted by water, remove the residue, put and melt the *yí táng* (malt sugar) in it, and take it in warm.

[Action] Warm the center and supplement deficiency, harmonize the exterior and relieve the tension.

[Indication] Deficiency-consumption and abdominal urgency, abdominal pain, prefer for warming or pressing, pain decrease when pressed, or throbbing in the heart, restlessness of vexation, lusterless complexion, wiry and astringent pulse, light tender tongue body, thin and white coating.

[Formula Analysis] Deficiency-consumption and abdominal pain, spasms of the abdominal pain, and frequent aching because of deficiency-cold of middle qi and [leads to] lack of warmth. In this formula, combined with *Guì Zhī Tāng*, *sháo yào* and *yí táng*. *Yí táng*, the chief medicine, is sweet, warm and moist, warms the center and supplements deficiency, and relieves tension and pain, *Important Formulas Worth a Thousand Gold Pieces for Emergency* (*Bèi Jí Qiān Jīn Yào Fāng*, 备急千金要方) says it as "supplements deficiency and cold, boosts qi and strength"; take *sháo yào* to restrain yin especially, combined with *guì zhī* to warm yang, both are deputy medicines; take *zhì gān cǎo* to assist, if combine with *sháo yào*, the combination of sour and sweet medicines can boost yin, relieve tension and pain, if combine with *guì zhī*, the combination of acrid and sweet medicines can support yang, warm the center and supplement deficiency; take *shēng jiāng*, *dà zǎo* as envoy medicines to supplement the spleen and stomach, combine with medicines to harmonize *ying* and *wei*. Combined into one formula, warms the center and supplements deficiency altogether, harmonizes the exterior and relieves tension, relieves and supplements yin and yang, harmonizes the function of the qi and blood. This formula does not use warming and powerful supplementations, but uses mild medicines to promote the spleen and stomach qi in the middle *jiao*, so it is called "*Xiǎo Jiàn Zhōng Tāng*".

[Clinical Application] The formula is modified from *Guì Zhī Tāng*, but *Guì Zhī Tāng* is good at releasing the flesh and induces sweating, harmonizes *ying-wei*, which treats the wind-strike exterior deficiency syndromes manifested with sweating and aversion to wind and disharmony between *ying* and *wei*; but this formula warms

the center and supplements deficiency, relieves exterior and tension, treats deficiency-cold of middle *jiao*, abdominal urgency and pain of deficiency-consumption syndromes. *Guì zhī* is the chief medicine in *Guì Zhī Tāng*, while *yí táng* is the chief medicine in this formula, because of the different proportions of medicines, and their functions and indications are different.

Dà Jiàn Zhōng Tāng (Major Center-Fortifying Decoction, 大建中汤)
Essentials from the Golden Cabinet (*Jīn Guì Yào Lüè*, 金匮要略)

[Ingredient]

Shǔ Jiāo (Pericarpium Zanthoxyli)　2 *he*, (6 g)

Gān Jiāng (Rhizoma Zingiberis)　4 *liang* (12 g)

Rén Shēn (Radix Et Rhizoma Ginseng)　2 *liang* (6 g)

[Usage]　Adopt 4 *sheng* water to boil the herbs till 2 *sheng* left, then remove the residue, put 1 *sheng jiao yí* (*yí táng*), boil till 1.5 *sheng* with a low fire, divide it and take it in warm, and after *yì chuī qǐng* (一炊顷) [Time required for cooking rice], take 2 *sheng* warm porridge later.

Modern Usage: Decocted by water, remove the residue, add *yí táng* (malt sugar)15 g and melt it, divide it into two times, and take it in warm.

[Action]　Warm the center and supplement deficiency, direct counterflow downward and relieve pain.

[Indication]　Debilitation of middle yang, yin cold accumulated inside, severe abdominal pain which refuses to press, vomiting and cannot eat, white and glossy tongue coating, deep and thready pulse, viscera cold, restless roundworms, severe upper abdominal pain [patient].

[Formula Analysis]　Debilitation of middle yang, which leads to the yin cold accumulate inside. In the formula, *shǔ jiāo*, the chief medicine, is very acrid and heat, warms the center and dispels cold, lowers qi and relieves pain, dispels roundworms and kills worms; *gān jiāng*, the deputy medicine, is very acrid and heat, warms the center and dispels cold, harmonizes stomach and arrests vomiting; yin cold and internal prevalence is due to deficiency of middle yang, take *gān jiāng*

as assistant medicine, is acrid and warm, supplements and boosts the spleen and stomach, upholds healthy qi; *yí táng*, the assistant and envoy medicine, fortifies the center and supplements deficiency, relieves urgency and pain, relieves the acrid and drying of [*shǔ*] *jiāo*, [*gān*] *jiāng*. Those four medicines together, can warming the center and supplementing deficiency, directing counterflow downward. This is a very supplementary and heat formula, which can warm and fortify viscera, dispel all yin cold, reinforce the middle yang, thus, it is called "*Dà Jiàn Zhōng Tāng*".

[Clinical Application]   The formula is to warm the center and supplement deficiency, direct counterflow downward and relieve pain. It is often used to treat abdominal pain, vomiting, patients of decline and debilitation of middle yang, cold yin and internal prevalence. The formula proves that the syndromes' cold yin is more serious than *Xiǎo Jiàn Zhōng Tāng*, so the functions of the formula to dispel cold and supplement deficiency are stronger than *Xiǎo Jiàn Zhōng Tāng*.

Section 2   Formulas that restores yang to rescue from counterflow

Formulas of restoring yang to rescue from counterflow mainly treat yin cold in the whole body, which is caused by the decline and debilitation of kidney yang. The true yang of the human body is in the kidney, if the kidney yang is deficient and debilitated, the yin cold is accumulated and prevails inside, which manifests with counterflow cold of the four limbs, listlessness, aversion to cold and lassitude, diarrhea with undigested food, mild, thin pulse and other symptoms, the warm and heat medicines must be used to restore yang to rescue from counterflow. If not rescued in time, yang will collapse and desert, manifested with unconscious, panting and hasting rising of qi, oily or leaking sweats, counterflow cold of the four limbs, faint pulse verging on expiry. Using the formula of restoring yang to rescue from counterflow as soon as possible, which can boost qi and rescue from desertion, might bring the patient's life back. The formula of restoring yang to rescue from counterflow mainly consists of acrid-warm, dryness-heat and sweet-warm, supplementing qi medicines, *fù zǐ*, *gān jiāng*, *ròu guì*, *rén shēn*, *zhì gān cǎo* and so on. *Sì Nì Tāng* (Frigid Extremities

Decoction, 四逆汤) and *Shēn Fù Tāng* (Ginseng and Aconite Decoction, 参附汤) are the representatives. But the decline and debilitation of yang qi can be different, and there are patients with edema due to yang deficiency, and failure of the kidney to receive qi, so when using yang-restoring to rescue from counterflow, need to combine with transforming qi and promoting urination, calming reception and prevailing yang, such as *Zhēn Wǔ Tāng* (True Warrior Decoction, 真武汤), *Hēi Xī Dān* (Galenite Elixir, 黑锡丹) and so on. Deficiency of yang with the exuberance of yin can progress into the syndrome of exuberant yin repelling yang. When diarrhea with undigested food, reversal cold of hands and feet, faint pulse-like almost disappear, but with fake heat, manifested with fever, red face and floating yang. When treating a true cold with false heat syndrome, do not be bewildered by false syndromes, we should grasp the truth and quickly use a formula to restore yang that can rescue the dangerous syndrome of floating deficiency yang, such as *Tōng Mài Sì Nì Tāng* (Channel-Unblocking for Frigid Extremities Decoction, 通脉四逆汤).

Sì Nì Tāng (Frigid Extremities Decoction, 四逆汤)
Treatise on Cold Damage (*Shāng Hán Lùn*, 伤寒论)

[Ingredient]

Gān Cǎo (Radix Et Rhizoma Glycyrrhizae)   2 *liang*, honey-fired (6 g)

Gān Jiāng (Rhizoma Zingiberis)   1.5 *liang* (4.5 g)

Fù Zǐ (Radix Aconiti Lateralis Praeparata)   1 grain, raw, skin-removed, cut into 8 pieces (9 g)

[Usage]   Adopt 1 *sheng* to boil till 1 *sheng* 2 *he*, remove the residue, take in warm. Strong [body constitution] people can take *dà fù zǐ*[①], 1 *mei*, and *gān jiāng* 3 *liang*.

Modern Usage: Decocted by water and take in warm.

[Action]   Restore yang to rescue from counterflow.

[Indication]   Yin cold and internal prevalence, decline and debilitation of yang qi, reversal cold of the hands and feet, aversion to cold and lying in curled-up

---

① *dà fù zǐ, hei shun pian* (黑顺片): pungentacrid, sweet and hot; Poisonous. Heart, kidney, spleen meridian.

posture, mental fatigue and tend to sleep, vomiting and abdominal pain, diarrhea with undigested food, or profuse sweating and yang collapse, deep pulse, or mild, thready and faint pulse, light tongue body, or black, glossy and moist coating.

[Formula Analysis] *Basic Questions-Discourse on Recession (Sù Wèn-Jué Lùn,* 素问·厥论*)* says,"if yang qi declined downward, that causes cold syncope." The main syndrome is reversal counterflow cold in the hands and feet, which is caused by the decline and debilitation of yang qi. *Basic Questions-Comprehensive Discourse on the Essentials of the Most Reliable (Sù Wèn-Zhì Zhēn Yào Dà Lùn,* 素问·至真要大论*)* says: "exuberant yin cold should be relieved with acrid-heat, assist with sweet-bitter". In the formula, *fù zǐ*, the chief medicine, is very acrid and heat, goes into the heart, spleen and kidney channel, which is the main medicine of restoring yang to rescue from counterflow to supplement life gate *(mìng mén*①*)* fire especially, goes into twelve channels, promotes all, maintains nothing after leaving; *gān jiāng*, the deputy medicine, is good at dispelling the exterior cold, helps chief medicine restore yang to rescue from counterflow; *zhì gān cǎo*, assistant and envoy medicine, is acrid and warm, boosts qi and warms yang, and can relieve the dryness of *fù zǐ* and *gān jiāng*. Using the three together, specializing in attack and fast-acting effects, can restore yang to cure a reversal cold of the hands and feet, so it is called *Sì Nì Tāng*.

[Clinical Application] The formula is a representative of restoring yang to rescue from counterflow, *Shāng Hán Lùn* takes it as the main formula to treat *shaoyin* syndrome. Take reversal cold of the hands and feet, mental fatigue and desire to sleep, mild and thready pulse as main points. The formula breaks yin cold and restores yang qi and can rescue feeble yang in a short time.

Shēn Fù Tāng (Ginseng and Aconite Decoction, 参附汤)
Sequel Recording of Sagely Beneficence (Jì Shēng Xù Fāng, 济生续方*)*[31]

[Ingredient]

Rén Shēn (Radix Et Rhizoma Ginseng)　0.5 *liang* (13 g)

---

① *mìng mén*, gate of vitality (命门).

Fù Zǐ (Radix Aconiti Lateralis Praeparata)　1 *liang*, blast-fried, skin-removed, (30 g)

[Usage]　Chew[cut] into three portions, water 2 *zhan*, *shēng jiāng*, 10 slices, boil it till eight-tenths left, remove the residue, and take in warm.

Modern Usage: Decocted by water, the amount can be decreased according to the original proportion.

[Action]　Restore yang, boost qi, and rescue from desertion.

[Indication]　Violent desertions of yang qi, reversal cold of the hands and feet, dizziness and short breathing, pale face, sweating and mild pulse, light tongue, thin and white coating.

[Formula Analysis]　Violent desertions of yang qi are yang collapse. In the formula, acrid-warm of *rén shēn* for powerful supplementation of original qi to consolidate acquired constitution; *fù zǐ*, very acrid and warm, warms and tonifyies original yang, powerfully supplements of pre-heaven (*xiān tiān*, 先天). The two medicines depend on each other, can boost the heart yang upward, warm the kidney downward, neutralize and supplement the spleen earth in the middle. The formula has strong and fast-acting effects, warms and supplements powerfully, which can inspire yang qi, boost qi, and rescue from desertion. It is the most suitable decoction for rescuing dying people.

[Clinical Application]

1. The formula is for restoring yang, boosting qi and rescuing from desertion. Clinics not only use it to treat violent desertion of yang qi, but also treat women of blood desertion and yang collapse who have violent flooding or postpartum profuse uterine bleeding; this is a rescue way for blood desertion.

2. Take this formula to restore yang and consolidate desertion, generally it can not replace ginseng with *dǎng shēn*. If ginseng cannot be found, 60–120 g of Codonopsis pilosula should be used; otherwise, a small amount is difficult to work.

Zhēn Wǔ Tāng (True Warrior Decoction, 真武汤)
Treatise on Cold Damage (*Shāng Hán Lùn*, 伤寒论)

[Ingredient]

Fú Líng (Poria)   *3 liang* (9 g)

Sháo Yào (Radix Paeoniae)   *3 liang* (9 g)

Shēng Jiāng (Rhizoma Zingiberis Recens)   *3 liang*, cut (9 g)

Bái Zhú (Rhizoma Atractylodis Macrocephalae)   *2 liang* (6 g)

Fù Zǐ (Radix Aconiti Lateralis Praeparata)   1 pcs, roasted, skin-removed, cut into 8pcs (9 g)

[Usage]   Adopt water 8 s*heng* to boil till 5 *sheng* left, remove the residue, and take in warm by 7 dosage 3 times a day.

Modern Usage: Decocted by water.

[Action]   Warm yang, Promot water.

[Indication]   The kidney yang declines, cause the water retention, the urine is unfavorable, the limbs are heavy and painful. Abdominal Pain, diarrhea or the limbs are swollen, the tongue is pale and smooth, and the pulse is slow.

[Formula Analysis]   The kidney is in charge of water metabolism, if the true yang of the kidney decline and debilitate, [thus]qi fails to regulate the water, and urine will be disturbed. The kidney governs water, therefore, *fù zǐ*, the chief medicine, which is very acrid and warm, warms the kidney and tonifys yang; spleen governs controlling water, therefore, take *fú líng*, *bái zhú* as deputy medicines to fortify the spleen and promote urination, *shēng jiāng*, warms and dispels water-cold qi; take *bái sháo* as an assistant mediuanl, which is bitter-sour and mild-cold, not only can relieve abdominal pain and promote urine, as *Shen Nong's Classic of the Materia Medica* (*Shén Nóng Běn Cǎo Jīng*, 神农本草经) says [*bái sháo*] "governs pathogenic qi and abdominal pain... relieves pain, promotes urine", and also can relieve the dryness of *fù zǐ* to warm yang and promote urination, but not hurt yin. Using all medicines together to warm kidney yang, dispel yin, and promote waterways to dispel water pathogens. *Zhēn Wǔ* (真武) is the True Warrior God who governs water in the north [in legend], this formula has the function of warming yang and promoting water, so it is called

71

Zhēn Wǔ Tāng.

[Clinical Application]　The formula is to treat the decline of *shaoyin*, and yang, water retention. According to the experience of professor Wang Mian-zhi[32], if there is abdominal dropsy, the dosage of *fú líng* can be increased; if less reception and abdominal distension, *chén pí, mù xiāng* can be put into moderately, to transform qi and help promote urination. In the formula, *shēng jiāng*, the dosage should be modified according to the original proportion and not be taken as a common medicine.

Hēi Xī Dān (Galenite Elixir, 黑锡丹)

Formulary of the Pharmacy Service for Benefiting the People in the Taiping Era (*Tài Píng Huì Mín Hé Jì Jú Fāng,* 太平惠民和剂局方)

[Ingredient]

Jīn Líng Zǐ (szechwan chinaberry fruit)　steaming, skin-removed, core-removed (30 g)

Hú Lú Bā (Common Fenu Greek Seed)　wine-soaked, fired (30 g)

Mù Xiāng (Radix Aucklandiae)　(30 g)

Fù Zǐ (Radix Aconiti Lateralis Praeparata)　roasted, skin-removed, knot-removed (30 g)

Ròu Dòu Kòu (Semen Myristicae)　stew (30 g)

Pò Gù Zhǐ (Fructus Psoralae)　wine-soaked, fired (30 g)

Chén Xiāng (Lignum Aquilariae Resinatum)　(30 g)

Huí Xiāng (Foeniculum vulgare)　fired (30 g)

Yáng Qǐ Shí (Actinolitum)　powdered, levigating, 1 *liang* (30 g)

Ròu Guì (Cortex Cinnamomi)　skin-removed, 0.5 *liang* (15 g)

Hēi Xī　2 *liang* (60 g)

Liú Huáng (Sulphur Transparent)　2 *liang* (60 g)

[Usage]　Original decoction take *hēi xī, liú huáng*, grind into powder, add the residue medicine into it, mix and grind them, and combine wine with it as the same big as *wú tóng zǐ* (Semen Firmianae), weather it without sun, then wipe them to make them glossy, take thirty to forty granules a time, take with salt-ginger soup or *Zǎo*

Tāng (*dà zǎo* soup) before taking a meal, women take the pills with *Ài Cù Tāng*.

Modern Usage: Combined with wine into pills, adults take 4.5 g every time, children take 1.5 to 3 g every time, take with warm boiled water or bland salt before taking a meal. Increase the dosage to 9 g if it is urgent.

[Action]   Warm and supplement kidney qi, calm reception and prevail yang.

[Indication]

1. Deficiency and decline of kidney yang, failure of the kidney to receive qi, lower deficiency and upper excess, phlegm congestion and panting, sweating and reversal cold of the hands and feet, light tongue and white coating, deep and thready pulse, or floating and rootless.

2. *Bēn Tún* (running piglet, 奔豚), qi rushing up to the chest, or ringing intestines and thin, unformed stool, or male *yang wěi*, the sea blood of female is deficient and cold, clear and thin leukorrhea.

[Formula Analysis]   Deficiency-cold of kidney yang, the failure of the kidney to receive qi, which is a lower deficiency, are the foundation of the disease; deficiency-cold of yang arises from internal, causing upper flooding of turbid yin, water flooding is phlegm, phlegm congestion in the chest, which is upper excess, the branch of the disease. In the formula, *hēi xī* and *liú huáng* are the chief medicines. *Hēi xī* is made from plumbum, sweet-cold and calm water, heavy in nature which is good at directing counterflow downward qi, draining phlegm-drool, relieving its tendency of phlegm congestion and panting; the kidney is viscus of water and fire and its, syndromes pertain to the exuberance of yin with the decline of yang, therefore take sour-warm of *liú huáng* to supplement fire and boost yang, warm *mìng mén* to dispel yin cold. Using the two medicines together, getting the meaning of mutual rooting of yin and yang and seeking yang within yin, are good at protecting true yin, warming true yang, receiving kidney qi, calming floating yang. Take *ròu guì* and *fù zǐ* as deputy medicines to warm and supplement *mìng mén*, take the fire back to the origin, *hú lú bā*, *pò gù zhǐ*, *huí xiāng* and *yáng qǐ shí* all can warm kidney and fortify yang, making yang congest and vigorous and then the problem will disappear automatically. Assist with *mù xiāng* to regulate qi if qi stagnation because of cold, qi will leak if deficient,

take *ròu dòu kòu* to consolidate the lower; if concern that pure yang things are too warm and dry that provoke mutual fire, take *jīn líng zǐ* as a paradoxical assistant, which is bitter and cold, and can clear the liver and rectify the spleen. Take *chén xiāng* as envoy, heavy texture and warm, to direct counterflow downward qi and receive kidney qi. Combined into a decoction, kidney qi can be warmed and supplemented, calming reception and floating yang altogether.

[Clinical Application] The formula is a representative of warming kidney, and receiving qi. Generations of doctors give the highest commentary on the decoction after having clinical practices. As Yu Chang said, "If encounter syndromes of yin fire counterflow upsurge, deserting true yang, panting and ringing phlegm, no decoction can make a difference except this. Chang [the author] uses...imitates every time, all make a difference", proving the formula has the function of rescuing dying. If there are cold feet and a sweating head like oil and beads, the yang is going to collapse and deficient desertion, and need to take *Hēi Xī Dān* with *Dú Shēn Tāng* or *Shēn Fù Tāng*.

Section 3　Formulas that warms the channels and dissipates cold

Formulas of warming the channels and dissipating cold are suitable for the syndromes caused by cold invading channels and blood stasis. This kind of disease is mainly caused by weakness of yin-blood, and the hurt of a cold pathogen; otherwise, caused by yang qi insufficient, yin-cold pathogen invades when deficient. So it is not good to use the decoction of acrid and heat; instead, use the decoction of warming the channels and dissipating cold medicines, such as *guì zhī, xì xīn, ròu guì, má huáng, jiāng tàn*and so on, combined with supplementing and boosting medicines, such as *dāng guī, bái sháo, shú dì, qǐ zǐ, lù jiǎo jiāo*. The representative decoctions are *Dāng Guī Sì Nì Tāng* (Chinese Angelica Frigid Extremities Decoction, 四逆汤), *Nuǎn Gān Jiān, Yáng Hé Tāng* (Harmonious Yang Decoction, 阳和汤).

Dāng Guī Sì Nì Tāng (Chinese Angelica Frigid Extremities Decoction, 当归四逆汤)
Treatise on Cold Damage (*Shāng Hán Lùn*, 伤寒论)

[Ingredient]

Dāng Guī (Radix Angelicae Sinensis)　3 *liang* (9 g)

Guì Zhī (Ramulus Cinnamomi)　3 *liang* (9 g)

Sháo Yào (Radix Paeoniae)　3 *liang* (9 g)

Xì Xīn (Radix Et Rhizoma Asari)　3 *liang* (4.5 g)

Gān Cǎo (Radix Et Rhizoma Glycyrrhizae)　2 *liang* (6 g), fired

Tōng Cǎo (Medulla Tetrapanacis)　2 *liang* (6 g)

Dà Zǎo (Fructus Jujubae)　25 *mei*, split (8 pcs)

[Usage]　Adopt 8 *sheng* to boil till 3 *sheng* left, then remove the residue, take 1 *sheng* in warm three times a day.

Modern Usage: Decocted by water.

[Action]　Warm the channels and dissipat cold, nourish the blood, and unblock channels.

[Indication]　Blood Deficiency with cold invaded, reversal cold of the hands and feet, thready and feeble pulse, light tongue and white coating. Suitable for the hurt of blood vessels caused by cold, lumbar, thigh, legs and feet pain.

[Formula Analysis]　Blood deficiency in the body, attacked by a cold pathogen, leads to congealing and stagnation in blood vessels, four limbs lack warm caring, so there is reversal cold of the hands and feet. The decoction is *Guì Zhī Tāng* which is no *shēng jiāng*, and more *dà zǎo*, put *dāng guī, xì xīn* and *mù tōng* in it. Blood deficiency and cold congealing, *dāng guī*, the chief medicine, supplements and harmonizes blood, warms and frees blood channels; take *guì zhī* to warms and frees channels, *sháo yào* to nourish blood and harmonize ying, they are deputy medicines; take *xì xīn* to warm the channels and dissipate cold, *mù tōng* to free and promote blood and channels, they are assistant medicines to regulate *zhì gān cǎo, dà zǎo* to supplement the spleen-qi, and *Míng Yī Bié Lù* records that *zhì gān cǎo* can "unblock channels, promote blood-qi". Combine all these into the decoction of warming the channels and dissipating cold, nourishing blood and unblocking vessels. In the

formula, *dāng guī*, the chief medicine, treats the reversal cold of the hands and feet syndrome caused by blood deficiency and cold stagnation, so it is called "*Dāng Guī Sì Nì Tāng*".

[Clinical Application]

1. The formula warms the channels and dissipates cold, nourishes blood, and unblocks vessels; mainly used to treat reversal colds of the hands and feet, painful limbs syndromes of blood deficiency, and existing colds. If women who are in blood deficiency and cold stagnation, which cause menstrual irregularities, delayed menstruation, menstrual abdominal pain, menstruation with a small amount and dark color, can also take this.

2. The earlier stage of chilblain, but still not an ulcer, can use this decoction to warm channels and dissipate cold, fumigation and washing or decocted.

Nuǎn Gān Jiān (Warm the Liver Decoction, 暖肝煎)
The Complete Works of [Zhang] Jing-yue (*Jǐng Yuè Quán Shū,* 景岳全书)

[Ingredient]

Dāng Guī (Radix Angelicae Sinensis)　2–3 *qian* (6–9 g)

Gǒu Qǐ (Fructus Lycii)　3 *qian* (9 g)

Xiǎo Huí Xiāng (Fructus Foeniculi)　2 *qian* (6 g)

Ròu Guì (Cortex Cinnamomi)　1, 2 *qian* (3–6 g)

Wū Yào (Radix Linderae)　2 *qian* (6 g)

Chén Xiāng (Lignum Aquilariae Resinatum)　1 *qian* (3 g) (or *mù xiāng*)

Fú Líng (Poria)　2 *qian*, (6 g)

[Usage]　Adopt water 1.5 *zhong* (45 ml), put *shēng jiāng* 3 to 5 slices in it, boil into seven-tenths, and take in warm after a meal.

Modern Usage: Put *shēng jiāng* 3–5 slices in it, decocted by water.

[Action]　Warm and supplement the liver and kidney, dispell cold, and move qi.

[Indication]　Liver and kidney yin-cold, lower abdomen pain, *shàn qì,* and other syndromes.

[Formula Analysis]　[when the patient'] liver and kidney are insufficient in

the body, and yin cold and internal prevalence, cold attacks lower *jiao*, *jueyin* loses to flow by qi. In the formula, *dāng guī* and *gǒu qǐ* are the chief medicines, warm and supplement the liver and kidney; *xiǎo huí xiāng* and *ròu guì* are the deputy medicines, warm the channels and dissipate cold; take *wū yào* and *chén xiāng* as assistant medicines to warm, free and regulate qi, *fú líng* to percolate and drain dampness with bland medicines; take *shēng jiāng* as envoy to warm and dispel water-cold qi. The formula treats origins by warming and supplementing the liver and kidney, treats branches by dispelling cold and moving qi, and combines origins and branches to make the function of warming the liver, so it is called "*Nuǎn Gān Jiān*".

[Clinical Application]　This formula is used for treating bulging disorders due to cold in the liver channel; hence comes the name. If lack of *chén xiāng*, Zhang Jing-yue[33]mentioned "[*chén xiāng*]can be replaced by *mu xīang*".

Yáng Hé Tāng (Harmonious Yang Decoction, 阳和汤)
Complete Collection of Patterns and Treatments in External Medicine (Wài Kē Zhèng Zhì Quán Shēng Jí, 外科证治全生集)[34]

[Ingredient]

Shú Dì (Rehmanniae Radix preparata)　1 *liang* (30 g)

Bái Jiè Zǐ (Semen Sinapis)　fired, ground　2 *qian* (6 g)

Lù Jiǎo Jiāo (Colla Cornus Cervi)　3 *qian* (9 g)

Ròu Guì (Cortex Cinnamomi)　skin-removed, powdered　1 *qian* (3 g)

Jiāng Tàn (Blast-fried ginger)　5 *fen* (1.5 g)

Má Huáng (Herba Ephedrae)　5 *fen* (1.5 g)

Shēng Gān Cǎo (Glycyrrhizae Radix)　1 *qian* (3 g)

[Usage]　Decocted.

Modern Usage: Decocted by water.

[Action]　Warm yang and supplement blood, dispell cold and free stagnation.

[Indication]　Yin abscess, abscess clinging to the bone, *liú zhù*, *hè xī fēng* (arthritis like crane knee, 鹤膝风), and others all are yin cold syndromes. Local swelling and no heads, white color or dark, not red nor heat, no thirsty, light tongue, white coating,

deep and thready pulse, or slow and thready pulse.

[Formula Analysis]　Yin abscess is mainly caused by qi and blood deficiency and cold, and cold consolidates phlegm to obstruct in muscles, sinew, bone, blood and vessels. In the formula, take *shú dì* as the chief medicine to nourish essence and blood especially, *Shen Nong's Classic of the Materia Medica* (*Shén Nóng Běn Cǎo Jīng*, 神农本草经) records it as "fill bone arrow, grow muscle, generate essence and blood, supplement insufficient five viscus, free blood, and vessels"; *lù jiǎo jiāo*, the deputy medicine, help yang to supplement bone arrow, fortify sinew and bone, *Běn Cǎo Gāng Mù* says it can also treat "sores, ulcers, swellings, toxin"; take *ròu guì* as assistant medicine to supplement fire of *mìng mén*, dispel yin cold, warm and free blood and vessels, ginger carbon, to break yin and restore yang to dissolve cold consolidation, and with a little *má huáng* to disperse and skip yang qi, open the interstitial space, removing the toxin of cold consolidation through the outer space, *bái jiè zǐ* to dispel phlegm and dissipate masses, treat phlegm of internal skin and outer membrane, only this can make it. Take *shēng gān cǎo* as an envoy medicine to relieve it by its sweetness, harmonize all medicines, limit the functionality of the acrid-heat of all medicines, and resolve toxins. The formula has the nourishment and cloying of *shú dì*, *lù jiǎo jiāo*, but gets diffusion and regulation of ginger, *ròu guì*, *má huáng*, supplement and no stagnation; though it has the acrid and dissipation of ginger, *ròu guì*, *má huáng*, it gets much nourishment and supplementation of *shú dì*, *lù jiǎo jiāo* so with diffusion and dispersion but does not hurt main, supplements with each other, so that their functions are all good. The proportion of the whole formula is fantastic, it has the functions of warming yang and supplementing blood, diffusing and regulating blood and vessels, dispersing cold and dispelling phlegm, making yin abscess disappeared, as yang harmony reverse suddenly, cold consolidation all dissolved, so it is called *Yáng Hé Tāng*.

[Clinical Application]　The formula is famous for treating surgery to obstruct sores and ulcers, and treats all yin abscesses mainly.

Chapter 6

Heat-Clearing Formulas

According to the principle, "when there is heat, treat it with cold; when there is warm, treat it with cool" in *Basic Questions-Comprehensive Discourse on the Essentials of the Most Reliable* (*Sù Wèn-Zhì Zhēn Yào Dà Lùn*, 素问·至真要大论), the formulas mainly consist of heat-clearing medicines, which can clear heat and purge fire, cool blood and resolve toxins, and treat for interior heat syndrome, are all called heat-clearing formula. It belongs to the clearing method of the eight methods.

Section 1　Formulas that clears heat from the qi level

Qi-clearing formula is suitable for the syndrome of heat at the qi level with symptoms like high fever, polydipsia, sweating, large surging or slippery rapid pulse, dry yellow coating or the symptoms of heat disturbing chest and diaphragm, and vexation. The formulas usually consisted of drugs for clearing heat and purging fire, like *shí gāo*, *zhī mǔ*, *zhú yè*, *huáng qín*, *zhī zǐ*, *etc.* Because heat evil easily consuming qi and damages yin, there are always medicines of benefit qi and nourishing yin in the formulas, like *rén shēn*, *mài dōng*, *gān cǎo*, *etc.* The representative formulas are *Bái Hǔ Tāng* (White Tiger Decoction, 白虎汤), *Zhú Yè Shí Gāo Tāng* (Lophatherum and Gypsum Decoction, 竹叶石膏汤), *Zhī Zǐ Chǐ Tāng* (Gardenia and Black Curd Beans Decoction, 栀子豉汤), *Liáng Gé Sǎn* (Diaphragm-Cooling Powder, 凉膈散), *etc.*

Bái Hǔ Tāng (White Tiger Decoction, 白虎汤)
Treatise on Cold Damage (Shāng Hán Lùn, 伤寒论)

[Ingredient]

Shí Gāo (Gypsum Fibrosum Praeparatum)   *1 Jin*, break (30 g)

Zhī Mǔ (Anemarrhena Asphodeloides Bunge)   6 *liang* (9 g)

Gān Cǎo (Radix Et Rhizoma Glycyrrhizae)   2 *liang*, honey-fired (6 g)

Jīng Mǐ (Oryza Sativa L)   6 *he* (15 g)

[Usage]   Adopt 1 *dou* water to boil the above herbs. After the rice is cooked, abandon the dregs and take 1 *sheng* of the decoction 3 times a day when it is warm.

Modern Usage: Decocted by water. After the rice is cooked, abandon the dregs and take the decoction when it is warm.

[Action]   Clear heat and promot fluid production.

[Indication]   *Yangming* heat syndrome, aversion to heat without cold, red face and rough breath, dry mouth with scorched tongue, polydipsia, profuse sweating, strongly surging pulse or floating, slippery and rapid pulse, deep red tongue with dry yellow coating.

[Formula Analysis]   This is an excessive heat syndrome caused by the inward penetration of heat, which transformed from the exterior cold pathogen or warm pathogen transmitting into qi level. *Shí gāo* is acrid, sweet in taste but cold in nature. Acrid can release muscle heat and cold can clear stomach fire. So *shí gāo* is good at clearing heat and purging fire, removing vexation and quenching thirst, and has the function of dispelling heat from the exterior. Therefore, it is the chief medicine. *Zhī mǔ*, the deputy medicine, which is bitter in taste and cold in nature with moisturizing quality, can not only clear the fire of the lung and stomach, but also enrich yin and moisten dryness. Matching *shí gāo* and *zhī mǔ* can strengthen the power of clearing heat, removing vexation, and quenching thirst. *Gān cǎo* and *jīng mǐ* can boost the stomach and engender fluids, harmonizing the center and clearing fire, which prevents the cold nature medicines not impair the spleen and stomach. Besides, *shí gāo* and *zhī mǔ* can strengthen the function of clearing heat and engendering fluids with *gān cǎo* and *jīng mǐ*'s help. The whole formula has only four flavors. But the

combination is precise and appropriate, specializing in clearing the heat of qi level of *yangming*, just like autumn wind brings the cool and the summer heat is cleared naturally. The White Tiger is the golden god of the west, so this formula is called White Tiger Decoction.

[Clinical Application] This is the main formula for treating *yangming* heat syndrome in *Treatise on Cold Damage* (*Shāng Hán Lùn*, 伤寒论) and the heat syndrome in qi level of lung and stomach in *Wēn Bìng Tiáo Biàn*. This fornula's main points of syndrome differentiation should be great body heat, great thirst, profuse sweating, and a large surging pulse.

Zhú Yè Shí Gāo Tāng (Lophatherum and Gypsum Decoction, 竹叶石膏汤) *Treatise on Cold Damage* (*Shāng Hán Lùn*, 伤寒论)

[Ingredient]

Zhú Yè (Folium Phyllostachydis Henonis) 2 *ba* (9 g)

Shí Gāo (Gypsum Fibrosum Praeparatum) 1 *jin* (30 g)

Bàn Xià (Rhizoma Pinelliae) half *sheng*, wash (9 g)

Rén Shēn (Radix Et Rhizoma Ginseng) 3 *liang* (9 g)

Gān Cǎo (Radix Et Rhizoma Glycyrrhizae) 2 *liang*, honey-fired (6 g)

Mài Mén Dōng (Radix Ophiopogonis) 1 *sheng*, discarding the pith (18 g)

Jīng Mǐ (Oryza Sativa L) half *sheng* (15 g)

[Usage] Adopt 1 *dou* water to boil the first 6 herbs. When there is 6 *sheng* left, add *jīng mǐ*. After the rice is cooked, abandon the rice. Take 1 *sheng* of the decoction, 3 times a day when it is warm.

Modern Usage: Decocted by water.

[Action] Clear heat and promot fluids production, boost qi, and harmonize the stomach.

[Indication] Febrile disease, heat evil has not been cleared, and damage to both qi and yin. The symptoms are fever and sweating, dry mouth and lips, polydipsia, infirmity, weak breath, qi counterflow to vomit, weak rapid pulse, and red tongue with less coating.

[Formula Analysis] The heat pathogen has not been cleared but immersed into the interior. This formula is comprised of *Bái Hǔ Tāng* and *Mài Mén Dōng Tāng*, *zhú yè* and *shí gāo*, and this formula can clear heat and remove vexation. According to *Truth-Seeking Herbal Foundation* (*Běn Cǎo Qiú Zhēn*, 本草求真)[35], *zhú yè* combined with *shí gāo* can clear the heat of the stomach and release polydipsia. Therefore, they are both the chief medicines. *rén shēn* and *mài mén dōng*, both deputy medicines, can boost qi and nourish yin. According to *Shen Nong's Classic of the Materia Medica* (*Shén Nóng Běn Cǎo Jīng*, 神农本草经), *mài mén dōng* is mainly treat for the expiration of stomach collateral and emaciation with short breath, *bàn xià*, the assistant medicine, can harmonize the stomach and direct qi downward to arrest vomiting. And when it combines with enough *mài mén dōng*, the effect is marvelous. Because *bàn xià* will not dry up with *mài mén dōng*'s help, *mài mén dōng* will not be greasy with *bàn xià*'s help. It best fits the formulas to clear heat and nourish yin, harmonize the stomach and direct qi downward. *gān cǎo* and *jīng mǐ*, the envoy medicine, can benefit the stomach and harmonize the center, and also prevent stomach impairment from the cold nature of *zhú yè* and *shí gāo*. All herbs combined can clear heat and harmonize the stomach, supplement deficiency without evil lingering, which is an effective formula to clear and supplement in parallel.

[Clinical Application] This formula can treat not only the later stage of the febrile disease that still has residual heat and *qi-yin* damage, but also the warm disease that the pathogenic factor is in the qi level and has damaged qi and yin, especially for the fever caused by summer heat or latent heat with *qi-yin* damaged.

Zhī Zǐ Chǐ Tāng (Gardenia and Black Curd Beans Decoction, 栀子豉汤)
Treatise on Cold Damage (*Shāng Hán Lùn*, 伤寒论)

[Ingredient]

Zhī Zǐ (Fructus Gardeniae)　14 pcs, split (9 g)

Xiāng Chǐ (Semen Sojae Praeparatum)　4 *he*, cotton wrapped (9 g)

[Usage] First, adopt 4 *sheng* water to boil *zhī zǐ* [4 cups of water and cook it down to 1/2 cups], add *xiāng chǐ*. When there is 1.5 *sheng* left [1/2 cups remain],

dischard the dregs and divide them into 2. Take 1 cup when it is warm. If vomiting, take the other cup after stopping vomiting.

Modern Usage: Decocted by water.

[Action] Clear heat and remove vexation.

[Indication] General fever with vexation, insomnia due to dysphoria, chest stuffiness and pain, but it is soft, not hard when pressed, with a yellowish tongue coating.

[Formula Analysis] External febrile disease, the pathogenic factor enters the interior, and the heat disturbs the chest and diaphragm. *Zhī zǐ*, bitter in taste and cold in nature, can clear heat and remove vexation. According to *Ming Yi Bie Lu*, *zhī zǐ* can treat the vexation of the heart. *xiāng chǐ* (*dòu chǐ*, 豆豉), bitter in taste and cold in nature, has the property of light and floating, and can disperse constraint-heat. According to *Míng Yī Bié Lù*, it can treat exogenous febrile disease with headache and aversion to cold or heat...vexation and agitation. The two medicines match each other, which is a good formula to clear and disperse the constraint-heat of the chest to treat dysphoria.

[Clinical Application] In *Treatise on Cold Damage* (*Shāng Hán Lùn*, 伤寒论), this formula is treating for the symptoms of insomnia due to dysphoria or even toss and turn with vexation caused by sweating, vomiting, purging when getting the febrile disease by cold. The later generations have developed the usage of this formula. When the pathogen of warm-heat disease enters the qi level early, and the heat disturbs the chest and diaphragm with the symptoms of fever, vexation, restless sleep, and yellowish coating, it can be used.

Liáng Gé Sǎn (Diaphragm-Cooling Powder, 凉膈散)
Beneficial Formulas from the Taiping Imperial Pharmacy (*Tài Píng Huì Mín Hé Jì Jú Fāng*, 太平惠民和剂局方)

[Ingredient]
Chuān Dà Huáng (Radix Et Rhizoma Rhei)   20 *liang* (600 g)
Pò Xiāo (Mirabilitum)   20 *liang* (600 g)

Gān Cǎo (Radix Et Rhizoma Glycyrrhizae)   20 *liang* (600 g), fired

Shān Zhī Zǐ Rén (Fructus Gardeniae)   10 *liang* (300 g)

Bò Hé Yè (Herba Menthae)   10 *liang* (300 g), stem removed

Huáng Qín (Radix Scutellariae)   10 *liang* (300 g)

Lián Qiào (Fructus Forsythiae)   2.5 *jin* (1250 g)

[Usage]   Grind all herbs into powder. Adopt 1 *zhan* water to boil 2 *qian* of the powder, and add 7 pieces of *zhú yè* and little honey. When there is 7 *fen* left, abandon the dregs. Take the decoction when it is warm after a meal. Children are supposed to take 0.5 *qian*, and the dose can be adjusted according to their age. Stop taking it if diarrhea appears.

Modern Usage: Grind all herbs into powder. Adopt water to boil 9–12 g of the powder one time, and add 3 g of *zhú yè* and little honey. Also, the ingredients can be decocted by water directly, and the dosage should be reduced in proportion to the original formula.

[Action]   Clear heat, drain fire and promote defecation.

[Indication]   The exuberant heat in the upper and middle *jiao*, vexation and thirst, red face with dry lips, mouth or tongue sore, vexing heat in the chest and diaphragm, pharyngalgia and emetic bleeding, constipation and dark urine, delirious speech and manic raving, or acute infantile convulsion, red tongue with yellow coating, slippery and rapid pulse.

[Formula Analysis]   The exuberant heat in the upper and middle *jiao*. Excessive heartfire flaming up and lung-heat fumigation in the upper *jiao*, and stomach-heat upward rushing in the middle *jiao*. This formula uses a large number of *lián qiào* to clear heat and resolve toxins, combined with *huáng qín* and *shān zhī* to clear heat and drain fire. *Bò hé* and *zhú yè* can disperse constraint fire. The above 5 herbs discharge heat from the upper. *dà huáng* and *pò xiāo*, salty in taste and cold in nature, can clear up the heat of the middle *jiao* by purgation. Besides, *gān cǎo* and honey can not only relieve the urgent purgation of *dà huáng* and *pò xiāo* which clear the heat of the middle *jiao*, but also can resolve the heat toxin, moisten the dryness and store the stomach fluid to protect healthy qi by relieving the urgent purgation.

This formula can clear heat and purge in parallel, and let the evil of fire and heat drain from *Yangming*, which reflects the treatment of clearing by purgation. According to the *Basic Questions-Comprehensive Discourse on the Essentials of the Most Reliable* (*Sù Wèn-Zhì Zhēn Yào Dà Lùn*, 素问·至真要大论), the pathogenic heat in the interior need to be treated by salty and cold with the assistance of sweet and bitter. This formula uses salty, cold, sweet and bitter, which is deeply conforming to that guidance. The formula can clear and discharge the pathogenic heat of the upper and middle *jiao*, so that the chest and diaphragm can be cleared and all the syndromes can be relieved. Therefore, it is called "Diaphragm-Cooling Powder".

[Clinical Application] According to the editor's clinical experience, this formula is also effective for throat swelling with redness, pain and even decay, persistent high fever, polydipsia, constipation, red tongue with dry yellow coating. If the decay of the throat is severe, use Tin-Like Powder to blow the throat at the same time.

Section 2　Formulas that clears the *ying* level and cools the blood

The formulas for clearing the *ying* level and cooling the blood are treating the syndromes that pathogenic heat has entered into the *ying* level or blood level. When the pathogenic heatenters into the *ying* level, the symptoms are general fever, especially at night, thirst or not, insomnia with vexation, unconsciousness, delirious speech, crimson and dry tongue, deficient and rapid pulse. The tendency of disease of heat in blood level is more severe than heat in *ying* level. Besides the above symptoms, it mainly appears as blood heat causing bleeding, like hematemesis, epistaxis, bloody stool, hematuria, or macules due to intense heat, dark crimson tongue, rapid pulse. Those formulas are comprised of salty-cold herbs like *shuǐ niú jiǎo, xuán shēn*, and sweet-cold herbs like *shēng dì huáng, mài dōng*. According to *Treatise on Epidemic Febrile Disease* (*Wài Gǎn Wēn Rè Piān*, 外感温热篇) written by Ye Tian-shi[36], the heat in *ying* level can be vented through the qi level...the heat in blood level will consume blood and cause bleeding, which need to cool the blood

and dissipate blood stasis. Therefore, when the pathogen is in the *ying* level, it is supposed to combine those herbs like *yín huā*, *lián qiào*, *zhú yè xīn*, to vent heat from the *ying* level through the qi level and clear it. When heat enters into blood level, it will consume blood and cause bleeding, which need to combine those herbs can cool blood and dissipate stasis to calm the blood and extinguish the fire, dispel stasis and engender blood, like *chì sháo*, *dān pí*. The representative formulas are *Qīng Yíng Tāng* (Ying Level Heat-Clearing Decoction, 清营汤) and *Xī Jiǎo Dì Huáng Tāng* (Rhinoceros Horn and Rehmannia Decoction, 犀角地黄汤).

Qīng Yíng Tāng (Ying Level Heat-Clearing Decoction, 清营汤)
Systematic Differentiation of Warm Diseases (*Wēn Bìng Tiáo Biàn*, 温病条辨)

[Ingredient]

Xī Jiǎo (Cornu Rhinocerotis)　3 *qian*, instead of cornu bubali (30 g)

Shēng Dì Huáng (Radix Rehmanniae)　5 *qian* (15 g)

Xuán Shēn (Radix Scrophulariae)　3 *qian* (9 g)

Zhú Yè Xīn (Folium Pleioblasti)　1 *qian* (3 g)

Mài Dōng (Radix Ophiopogonis)　3 *qian* (9 g)

Dān Shēn (Radix Et Rhizoma Salviae Miltiorrhizae)　2 *qian* (6 g)

Huáng Lián (Rhizoma Coptidis)　1.5 *qian* (4.5 g)

Yín Huā (Flos Lonicerae Japonicae)　3 *qian* (9 g)

Lián Qiào (Fructus Forsythiae)　2 *qian*, including core (6 g)

[Usage]　Adopt 8 cups of water to boil all the herbs until there are 3 cups left. Take the decoction 3 times a day.

Modern Usage: Decocted by water.

[Action]　Clear the *Ying* level and resolve toxins, vent heat, and nourish yin.

[Indication]　The warm pathogen transmits into the *Ying* level initially, causing general fever, especially at night, thirst or not, insomnia with vexation, unconsciousness sometimes, crimson and dry tongue, deficient and rapid pulse, or faint macules.

[Formula Analysis]　The warm pathogen is not cleared up in the qi level,

and gradually transmits into the *ying* level. According to the *Basic Questions-Comprehensive Discourse on the Essentials of the Most Reliable* (*Sù Wèn Zhì Zhēn Yào Dà Lùn*, 素问·至真要大论), "if the heat has encroached upon the interior, that is treated with salty [flavor] and cold [qi]. Assist with sweet and bitter [flavor]". *xī jiǎo* now it will be replaced by cornu bubali, salty in taste and cold in nature, can enter the heart channel, clear the *ying* level, resolve toxins, and discharge heat from the blood. So it is the chief medicine. Intense heat damages yin-fluid, so the deputy medicines are *shēng dì huáng, xuán shēn, mài dōng*. Use sweet-cold and salty-cold herbs in parallel to clear the heat in the *ying* level by nourishing yin and engendering fluid. *huáng lián*, bitter in taste and cold in nature, can clear heart heat, drain fire and resolve toxins. *dān shēn*, bitter in taste and a little cold in nature, can clear heat, cool the blood and remove vexation. *yíng huā* and *lián qiào* used in parallel can clear heat and resolve toxins. The bove four herbs are all assistant medicines. Moreover *zhú yè xīn*, the envoy medicine, with acrid, bland and sweet in taste and cold in nature, is good at clearing heart-heat. In addition, *yíng huā, lián qiào* and *zhú yè xīn*, all cold in nature and light in property, can vent and discharge the evil to vent heat-evil from the *ying* level through the qi level and clear it. Combining all the medicines can clear the *ying* level, resolve toxins, vent heat and nourish yin. It is the main formula for treating heat-damaging *ying-yin* [营阴].

[Clinical Application]   This formula treats the syndrome that warm-heat pathogens enter the *ying* level. It also can be used for the syndrome that the pathogens enter the *ying* level initially while not being completely cleared in the qi level. It can clear both *qi* and *ying* levels. If the symptoms of convulsive syncope or limbs convulsion, it is because the heat in the *ying* level causes stirring wind and we can add *gōu téng, dān pí, líng yáng jiǎo*, or little Purple Snow Elixir to clear heat and extinguish wind.

Xī Jiǎo Dì Huáng Tāng (Rhinoceros Horn and Rehmannia Decoction, 犀角地黄汤)

Valuable Prescriptions of Emergency (*Bèi Jí Qiān Jīn Fāng*, 备急千金方)[37]

[Ingredient]

Xī Jiǎo (Cornu Rhinocerotis)　instead of cornu bubali (30 g)

Shēng Dì Huáng (Radix Rehmanniae)　5 *qian* (15 g)

Sháo Yào (Radix Paeoniae)　3 *liang* (9 g)

Mǔ Dān Pí (Cortex Moutan)　2 *liang* (6 g)

[Usage]　Ground all the herbs into pieces. Adopt 9 *sheng* water to boil until there is 3 *sheng* left. Divide the decoction 3 times to take.

Modern Usage: Decocted by water.

[Action]　Clear heat and nourish yin, cool the blood, and dissapate blood stasis.

[Indication]

1. The warm and heat pathogens enter into the blood level deeply and intense heat cause bleeding, which appears as hematemesis, epistaxis, bloody stool and hematuria, or unconsciousness and delirious speech, crimson spotted tongue, rapid pulse.

2. Retention of blood and stasis, excessive joy like going mad, desire to rinse the mouth with water but no desire to swallow, no abdominal fullness but feeling fullness, black stool, and easily defecating.

[Formula Analysis]　The warm and heat pathogens enter the blood level deeply and cause bleeding. *Xī jiǎo*, salty in taste and cold in nature, can clear heat, cool blood and resolve toxins. According to *The Grand Compendium of Materia Medica* (*Běn Cǎo Gāng Mù*, 本草纲目), it can treat hematemesis, epistaxis, bloody stool, hematuria, blood amassment by cold damage, mania and incoherent speech, jaundice and macules...drain the liver and cool the heart, clear stomach and resolve toxins. *Shēng dì huáng*, sweet in taste and cold in nature, can nourish yin and clear heat, cool the blood, and stanch bleeding. So the above two herbs are both the chief medicines. *Chì sháo*, bitter in taste and a little cold in nature, can regulate *ying* and discharge heat, cool the blood and dissipate blood stasis. *Mǔ dān pí*, acrid and bitter,a

little cold in nature, can drain the fire hiding in the blood, cool the blood and dissipate stasis. The two herbs are both deputy medicines. They can not only strengthen *xī jiǎo* and *shēng dì huáng*'s function of cooling blood, but also prevent the blood from stagnation, which makes stanch bleeding without stasis. The heat enters the blood level, consumes the blood and causes bleeding. If the heat lingers, the blood will still restless; without enriching yin, the fire can not be extinguish, without dissolving the stasis, the new blood can not engender. This formula can nourish yin while clearing the heat, which makes heat cleared, blood harmonization without the worry of consuming blood. In addition, it dissipates blood stasis while cooling the blood, which makes stanch bleeding without stasis. Although there are only four herbs, it has a particular function with good effect by the precise combination of medicines.

[Clinical Application]   This formula is primarily designed for the pathogens of warm and heat blazing in the blood level. It is an crucial formula to treat kinds of blood loss due to heat invading the blood level. It is better to use fresh *shēng dì huáng* than the dry one because the fresh one's function of clearing heat, cooling the blood, and stanching bleeding is better. As for the *sháo yào* in the formula, *chì sháo* is always the first choice because its function of cooling blood and dissipating stasis is better than *bái sháo*. However if the damage to yin and blood is severe, *bái sháo* can also be used.

Section 3   Formulas that clears heat and resolves toxins

The formulas for clearing heat and resolving toxins are suitable for the syndromes of an epidemic, warm toxins, sores, ulcers and furuncle toxins. An externally-contracted pathogen causes epidemic and warm toxins with strong infectiousness. The symptoms are always vexation, agitation and mania, intense heat causing macules or red swollen head and face, thirst, sore throat, *etc.* The symptoms of sores, ulcers and furuncle toxins are various because of the differences in the disease location. In a word, the heat toxin can be whole the body or localized, in the qi level or blood level. We need to take concrete analysis according to the patient's

clinical manifestation. The formulas in this section are comprised of the herbs that can clear heat and resolve toxins, like *huáng lián, huáng qín, huáng bǎi, zhī zǐ, yín huā, lián qiào, bǎn lán gēn, xuán shēn, pú gōng yīng, zǐ huā dì dīng, etc.* Besides, according to the specific symptoms, we can combine herbs that can cool blood, move qi, scatter wind. The representative formulas are *Huáng Lián Jiě Dú Tāng* (Coptis Toxin-Resolving Decoction, 解毒汤), *Qīng Wēn Bài Dú Yǐn* (Epidemic-Clearing Toxin-Resolving Beverage, 清瘟败毒饮), *Pǔ Jì Xiāo Dú Yǐn Zi* (Universal Relief Toxin-Removing Beverage, 普济消毒饮), *Xiān Fāng Huó Mìng Yǐn* (Immortal Formula Life-Giving Beverage, 仙方活命饮), *etc.*

Huáng Lián Jiě Dú Tāng (Coptis Toxin-Resolving Decoction, 黄连解毒汤) *Arcane Essentials from the Imperial Library* (*Wài Tái Mì Yào,* 外台秘要) [38] *quoting Cui's formula*

[Ingredient]

Huáng Lián (Rhizoma Coptidis)   3 *liang* (9 g)

Huáng Qín (Radix Scutellariae)   2 *liang* (6 g)

Huáng Bǎi (Cortex Phellodendri Chinensis)   2 *liang* (6 g)

Zhī Zǐ (Fructus Gardeniae)   14 *mei*, Broken (9 g)

[Usage]   Cut all the herbs and adopt 6 *sheng* water to boil until there is 2 *sheng* left. Divide the decoction, take in two doses.

Modern Usage: Decocted by water.

[Action]   Drain fire and resolve toxins.

[Indication]   All the excess fire-heat syndromes, mania and vexation, dry mouth and throat, great fever with retching, disordered speech, insomnia, hematemesis and epistaxis, even appearing macules, carbuncle and furuncle toxin, yellow greasy coating, rapid solid pulse.

[Formula Analysis]   The pathogen of fire-heat toxin is full of the *sanjiao*. Intense fire-heat is accumulaties and becomes a toxin, so resolving the toxin must first drain the fire. Draining fire is the so-called toxin resolution. This formula uses a large dosage of *huáng lián*, the chief medicine, to drain the fire of the heart and middle *jiao*.

Huáng qín can drain the fire in the upper *jiao*, and *huáng bǎi* can drain the fire in the lower *jiao*. *Zhī zǐ* can drain all the fire of *san jiao* by guiding the heat to be drained through the bladder. The above three are the assistant medicines. These medicines, conformed to direct repulsion with bitter-cold medicines, can remove the fire evil and resolve the heat toxin. Therefore, the formula was named.

[Clinical Application]

1. This is the representative formula to treat the pathogen of fire-heat toxin filling the *san jiao* so that using *huáng lián*, *huáng qín*, *huáng bǎi* and *zhī zǐ* those great bitter and cold medicines. It is suitable for intense heat toxin without liquid damage, yellow greasy coating, and strong rapid pulse. If the heat has damaged fluid and the tongue is crimson with a rapid solid pulse, we can not use this formula because the bitter-cold herbs easily transforming into dryness to yin-damage.

2. During the clinical application, this formula is always combined with *yíng huā* and *lián qiào* to strengthen the function of clearing heat and resolving toxins. If treating the sores, ulcers and furuncle toxins, it is better to add *pú gōng yīng*, *zǐ huā dì dīng*, *lù dòu yī*, *gān zhōng huáng*, etc. If defecation is not smooth or causes constipation, we can add *dà huáng* to promote defecation and let the heat toxin drained by urine and stool. If the formula is made into water pills, it is called *zhī zǐ jīn huā dān* according to *The Complete Works of [Zhang] Jing-yue* (*Jǐng Yuè Quán Shū*, 景岳全书). The decoction is for urgent conditions while the pill is for moderate conditions. There is a slight difference.

Qīng Wēn Bài Dú Yǐn (Epidemic-Clearing Toxin-Resolving Beverage, 清瘟败毒饮)
Achievements Regarding Epidemic Rashes (*Yì Zhěn Yì Dé*, 疫疹一得)[39]

[Ingredient]

Shí Gāo (Gypsum Fibrosum)　large dose 6–8 *liang,* mid dose 2–4 *liang,* small dose 0.8–1.2 *liang* (24–250 g)

Shēng Dì (Radix Rehmanniae)　large dose 0.6–1 *liang,* mid dose 2–5 *qian,* small dose 2–4 *qian* (12–30 g)

Xī Jiǎo (Cornu Rhinocerotis)　large dose 6–8 *qian,* mid dose 3–5 *qian,* small

dose 2–4 *qian*, instead by *shuǐ niú jiǎo* (30–60 g)

Huáng Lián (Rhizoma Coptidis)   large dose 4–6 *qian*, mid dose 2–4 *qian*, small dose 1–1.5 *qian* (3–18 g)

Zhī Zǐ (Fructus Gardeniae)   (9 g)

Jié Gěng (Radix Platycodonis   (6 g)

Huáng Qín (Radix Scutellariae)   (9 g)

Zhī Mǔ (Rhizoma Anemarrhenae)   (9 g)

Chì Sháo (Radix Paeoniae Rubra)   (9 g)

Xuán Shēn (Radix Scrophularia)   (15 g)

Lián Qiào (Fructus Forsythiae)   (9 g)

Gān Cǎo (Radix Et Rhizoma Glycyrrhizae)   (6 g)

Dān Pí (Cortex Moutan)   (9 g)

Zhú Yè (Folium Phyllostachydis Henonis)   (15 g)

[The original book does not write the dose of above 10 herbs]

[Usage]   Firstly, boil the *shí gāo* [boiling 10–15 mins] and add all the rest herbs. Mix *xī jiǎo* and cuttlefish juice. Take them together.

Modern Usage: Decocted by water.

[Action]   Clear heat from the qi level and cool blood, drain fire and resolve toxins.

[Indication]   Heat toxin of an epidemic, blazing of both qi and blood, intense headache as splitting, mania and vexation, dry mouth with throat pain, great fever with belching, disordered speech and insomnia, hematemesis and epistaxis, macules due to intense heat, spotted tongue with parched lips. The pulse is deep and sink, or deep thin and rapid, or deep rapid, or floating rapid.

[Formula Analysis]   Epidemic is a kind of warm-heat disease caused by an epidemic pathogen, with strong infectiousness. This formula is formed by *Bái Hǔ Tāng*, *Xī Jiǎo Dì Huáng Tāng*, and *Huáng Lián Jiě Dú Tāng* with modifying. Only a hefty dose of cold herbs can cool the blazing of both qi and blood, deal with the fullness of heat toxin. The formula uses a hefty dose of *shí gāo* as the chief medicine to clear the stomach heat. The stomach is the sea of water and grain, and the source

of qi and blood production. Moreover, the qi of twelve meridians comes from the stomach. Besides, *yangming* is a meridian with much qi and blood. If the heat of the *yangming* stomach meridian is cleared, the fire of the twelve meridians will be dissipated and the intense heat will also retreat. *Xī jiǎo*, *huáng lián* and *huáng qín* can clear the fire of heart and lung in the upper *jiao*. *Dān pí*, *zhī zǐ* and *chì sháo* can clear the fire of the liver meridian. *Shēng dì* and *zhī mǔ* can clear heat and rescue yin. The above eight herbs are all deputy medicines. *Lián qiào* can clear heat and resolve toxins. *Xuán shēn* can nourish yin and resolve toxins. *Zhú yè* can clear the heart heat and remove vexation. *Jié gěng* can make the function of herbs apply on the upper. The above four herbs are all assistant medicines. *Gān cǎo*, the envoy medicine, can resolve the heat toxin, regulate all the herbs and harmonize the stomach qi. All herbs are used together to clear the heat in qi level, cool blood, drain fire and resolve toxins. Because this formula treats the heat toxin of epidemic especially, it is called "Epidemic-Clearing Toxin-Resolving Beverage".

[Clinical Application]　　The formula treats the heat toxin of an epidemic filling the whole body and the blazing of the qi and blood. We should grasp the dosage of each herb according to the severity of the disease in the clinic. If the heat toxin is potent and the diseases stage is severe, it is supposed use a large dosage of herbs. Meanwhile, the formula is so cold that the patient with mild disease can take it in small dosages in order to not impair the stomach qi.

Pǔ Jì Xiāo Dú Yǐn Zi (**Universal Relief Toxin-Removing Beverage**, 普济消毒饮子)
Dong-Yuan's Tried and Tested Formulas (*Dōng Yuán Shì Xiào Fāng,* 东垣试效方)[40]

[Ingredient]

Huáng Lián (Rhizoma Coptidis)　　5 *liang* (15 g)

Huáng Qín (Radix Scutellariae)　　5 *liang* (15 g)

Jú Hóng (Exocarpium Citri Rubrum)　　2 *qian* (6 g)

Xuán Shēn (Radix Scrophulariae)　　2 *qian* (6 g)

Gān Cǎo (Radix Et Rhizoma Glycyrrhizae)　　2 *qian* (6 g)

Lián Qiào (Fructus Forsythiae)　　1 *qian* (3 g)

Shǔ Zhān Zǐ (Fructus Arctii) 1 *qian* (3 g)

Bǎn Lán Gēn (Radix Isatidis) 1 *qian* (3 g)

Mǎ Bó (Lasiosphaera Seu Calvatia) 1 *qian* (3 g)

Bò He (Herba Menthae) 1 *qian* (3 g)

Bái Jiāng Cán (Bombyx Batryticatus) 7 *fen* (2 g)

Shēng Má (Rhizoma Cimicifugae) 7 *fen* (2 g)

Chái Hú (Radix Bupleuri) 2 *qian* (6 g)

Jié Gěng (Radix Platycodonis) 2 *qian* (6 g)

[One formula is without *bò he* but adding *rén shēn 3 qian*]

[Usage] Grind all the herbs into powder and divide them into 2 parts: one part is mixing with hot water and taking it regularly. And make the other part into a pill with honey, and melt it in the mouth.

Modern Usage: Decocted by water, the dosage can be modified according to the original proportion.

[Action] Clear heat and resolve toxins, disperse wind and dissipate evil.

[Indication] Swollen-head infection. At first, there is fever and aversion to cold, heavy feeling of limbs. Then, the head and face become red and swollen, the eyes cannot open, throat discomfort, thirst with tongue dryness, yellow coating, floating rapid and strong pulse.

[Formula Analysis] Swollen-head infection, also named *Dà Tóu Tiān Xíng* [大头天行], is caused by the pathogen of wind-heat epidemic toxin congesting the upper *jiao* and attacking the head and face. The formula uses *huáng lián* and *huáng qín* as the chief medicines to clear and drain the heat toxin of the upper *jiao*, *xuán shēn* can nourish yin and engender fluid, drain fire and resolve toxins, soften hardness and dissipate masses, *jú hóng* can rectify qi and dissolve phlegm, *gān cǎo* can drain fire and resolve toxins. The above three herbs are all deputy medicines. *lián qiào*, *bǎn lán gēn and mǎ bó* can clear heat and resolve toxins. Besides, *lián qiào* also can dissipate masses and disperse swelling. Moreover, *mǎ bó* also can clear and relieve the throat. *Shǔ zhān zǐ*, *bò he*, *bái jiāng cán* can scatter and dissipate wind-heat. Also, *shǔ zhān zǐ* and *bái jiāng cán* can clear and relieve the throat, dissipate masses

and disperse swelling. The above six are assistant medicines. *shēng má* and *chái hú* can raise and lift clear yang, scatter and dissipate wind heat. *Jié gěng can* clear and relieve the throat, and make the function of herbs apply to the upper. The three herbs are envoy medicines. The formula includes clearing and dissipating, descending and ascending, can clear heat and resolve toxins, scatter wind, and dissipate evil. When swollen-head infection is prevalent, taking this formula can relieve it universally and remove the warm toxin. Therefore, this formula is called "Universal Relief Toxin-Removing Beverage".

[Clinical Application] This is the regular formula to treat the swollen-head infections. The original formula notes that if the stool is hard, it is supposed to add 1–2 *qian dà huáng* simmered with rice wine to promote defecation. Moreover, the effect is pretty good. If the patient has a deficiency of healthy qi, one can add some *dǎng shēn* appropriately to reinforce healthy qi to dispel evil.

Xiān Fāng Huó Mìng Yǐn (Immortal Formula Life-Giving Beverage, 仙方活命饮)
Fine Formulas for Women with Annotations and Commentary (Jiào Zhù Fù Rén Liáng Fāng, 校注妇人良方)[41]

[Ingredient]

Bái Zhǐ (Radix Angelicae Dahuricae)

Bèi Mǔ (Bulbus Fritillaria)

Fáng Fēng (Radix Saposhnikoviae)

Chì Sháo (Radix Paeoniae Rubra)

Dāng Guī (Radix Angelicae Sinensis)

Gān Cǎo (Radix Et Rhizoma Glycyrrhizae)

Zào Jiǎo Cì (Spina Gleditsiae)   fried

Chuān Shān Jiǎ (Squama Manitis)   honey-fried

Tiān Huā Fěn (Radix Trichosanthis)

Rǔ Xiāng (Olibanum)

Mò Yào (Myrrha)

The above all are 1 *qian* (3 g)

Jīn Yín Huā (Flos Lonicerae Japonicae)

Chén Pí (Pericarpium Citri Reticulatae)

The above two are both 3 *qian* (9 g)

[Usage] Adopt a big bowl of rice wine to decoct all the herbs and take it when it is almost hot.

Modern Usage: Decocted by water, or half water with half rice wine.

[Action] Clear heat and resolve toxins, disperse swelling and promote suppuration, invigorate blood to relieve pain.

[Indication] Initial toxins of sores and swelling, red swelling and pain, general fever and aversion to cold, thin white or yellowish coating, rapid and strong pulse, which belong to yang syndrome.

[Formula Analysis] The congestion of heat toxin and stagnation of qi and blood causes the toxins of sores and swelling. The formula uses *jīn yín huā*, the holy herb for carbuncles, to clear heat, resolve toxins, disperse sores and carbuncles. According to *The Grand Compendium of Materia Medica* (*Běn Cǎo Gāng Mù*, 本草纲目), it can treat swelling toxins, carbuncle...clear heat, and resolve toxins. So *jīn yín huā* is the chief medicine, *fáng fēng* and *bái zhǐ* can dispel wind and disperse swelling, *dāng guī* and *chì sháo* can invigorate blood and unblock the collaterals, *rǔ xiāng* and *mò yào* can dissipate stasis to relieve pain, *chén pí* can rectify qi to resolve stagnations. The above six herbs are deputy medicines, *bèi mǔ* and *tiān huā fěn* can clear heat and dissolve phlegm, dissipate masses and disperse swelling, *gān cǎo* can drain fire and resolve toxins, dissipate carbuncle and disperse swelling. The above three herbs are the assistant medicines, *chuān shān jiǎ* and *zào jiǎo cì* can disperse swelling and promote suppuration. Futhermore, their property is moving and dispersing, which can go to the lesion directly. Rice wine can invigorate blood and unblock the collaterals to motivate the herbs' potential. The above three are the assistant medicines. All the herbs used together can clear heat and resolve toxins, disperse swelling, promote suppuration and invigorate blood to relieve pain.

[Clinical Application]

1. This is the preferred formula for treating initial sores and swelling toxins. All the symptoms of initial sores and swelling toxin that red swelling and pain belong to excess yang syndrome can use the formula. If the pus has not formed, taking it can dissipate the sores. If the pus has formed, taking it can promote ulceration. Therefore *Golden Mirror of the Medical Tradition* (*Yī Zōng Jīn Jiàn*, 医宗金鉴) admires this formula as the holy medicine for sores and carbuncles, and the first formula for external disease.

2. If the pain of sores or swelling toxin is severe, we can reduce *rǔ xiāng* and *mò yào*. If the red swelling pain is severe, we can add *zǐ huā dì dīng*, *pú gōng yīng*, and *lián qiào*. If the patient combine with constipation, add *dà huáng*. If great heat and thirst with fluid damaged, we need to remove *fáng fēng*, *bái zhǐ* and *chén pí*.

Wǔ Wèi Xiāo Dú Yǐn (Five Ingredients Toxin-Removing Beverage, 五味消毒饮)
Golden Mirror of the Medical Tradition (*Yī Zōng Jīn Jiàn*, 医宗金鉴)

[Ingredient]

Jīn Yín Huā (Flos Lonicerae Japonicae)   3 *qian* (20 g)

Yě Jú Huā (Flos Chrysanthemi Indici)

Pú Gōng Yīng (Herba Taraxaci)

Zǐ Huā Dì Dīng (Herba Violae)

Zǐ Bèi Tiān Kuí Zǐ (Radix Semiaquilegiae)

The above four are all 1.2 *qian* (9 g)

[Usage]   Adopt 2 *zhong* water to boil all the herbs. When it is about to boil to eight-tenths, add half *zhong* of lime-free wine [无灰酒]. Take it after boiling it 2 or 3 times. Decoct the dregs in the same way and take it. Cover the quilt until sweating.

Modern Usage: Boil with water, adds 1 or 2 spoons of rice wine and take it.

[Action]   Clear heat, resolve toxins and dissipate swelling.

[Indication]   Various furuncle toxins, local redness, swelling, hotness and pain. At first, it is like a millet, with hard roots as deep as nails. Red tongue with yellow coating and strong rapid pulse.

[Formula Analysis]   The *Basic Questions-Discourse on the Generation of Qi and Communication with Heaven* (*Sù Wèn-Shēng Qì Tōng Tiān Lùn*, 素问·生气通天论) said that "In case of overintake with rich food, the feet generate large boils (furuncle)". The furuncle toxin is caused by the attack of warm-heat fire toxin and eating much greasy and surfeit flavor food which makes the heat accumulate in the interior and stagnation of qi and blood. The formula uses *jīn yín huā* as the chief medicine to clear heat and resolve toxins, cool blood and dissipate swelling. *Yě jú huā* and *zǐ bèi tiān kuí zǐ* are good at resolving the furuncle toxin. *Pú gōng yīng* and *zǐ huā dì dīng* can clear heat, resolve toxins, and dissipate swelling. The above four herbs are all assistant medicines. Little rice wine can promote the herbs' potential and blood circulation, which is the envoy medicine. This formula's five herbs are all good at clearing heat and resolving toxins. So the formula is named "Five Ingredients Toxin-Removing Beverage".

[Clinical Application]   This formula effectively treats furuncle and swelling toxins. According to the experience of Professor Yue Mei-zhong[42], the curative effect will be better if it adds *chóng lóu*, *bàn zhī lián* and *fěn gān cǎo*.

Section 4   Formulas that clears *zang-fu* heat

The clearing *zang-fu* heat formula applies to the syndrome of abnormal exuberance in *zang-fu*. Due to the *zang-fu* on which pathogenic heat focuses on the clinical manifestation. Moreover, the formula consists of different kinds of heat-clearing medicine due to the characteristics of *zang-fu*. For example, clearing heart fire use *huáng qín*, *huáng lián*, *zhú yè* mainly, clearing spleen and stomach fire uses *shí gāo* mostly, clearing liver heart uses *lóng dǎn cǎo*, *huáng qín*, *huáng lián*, *hēi shān zhī* mostly, clearing lung heat uses *lú gēn*, *sāng bái pí* mainly, clearing large intestine uses *huáng qín*, *bái tóu wēng* mostly. There are typical formulas such as *Xiè Xīn Tāng* (heart-draining decoction, 泻心汤), *Dǎo Chì Sǎn* (red-guiding powder, 导赤散) for clearing heart fire, *Lóng Dǎn Xiè Gān Tāng* (gentian liver-draining decoction, 龙胆泻肝汤), *Zuǒ Jīn Wán* (left metal pill, 左金丸) for clearing liver fire, *Qīng Wèi*

Săn (stomach-heat-clearing powder, 清胃散) clearing stomach fire, *Wĕi Jìng Tāng* (phragmites stem decoction, 苇茎汤), *Xiè Bái Săn* (white-draining powder, 泻白散) for clearing lung fire, *Sháo Yào Tāng* (peony decoction, 芍药汤), *Gé Gēn Huáng Qín Huáng Lián Tāng* (Pueraria, Scutellaria, and Coptis decoction, 葛根黄芩黄连汤), *Bái Tóu Wēng Tāng* (pulsatilla decoction, 白头瓮汤) for clearing large intestine fire. These formulas belong to the therapeutic method of "treat heat with cold", "treat excess with drainage", *Basic Questions-Comprehensive Discourse on the Essentials of the Most Reliable* (*Sù Wèn-Zhì Zhēn Yào Dà Lùn*, 素问·至真要大论).

Xiè Xīn Tāng (Heart-Draining Decoction, 泻心汤)
Essentials from the Synopsis of Golden Chamber (*Jīn Guì Yào Lüè*, 金匮要略)

[Ingredient]

Dà Huáng (Radix Et Rhizoma Rhei)   2 *liang* (6 g)

Huáng Lián (Rhizoma Coptidis)   1 *liang* (3 g)

Huáng Qín (Radix Scutellariae)   3 *liang* (9 g)

[Usage]   Three herbs in the original formula with 3 *sheng* water boiled into 1 *sheng*, then drink them immediately.

Modern usage: Decocted with water.

[Action]   Purge fire and clear heat.

[Indication]   For patients with internal blazing of heart and stomach fire, force moving of blood, spitting of blood and bleeding, constipation and bloody urine, yellow and greasy coating. Moreover, this formula can also treat symptoms like accumulated heat in *Sanjiao*, redness swelling, the pain in the eye, aphtha of the mouth and tongue, abscesses.

[Formula Analysis]   Internal blazing of the heart and stomach fire that damages yang collateral and causes bleeding. This formula use *dà huáng* as the chief medicine for draining fire and heat by its bit taste and the moving stasis ability. Like Tang Rong-chuan once said, "*Dà Huáng*, this herb can bring forth the fresh through the stale...promote descending without pathogens lingering." Use *huáng lián, huáng qín* as deputy medicine for their function of purging fire and clearing heat which can

cooperate with *dà huáng* to make the fire subdued, heat cleared, and the bleeding stopped by itself. This formula is excellent for treating to treat blood heat and blood-spitting, which can stop bleeding without lingering pathogens.

[Clinical Application] This formula recorded as to treat "heart qi insufficiency, blood spitting and bleeding from the *Synopsis of Golden Chamber* (Jīn Kuì Yào Lüè, 金匮要略). Heart qi insufficiency is caused by heat in excess, and this formula can stop bleeding by purging fire and clearing heat. Purging the heart that is draining fire and promotes bleeding is equivalent to stopping it. And this formula can treat vicarious menstruation and lochia after delivering a baby because of heart fire blazing and bleeding. According to the late Japanese famous doctor Otsuka Keisetsu[43]'s experience, "taking medicine cold when the patient is bleeding is preferred."

Dăo Chì Săn (Red-Guiding Powder, 导赤散)
Craft of Medicines and Patterns for Children (*Xiăo Ér Yào Zhèng Zhí Jué,* 小儿药证直诀)

[Ingredient]
Xiān Dì HuángHuáng (Fresh Radix Rehmanniae Recens)
Mù TōngTōng (Caulis Akebiae)
Gān Căo (Fresh Radix Tenuis Glycyrrhizae)
Shāo Shāo (Fresh Radix Tenuis Glycyrrhizae)
All the herbs equal distribution

[Usage] Grind herbs into a powder, then take 3 *qian* of the powder with 1 *zhan* water and *zhú yè* and decoct them into 5 *fen*, drink it warmly after a meal.

Modern usage: Add modest *zhú yè* and decoct it with water. Its dosage changes the ratio of the original formula.

[Action] Clear heart [fire] and promote urination.

[Indication] People who have heat in heart meridian, red face, vexation and agitation, thirst and want to drink cold, aphtha in mouth and tongue, or the heat moved to the small intestine and have bloody difficult and painful urination, red tongue tip

with rapid pulse.

[Formula Analysis] Heat stagnates in the heart meridian and turns into fire flames upward. There is an interior-exterior relationship between the heart and the small intestine, and heat in the heart will move to the small intestine. *Xiān dì huáng* in this formula is used as chief medicine for clearing heat, cooling the blood and nourishing yin because of the taste of sweet, bitter and cold, which can clear heart heat, cool heart blood and nourish heart yin, and kidney fluid which can coordinate heart fire and then the heat in the heart is cleared by itself, *mù tōng* is used as deputy medicine for subduing fire and promoting urination because of its taste of bitter and cold which can get the heat in heart out of the small intestine, and when cooperating with *xiān dì huáng*, it can promote urination without damaging yin. *Zhú yè* is used as an assistant medicine for clearing heart fire, promoting urination and releasing vexation because of its taste of acrid, bland, and natural are sweet and cold. *Gān cǎo shēng, gān cǎo shāo* is used as an envoy medicine for clearing heat, draining fire, relaxing the tension and stopping pain. With these four herbs, heart fire can be cleared, yin can be nourished, urination can be promoted and heat can be removed. Because red belongs to the heart and this formula can eliminate the heat from the heart and the small intestine by urine, this formula is called *Dǎo Chì Sǎn*.

[Clinical Application]

1. This formula guides out excess heart fire via the small intestine, which is the typical formula for clearing heart fire and promoting urination. After this, there has a saying:"one formula uses *huáng qín* instead of *gān cǎo*; another formula uses *dēng xīn cǎo*." According to the clinical experience of the editor, if the patient has the exuberance of heart fire, adding *huáng qín*; if the patient has short and dark urine, adding *dēng xīn cǎo* is better.

2. In this formula, *hàn lián cǎo, bái máo gēn, xuè yú tàn, chē qián zǐ, ē jiāo zhū* which have the function of reinforcing the cooling function and stop bleeding, promoting urination and relieving strangury, can be used to treat bloody strangury.

Lóng Dǎn Xiè Gān Tāng (Gentian Liver-Draining Decoction, 龙胆泻肝汤)
Medical Formulas Collected and Analyzed (*Yī Fāng Jí Jiě,* 医方集解)[44]

[Ingredient]

Lóng Dǎn Cǎo (Radix et Rhizoma Gentianae)　stir-bake with rice-wine (6 g)

Huáng Qín (Radix Scutellariae)　dry-fried (6 g)

Zhī Zǐ (Fructus Gardeniae)　stir-bake with wine (9 g)

Zé Xiè (Rhizoma Alismatis)　(9 g)

Mù Tōng (Caulis Akebiae)　(6 g)

Chē Qián Zǐ (Semen Plantaginis)　(9 g)

Dāng Guī (Radix Angelicae Sinensis)　washing with rice wine

Shēng Dì Huáng (Fresh Radix Rehmanniae Recens)　stir-bake with wine (12 g)

Chái Hú (Radix Bupleuri)　(4.5 g)

Gān Cǎo (Radix et Rhizoma Glycyrrhizae)　slices are used after cleansing (3 g)

[Usage]　The original book does not record the administration.

Modern Usage: Decocted with water. Alternatively, it can be made into pills, taken 6 g with warm water, and twice a day.

[Action]　Clear liver fire, eliminate damp-heat.

[Indication]

1. Patients with excess fire in liver and gallbladder, [manifested as] hypochondriac pain and headache, bitter mouth and red eyes, deaf and ear swelling.

2. Patients with damp-heat pouring downward in liver meridian, [leads to] turbid and dribbling urine, vaginal itching and swelling, sinew atrophy and damp perineum, bloody and white leukorrhea, red side of the tongue with yellow greasy coating, and strong rapid wiry pulse.

[Formula Analysis]　*Lóng dǎn cǎo* in this formula is used as the chief medicine aim for clearing excess fire of liver and gallbladder, it is bitter and cold. *Huáng qín* and *zhī zǐ* are used as deputy medicine for clearing heat and drying dampness which can help *lóng dǎn cǎo* drain liver fire and clear damp-heat because

their taste of cold and bitter, *zé xiè*, *mù tōng*, *chē qián zǐ* are used as assistant medicine for clearing damp-heat and make excess fire and damp-heat go through urination. The liver is the viscera for storing blood; if the liver fire flames, the yin blood will be damaged. If added too much bitter and dry medicine, the yin blood will be damaged as well, so *dāng guī* and *shēng dì huáng* is used to nourish liver blood and dispel pathogen without damaging the healthy qi, *chái hú*, which is the channel medicine of the liver, is used as envoy medicine for governing free activity of the liver qi, and *gān cǎo* is used as an envoy medicine as well for harmonizing the actions of all medicines in a formula and preventing the stomach from such bitter and cold medicine. The advantage of this formula is that it combines nourishing and reduction perfectly, which can drain liver fire, clear damp heat, and avoid damaging yin blood by this bitter and cold medicine.

[Clinical Application]

1. This formula can clear liver and gallbladder fire and drain damp heat. Anyone with an excess fire in the liver and gallbladder or damp heat in the liver meridian without damaging fluid can use this formula to direct repulsion with bitter-cold medicines.

2. The medicine in this formula is too bitter and cold which will hurt the spleen and stomach, so the use of the formula should be stopped when the patient recovers. *Lóng dǎn cǎo* and *zhī zǐ* are fried with alcohol, and *huáng qín* is dry-fried to avoid damaging stomach qi with bitter and cold medicine. Futhermore, the dosage of *lóng dǎn cǎo* should not be too big, which should be between 3 g to 6 g.

Zuǒ Jīn Wán (Huí Lìng Wán) (Left Metal Pill, 左金丸)
Essential Teachings of [Zhu] Dan Xi (Dān Xī Xīn Fǎ, 丹溪心法)

[Ingredient]

Huáng Lián (Rhizoma Coptidis)　6 *liang* (180 g)

Wú Zhū Yú (Fructus Evodiae)　1 *liang* (30 g)

[Usage]　Grind the medicines into a powder, make them into pills with water or process it into cakes, then steam, take 50 pills with rice soup.

Modern Usage: Grind the medicine in the original formula into a powder, make it into pills with water. Or makes into pills, take 2–3 g with warm water. Or decoct with water and its dosage changes at the ratio of the original formula.

[Action] Clear liver heat and drain fire, direct counterflow downward and arrest vomiting.

[Indication] Patient with liver fire invading the stomach, hypochondriac pain, gastric stuffiness and belching, acid regurgitation and vomiting, bitter taste in the mouth with red side of the tongue and yellow coating, wiry and rapid pulse.

[Formula Analysis] This formula can clear liver fire. *Huáng lián* in this formula is used as chief medicine for clearing heart fire because of its taste of bitter and cold, because the heart is the son of the liver, when the heart fire is cleared, the liver fire is calmed, which is the way of "excess syndrome should clear the son [according to five elements]". And *wú zhū yú* is used as deputy medicine for soothing the liver and resolving constraint, direct counterflow downward and arrest vomiting and preventing stomach qi from the bitter and cold of *huáng lián* while avoiding *huáng lián* directing repulsion with bitter-cold medicines to mutual repelling of fire flaming because of its taste of great acrid and heat. The dosage of *wú zhū yú* is 1/6 of *huáng lián*, so the *wú zhū yú* will not do harm to clearing liver fire but can be assistant. Those two medicines, heat and cold, being opposite and complementary, clear liver and drain fire, direct counterflow downward and arrest vomiting together. *Huáng lián* is put in an vital position to clear fire, which can restrict metal that helps metal back to restrict wood normally, and then the liver can calm. Support metal control wood, so this formula is called "*Zuǒ Jīn*".

[Clinical Application] This formula treats the excess hypochondriac pain caused by liver fireflaming. If the hypochondriac pain is caused by insufficient liver blood, nourishing blood and softening the liver method is needed to replace this treatment. If the patient has syndrome-like acid regurgitation and vomiting because of deficiency-cold of the spleen and stomach, this formula is unsuitable.

Qīng Wèi Săn (Stomach-Heat-Clearing Powder, 清胃散)
Secrets from the Orchid Chamber (*Lán Shì Mì Cáng*, 兰室秘藏)[45]

[Ingredient]

Dāng Guī (Radix Angelicae Sinensis) (6 g)

Huáng Lián (Rhizoma Coptidis) If it does not have good quality, 2 *fen* should be added and double the dosage in summer (4.5 g)

Xiān Dì Huáng (Fresh Radix Rehmanniae Recens) processed with rice wine, 3 *fen* (12 g)

Mǔ Dān Pí (Cortex Moutan) 5 *fen* (9 g)

Shēng Má (Rhizoma Cimicifugae) 1 *qian* (6 g)

[Usage] Grind herbs into powder, decoct them with 1.5 *zhan* water into 1 *zhan*, remove the sediment, and take medicine coldly.

Modern Usage: Decocted with water.

[Action] Clear and drain the stomach fire and cool the blood.

[Indication] The heat accumulated in the stomach [in the end] rushing upward, [manifested as] toothache which causes a headache, hot feeling in the face, prefer cool feeling and averse to hot [drinks], ulcerated gums, or bleeding gums, or mouth, lips, cheek swelling and pain, bad and hot breath, mouth parched and tongue scorched, with red tongue and yellow coating, large, slippery and rapid pulse.

[Formula Analysis] *The Spiritual Pivot-Channel* (*Líng Shū-Jing Mai*, 灵枢·经脉) says: "the foot *yangming* stomach channel... it enters the upper gum and turns downward along the nose's lateral side. Re-emerging, it curves around the lips and descends to meet RN24 (*chéng jiāng*) [at the mentolabial groove]. Then it runs posterolaterally across the lower portion [of the cheek] at ST5 (*dà yíng*). Winding around ST6 (*jiá chē*) [Which is the angle of the mandible], it ascends in front of the ear. Then it follows the anterior or hairline and reaches the forehead." "The large intestine channel of the channel-*yangming*...passes through the cheek and enters the gums of lower teeth". *Huáng lián* in this formula is used as chief medicine for clearing fire and heat; *xiān dì huáng* and *mǔ dān pí* are used as deputy medicine for cooling blood and clearing heat; *dāng guī* is used as assistant medicine for nourishing

yin blood and removing yang heat; *shēng má*, which is used as envoy medicine for resolving *yangming* heat toxin and raising the stomach qi and clearing yang, ascending of the clearing making the descending of heat and soothing the swelling, stopping the pain. Combined with all these medicines, clearing stomach qi, draining fire and cooling the blood can achieve.

[Clinical Application]

1. This formula is designed for stomach fire flaming and toothache, and now it can be used to treat patient with stomach heat syndrome and blood heat and fire constraint. According to *Medical Formulas Collected and Analyzed* (*Yī Fāng Jí Jiě*, 医方集解), "adding *shí gāo* can strengthen the power of clearing stomach fire and other medicine can be added depending on the patient's syndromes".

2. If the excessive heat damages fluid, *mài dōng, huā fěn* can be added. If the patient has constipation, *dà huáng* can be added to guide heat downward which is very effective.

Yù Nǚ Jiān (Jade Lady Decoction, 玉女煎)
The Complete Works of [Zhang] Jing-yue (*Jǐng Yuè Quán Shū*, 景岳全书)

[Ingredient]

Shí Gāo (Gypsum Fibrosum)　3–5 *qian* (9–15 g)

Shú Dì Huáng (Radix Rehmanniae Praeparata)　3 *qian* or 1 *liang* (9–30 g)

Mài Dōng (Radix Ophiopogonis)　2 *qian* (6 g)

Zhī Mǔ (Rhizoma Anemarrhenae)　0.5 *qian* (4.5 g)

Niú Xī (Radix Achyranthis Bidentatae)　0.5 *qian* (4.5 g)

[Usage]　Decocted 1.5 *zhan* water into 7 *fen* and take medicine warm or cold. Modern Usage: Decocted with water.

[Action]　Clear stomach heat, enrich kidney yin.

[Indication]　Patient with the insufficiency of *shaoyin* and excess of *yangming*, vexing heat and thirst, headache, toothache, blood vomiting and blood loss, with surging floating and slippery pulse, deficient and large pulse if taken heavily, crimson tongue, dry and yellow coating.

[Formula Analysis] This is the *yangming* stomach heat damages fluid meanwhile shaoyin yin deficiency consuming fluid. *Shí gāo*, acrid taste, sweet and [very] cold, in this formula can clear excessive *yangming* stomach fire; *shú dì huáng* can nourish the deficiency of *shaoyin* kidney water. They are both used as chief ingredients. *Zhī mǔ*, one of the deputies, can help *shí gāo* clear the stomach fire without concerning that the bitter and dry medicine will damage the fluid for its tastes bitter and cold, nourish and moisten. *Mài dōng* is used as an assistant medicine for nourishing the yin of the lung and stomach because of its taste of sweet and cold, which used with *shú dì huáng* can nourish the water and clear the fire by the meaning of mutual generation between metal and water. *Niú xī* is used as an envoy medicine for nourishing kidney yin, guiding the blood downward and getting the fire down. Combined with all of these ingredients, the effect of clearing heat and strengthening the water can achieve.

[Clinical Application] This formula treats the syndromes like vexing heat, thirst, headache, toothache, blood vomiting, lose and so on which are caused by deficiency of water and excess fire. The original book records that: "If the fire flame, *zhī zǐ*, *dì gǔ pí* can be added; if there is much sweating with extremely thirsty, 14 grains *wǔ wèi zǐ* should be added; if there is difficult urination or the fire can not goes down, 1.5 *qian zé xiè* or *fú líng* (*yún líng*; *yún fú líng*) can be added; if the patient has a deficiency of lung and kidney because of damage of qi caused by essence, *rén shēn* can be added.

According to the editor's clinical experience, this formula uses *shēng dì* instead of *shú dì huáng*, which can strengthen the effect of clearing heat. If blood loss by the excessive heat, a large amount of *shēng dì* can be added with *chì sháo*, *mǔ dān pí* and *bái máo gēn*.

Wěi Jìng Tāng (Phragmites Stem Decoction, 苇茎汤)
Valuable Prescriptions of Emergency (*Bèi Jí Qiān Jīn Yào Fāng*, 备急千金要方)

[Ingredient]

Lú Gēn (Rhizoma Phragmitis) cut, 2 *sheng*, with 2 *dou* and boil into 5 *sheng*, (30–60 g)

Yì Yǐ Rén (Semen Coicis)   half *sheng* (15–30 g)

Guā Lóu (Fructus Trichosanthis)   half *sheng* (15–30 g)

Táo Rén (Semen Persicae)   30 *mei* (9 g)

[Usage]   Chew[cut] herbs, boil them with Phragmites soup into 2 *sheng* and drink 1 *sheng*. The patient will vomit the pus and blood after taking it.

Modern Usage: Decocted with water.

[Action]   Clear lung heat and dissolve phlegm, dispel stasis, and discharge pus.

[Indication]   Patients who have lung abscess, mild fever, cough, even with foul-smelling sputum or pus and blood, mild chest pain, dry mouth and throat but no desire for drink, vexation and agitation, dry, scaly skin of the chest, with slippery and rapid pulse, yellow and greasy coating.

[Formula Analysis]   Wind-heat attacks from the exterior (or wind-cold constraint [inside] transforming into fire), internal phlegm and heat combined, external and internal pathogen combined and lingered in the lung, which causes the phlegm-heat and static blood stagnate, and lead to lung abscess. *Lú gēn* in this formula is used as chief medicine to clear lung heat, relieve vexation and thirst, used in large dosages to treat lung abscess, *yì yǐ rén* in this formula is used as deputy medicine to clear heat and drain dampness, dissolve phlegm and drain pus for its taste of sweet, bland and slightly cold; and *guā lóu* is used as deputy medicine as well to dissolve phlegm and drain pus which is the effective medicine to treat internal abscess for its taste of sweet and cold which can clear heat, *táo rén* in this formula is used as assistant medicine to moisten the lung to relieve cough, dissolve stasis for its taste of bitter, sweet and smooth. This formula has only four herbs, which is quite plain but the effect can clear heat, dissolve phlegm and pus. This formula has the characteristic of "heavy but not severe, mitigative but not exhausting".

[Clinical Application]

1. This formula is designed for treating lung abscesses, can be used regardless of the patients period. After taking this formula, the patient in the early stage can dissipate the abscess, and patient in the later period can dissolve phlegm and pus, the lung can recover its function and the patient can be healed.

2. When the abscess is forming and the patient manifests as heat toxin stasis and masses with fishy phlegm, this formula can combine with *Xī Niú Wán* to resolve toxins and dissolve stasis. When the abscess is festering and the patient vomits and coughs out blood with pus-like porridge, this formula can be used with *jié gěng, gān cǎo, xiàng bèi mǔ, yú xīng cǎo* to strengthen the effect of clearing heat, resolving toxins and dissolving phlegm and pus.

Xiè Bái Sǎn (White-Draining Powder, 泻白散)
Craft of Medicines and Patterns for Children (*Xiǎo Ér Yào Zhèng Zhí Jué*, 小儿药证直诀)

[Ingredient]

Dì Gǔ Pí (Cortex Lycii)

Sāng Bái Pí (Cortex Mori) dry-fried

Each of them uses 1 *liang* (30 g)

Zhì Gān Cǎo (Radix et Rhizoma Glycyrrhizae Praeparata cum Melle) 1 *qian* (3 g) [zhou Xue-hai's replica said, "in *Materia Medica of Combinations* (*Jù Zhēn Běn Gān Cǎo*, 聚珍本甘草), it use 0.5 *liang*."]

[Usage] Grind the herbs into powder by filing or pounding, add *jīng mǐ* (*Nonglutinous rice*) 1 *cuo* [5–10g], decoct it into 7 *fen* with 2 *zhan* water. Take medicine before a meal.

Modern Usage: Add *jīng mǐ* 1 *cuo* [5 g], decoct with water. Its dosage changes the ratio of the original formula.

[Action] Drain lung fire and clear heat, relieve cough, and calm panting.

[Indication] Patients who have lurking fire due to constrained heat in the lung with cough or even wheezing, lurking heat in the lung makes the skin hot to the touch, especially between the 3:00 pm–5:00pm, red tongue with a yellow coating, thready and rapid pulse.

[Formula Analysis] The lung governs the qi, which needs purification and descent. *Sāng bái pí* in this formula is used as chief medicine to drain lung fire and clear heat, relieve cough, and calm panting for its taste of sweet and cold; *dì gǔ pí* is

used as deputy medicine to help chief medicine drain the lurking lung fire which is very good at reducing the fever for its taste of sweet, bland and cold, *zhì gān căo* can moisten the lung to relieve cough, nourish the stomach and harmonize the center with *jīng mǐ* which can supplement qi of spleen and lung and prevent from the damage of stomach caused by *sāng bái pí* and *dì gǔ pí*'s cold and cool. These two medicines are both assistant and envoy medicine. These four herbs can drain lung fire and clear heat, relieve cough and calm panting without damaging healthy qi. So this formula is suitable for the patient with latent fire in the lung while the healthy qi which has not been damaged too much. This formula is so-called: "White-Draining" because the lung is [corresponding to] white and this formula can drain the latent fire in the lung.

[Clinical Application]   This formula is used to treat cough and panting caused by the latent fire in the lung and qi counterflow without descending. If the heat in the lung meridian is severe, then the power of clearing heat of this formula is not enough, *huáng qín* and *zhī mǔ* should be added to strengthen the effect of drain lung fire and clear heat; a patient who has severe cough can add *xìng rén*, *chuān bèi mǔ* and *guā lóu pí* to moisten the lung to relieve cough; a thirsty patient can add *tiān huā fěn* to promote fluid production to quench thirst.

Sháo Yào Tāng (Peony Decoction, 芍药汤)
*Collection of Writings on the Mechanism of Disease, Suitability of Qi, and the
Safeguarding of Life as Discussed in the 'Basic Questions' (Sù Wèn-Bìng Jī Qì
Yí Bǎo Mìng Jí,* 素问·病机气宜保命集)[46]

[Ingredient]

Sháo Yào (Radix Paeoniae)   1 *liang* (15 g)

Dāng Guī (Radix Angelicae Sinensis)   0.5 *liang* (9 g)

Huáng Lián (Rhizoma Coptidis)   0.5 *liang* (9 g)

Bīng Láng (Semen Arecae)   2 *qian* (6 g)

Mù Xiāng (Radix Aucklandiae)   2 *qian* (6 g)

Gān Căo (Radix et Rhizoma Glycyrrhizae)   dry-fried 2 *qian* (6 g)

Dà Huáng (Radix Et Rhizoma Rhei)   3 *qian* (6 g)

Huáng Qín (Radix Scutellariae) 0.5 *liang* (9 g)

Ròu Guì (Cortex Cinnamomi) 2.5 *qian* (1.5 g)

[Usage] In the original book, Chew [cut] herbs and boil half dosage of them with 2 *zhan* water into 1 *zhan*, and take it warm after the meal. If the patient has diarrhea with blood, *dà huáng* should be added gradually; if the patient has diarrhea after sweating, half *liang* [30 g] *huáng bǎi* should be added and decocted with water as well.

Modern Usage: Decocted with water.

[Action] Move blood and regulate qi, clear heat and resolve toxins.

[Indication] Patients with dysentery caused by damp-heat manifested as abdominal pain, stool with pus and blood, white and red, abdominal urgency with tenesmus, burning sensation in the anus, slippery and rapid pulse, and yellow and greasy coating.

[Formula Analysis] This syndrome is caused by dampheat epidemic toxin accumulated in the intestine. *Sháo yào* (in this formula is play an vital role to harmonize blood and relieve the abdominal pain, which is called: "suitable for pathogenic qi and abdominal pain" in *Shen Nong's Classic of the Materia Medica* (*Shén Nóng Běn Cǎo Jīng*, 神农本草经), and is called: "[it] suitable for [treating] diarrhea and dysentery, abdominal pain and rectal heaviness" in *The Grand Compendium of Materia Medica* (*Běn Cǎo Gāng Mù*, 本草纲目), so this herb is the chief medicine, *dāng guī*, as deputy medicine which good at moving blood, combined with *sháo yào* (can harmonize *ying*, treat dysentery and abdominal pain; with *huáng lián* and *huáng qín* to clear heat and dry dampness and resolve toxins, *bīng láng* and *mù xiāng* are used to regulate qi and remove stagnation, *dà huáng* is used to clear damp-heat and remove stagnation, move blood, which are assistant medicine, *ròu guì* is used as paradoxical assistant medicine because its taste of acrid and warm can move blood while avoid large cold and bitter [herbs] damaging the stomach; *gān cǎo* is used as envoy medicine to relieving spasm and pain and harmonize all of these herbs. *Sháo yào* combined with *gān cǎo* are very good at relieving pain; *dà huáng* combined with *bīng láng* and *mù xiāng* can enhance the impact of removing stagnation which is

called the way of "treating incontinent syndrome with dredging method"; *dà huáng* combined with *ròu guì* can strengthen the effect of moving blood, *ròu guì* combined with *dà huáng* can avoid the potential hazard about acrid and heat will increase the fire. Liu He-jian once said, "moving blood, then the bloody purulent stool can be cured; regulating qi, then tenesmus can relieve."

[Clinical Application]

This formula is used to treat dysentery caused by damp-heat. If the patient has severe heat, *ròu guì* should be removed; if the patient has dysentery with lots of red pus and less white, or even has fresh purple pus and blood only, despite removing *ròu guì*, *dà huáng* should be changed into *dà huáng tàn* using *mǔ dān pí tàn* and *jīn yín huā* to cool blood and stop bleeding.

Gě Gēn Huáng Qín Huáng Lián Tāng (Pueraria, Scutellaria, and Coptis Decoction, 葛根黄芩黄连汤)
Treatise on Cold Damage (Shāng Hán Lùn, 伤寒论)

[Ingredient]

Gě Gēn (Radix Puerariae Lobatae)   half *jin* (15 g)

Gān Cǎo (Radix Et Rhizoma Glycyrrhizae)   2 *liang*, dry-fried with liquid adjuvant (6 g)

Huáng Qín (Radix Scutellariae)   3 *liang* (9 g)

Huáng Lián (Rhizoma Coptidis)   3 *liang* (9 g)

[Usage]   Boil *gé gēn* firstly with 8 *sheng* water, then take 2 *sheng* away and add other herbs, boil into 2 *sheng*, remove the sediment, take it warmly.

Modern Usage: Decocted with water.

[Action]   Clear the interior and release the exterior.

[Indication]   The exterior-heat syndrome was not relieved but entered inside and led to generalized fever with diarrhea, heat vexation in the chest, thirst, panting and sweating, a red tongue with yellow tongue coating, rapid or skipping pulse.

[Formula Analysis]   At the early stage of exterior syndrome, the pathogen contracted in *taiyang*, the exterior-releasing method should be used. *Gé gēn* in this

formula is used as chief medicine to release the flesh, and ascend the clear yang of the spleen and stomach to stop diarrhea; *huáng qín* and *huáng lián* are used as assistant medicines to clear the internal heat, strengthen the intestine and stop diarrhea; *gān cǎo*, harmonize the center and coordinate all of the herbs. These herbs form this formula of clearing internal heat and simultaneously releasing the exterior. The original formula boils *gě gēn* first and adds other herbs, which aim to gentle the power of release fleshy and enhance the power of clear interior heat. This is the three-seven law [three-tenths focus on the exterior, seven-tenths on the interior].

[Clinical Application] This formula is the typical formula to treat a generalized fever with diarrhea, which is centered on clearing interior heat. However, it can relieve the exterior pathogen and clear the interior heat of the stomach and intestine. As for heat diarrhea and heat dysentery, no matter with the exterior pathogen or not, this formula can be used. If the patient combines with vomit, *bàn xià* and *zhú rú* can be added to downbear counterflow; if the patient has food stagnation, *shān zhā* and *shén qū* can be added to promote digestion; if manifested as abdominal distension and pain, *mù xiāng* and *bái sháo* should be added to relax the tension and stop the pain.

Bái Tóu Wēng Tāng (Pulsatilla Decoction, 白头瓮汤)
Treatise on Cold Damage (*Shāng Hán Lùn*, 伤寒论)

[Ingredient]

Bái Tóu Wēng (Radix Pulsatillae)   2 *liang* (12 g)

Huáng Bǎi (Cortex Phellodendri Chinensis)   (9 g)

Huáng Lián (Rhizoma Coptidis)   3 *liang* (9 g)

Qín Pí (Cortex Fraxini)   3 *liang* (9 g)

[Usage]   Boil the herbs with 7 *sheng* water into 2 *sheng*, remove the sediment, take 1 *sheng* warm. If it does not work, and take another 1 *sheng* decoction.

Modern Usage: Decocted with water.

[Action]   Clear heat and resolve toxins, cool blood and alleviate dysenteric disorders.

[Indication] Heat dysentery and tenesmus, thirst and desire for drinks, abdominal pain, diarrhea with pus and blood, burning sensation around the anus, a red tongue with yellow coating, wiry and rapid pulse.

[Formula Analysis] *Treatise on Cold Damage* (*Shāng Hán Lùn*, 伤寒论) said that: "*Bái Tóu Wēng Tāng* will be the remedy for diarrhea with fever, and tenesmus." and "Diarrhea with thirst will serve as proof of interior heat. In such a case, Pulsatilla Decoction should be adopted." *Bái Tóu Wēng* is the principal medicine for treating dysenteric disorders, which is recorded: "it can stop toxic diarrhea" in *Miscellaneous Records of Famous Physicians* (*Míng Yī Bié Lù*, 名医别录) to treat heat toxin and bloody diarrhea for its taste of bitter and cold. *Huáng Lián* and *huáng bǎi* are assistant medicines to clear heat, dry dampness and treat dysenteric disorders, *qín pí* is used as assistant medicine as well to clear heat, dry dampness and stop diarrhea for its taste of bitter, cold and astringent natures. All these herbs have the effect of clearing heat and resolving toxins, cooling blood, and stopping diarrhea.

[Clinical Application] This formula is the typical formula that is used to treat heat toxins and bloody diarrhea. If the patient is in critical condition with purple pus and bloody stool, fever and thirst, severe abdominal pain, red and crimson tongue, large and rapid pulse, which belongs to epidemic toxin dysentery, *chì sháo*, *mǔ dān pí* and *jīn yín huā* should be added into this formula.

Section 5 Formulas that clears heat and dispels summer-heat

The clearing heat and dispelling summer-heat formula apply to the summer-heat syndrome, which appears in late summer. The primary syndromes are fever, vexation, thirst, sweating, tiredness, and deficient pulse. *The Basic Questions-Discourse on Heat* (*Sù Wèn-Rè Lùn,* 素问·热论) says: "Febrile disease that begins with cold factors is termed *Bing Wen* (病温) when occurring before the summer solstice. When it occurs during or after the summer solstice, we call it *Shu Bing* (暑病)." However, in the summer period, the summer-heat [qi] goes down while the dampness [on the ground] steams upward, which colluds together, leads to disease. So it is called that:

"summer-heat is inevitably accompanied by dampness." Summer-heat is the yang and heat pathogen that easily damages qi and consumes body fluid, resulting in the syndrome of qi and fluid deficiency. If the patient has severe fever, vexation and thirsty, profuse sweating, it needs to clear summer-heat by boost qi and promote fluid production such as *Bái Hǔ Jiā Rén Shēn Tāng* (White Tiger Decoction Plus Ginseng, 白虎加人参汤) (clearing heat formula); but if the patient also has exterior cold which is caused by enjoying the cold beverages or cool off [less clothes or exposure in the air condition] excessively, manifested as hyperpyrexia and headache, aversion to cold but without sweating, the drain summer heat and release the exterior formula such as *Xiāng Rú Yǐn* (Mosla Beverag, 香薷饮) (exterior-releasing formula) can be used; if the patient is attacked by summer-heat with dampness that needs to clear summer-heat and drain dampness, which is mentioned in *Miscellaneous Writings of Famous Physicians of the Ming Dynasty* (*Míng Yī Zá Zhù*, 明医杂著)[47] "the best method of clearing summer heat is to clear heart fire and promote urination." such as *Liù Yī Sǎn* (Six-to-One Powder, 六一散); as the summer heat can damages qi and consumes fluid, the treatment should focus on reinforcing qi and tonifying fluid production such as *Qīng Shǔ Yì Qì Tāng* (Summer heat-Clearing Qi-Boosting Decoction, 清暑益气汤).

The prerequisite for dispelling summer heat medicines is knowing whether there is a combination syndrome or not. If the patient has a summer heat pathogen with dampness, but the heat is more severe than the dampness. It means the too warm and dry medicines should not be chosen to avoid consuming the body fluid. Conversely, if the dampness exceeds the heat, the nourishment and moistening with sweet-cold medicines should be used carefully to prevent lingering dampness pathogens.

Liù Yī Sǎn (Six-to-One Powder, 六一散) (original *Yì Yuán Sǎn*, 益元散) *Direct Investigation of Cold Damage* (*Shāng Hán Zhí Gé*, 伤寒直格) [48]

[Ingredient]

Huá Shí (Talcum)   6 *liang*, white and fine, in good quality 6 *liang* (180 g)

Gān Cǎo (Radix et Rhizoma Glycyrrhizm ae)   1 *liang* (30 g)

[Usage]   Grind herbs into powder, take 3 *qian* with honey and warm water [or

without honey] three times a day. Alternatively take with cold spring water.

[Action]   Clear summer heat, resolve dampness.

[Indication]   The combination of summer heat injuring the qi and dampness obstructing the interior gives rise to damp-heat, manifested as vexation, thirst, inhibited urination, vomiting, diarrhea, yellow and greasy coating. Or if it [damp-heat] blocks in the bladder, various types of painful urinary dribbling may present, like reddish urine, difficulty and painful urination, dribbling urinary obstruction, and urolitic stranguria.

[Formula Analysis]   Summer heat is the yang and heat pathogen, [according to five elements] the summer heat qi corresponding to the heart. In this formula, *huá shí* is used as chief medicine to clear summer heat, drain dampness and relieve strangury for its taste of sweet, bland, and its heavy [nature] which can go downward, the slippery [nature] which can unblock the orifices. In *Shen Nong's Classic of the Materia Medica* (*Shén Nóng Běn Cǎo Jīng*, 本草纲目) says: "it can treat fever and diarrhea, inhibited lactation, dribbling urinary block and relieve strangury". And few *gān cǎo* is used as assistant medicine to harmonize the center qi and mitigate *huá shí*. Through the cooperation of these two medicines which can clear summer heat and drain dampness, the hiding summer heat and dampness will be expelled from the urine; also, the fever is removed, the thirst is released and the diarrhea is stopped. In *Miscellaneous Writings of Famous Physicians of the Ming Dynasty* (*Míng Yī Zá Zhù*, 名医杂录) says: "the method of clearing summer heat is to clear heart fire and promote urination", this is fits the meaning of this formula. It is an important method of treating summer heat pathogen with dampness. This formula is made by six *liang huá shí* and one *liang gān cǎo* in powder, so it is called: "*Liù Yī Sǎn* " and it also means "one heaven produces water, six ground carry and correspond it."

[Clinical Application]

1. This is the best formula that can treat summer heat with dampness, and clinically it needs to add *huò xiāng, pèi lán, qīng hāo, tōng cǎo, xī guā pí, zhú yè*.

2. If the patient has inhibited voidings of reddish urine, dribbling urinary block, and stranguria, needs to add *chē qián zǐ, zé xiè, biǎn xù, qú mài*; if the patient has stone

gonorrhea, it needs to add *jīn qián cǎo, hǎi jīn shā, shí wéi, dōng kuí zǐ* to relieve strangury and expel stones; if the patient has blood gonorrhea, it needs to add *cè bǎi yè, chē qián cǎo, ǒu jié*, which is called as *Sān Shēng Yì Yuán Sàn* (three fresh medicines boost original qi powder, 三生益元散).

Qīng Shǔ Yì Qì Tāng (Summer-heat-Clearing Qi-Boosting Decoction, 清暑益气汤)
Warp and Woof of Warm-febrileDiseases (*Wēn Rè Jīng Wěi*, 温热经纬)[49]

[Ingredient]

Xī Yáng Shēn (Radix Panacis Quinquefolii)   (4.5 g)

Shí Hú (Caulis Dendrobii)   (12 g)

Mài Dōng (Radix Ophiopogonis)   (9 g)

Huáng Lián (Rhizoma Coptidis)   (3g)

Zhú Yè (Folium Phyllostachydis Henonis)   (6 g)

Hé Gěng (Petiolus Nelmbinis)   (12 g)

Zhī Mǔ (Rhizoma Anemarrhenae)   (6 g)

Gān Cǎo (Radix Et Rhizoma Glycyrrhizae)   (3 g)

Jīng Mǐ (Oryza Sativa L)   (15 g)

Xī Guā Pí (Exocarpium Citrulli)   (30 g)

[the original formula doesn't record the dosage]

[Usage]   The original book does not record the administration.

Modern Usage: Decocted with water.

[Action]   Clear summer heat and boost qi, nourish yin, and promote fluid production.

[Indication]   Patient who has been attacked by summer heat with qi and fluid injured, fever and sweating, vexation thirsty, fatigued limbs, lassitude, deficient but rapid pulse.

[Formula Analysis]   Summer heat pathogen is the yang pathogen which is relatively easy to consume qi and fluid. This formula uses *xī yáng shēn* as chief medicine to nourish yin and promote fluid production of it bitter, sweet taste and

117

cool nature. *Shí hú* and *mài dōng* are used as deputy medicines to nourish yin and clear heat for their taste of sweet and cold, which also can promote fluid production. *huáng lián* and *zhú yè* are used to clear heart fire and relieve vexation, *huáng lián*'s taste is bitter and cold, *zhú yè* is acrid, bland, sweet and cold. *Hé gěng* is used to clear summer heat and move qi to soothe the chest. *Zhī mǔ* is used to enrich yin and clear fire for its taste bitter cold, and good at nourishing and moistening the *yin*. *Xī guā pí* is used to clear summer heat. These medicines are used as assistant medicines. *Gān cǎo* and *jīng mǐ* are used as envoy medicines to reinforce the stomach and harmonize the middle. All of these medicines in this formula have the effect of clearing summer heat, reinforcing qi, enriching yin and promoting fluid production which is the reason why it is called: "*Qīng Shǔ Yì Qì Tāng*".

[Clinical Application] This formula is used to treat a patient who has been attacked by summer heat, the qi and fluid being injured, manifested with fever and sweating, vexation, thirst, fatigued limbs, deficient and rapid pulse, white thin and dry coating, red tongue. The critical differentiation point is the disease occurred in summer.

In this formula, the dosage of *huáng lián* should be controlled to avoid bitterness and cold, which change into dryness and damage the fluid.

Section 6   Formulas that clears deficiency-heat

The clearing deficiency-heat formula applies to the syndromes of the late period of febrile disease, which has heat pathogen and yin fluid consumption; the heat staying in yin will cause a feeling of hot in nightfall but dissapear in the morning, with red tongue and few coating without sweating. At the same time, the fever is reduced or has steaming bone fever, red lips and flushed cheeks, thin and night sweat because of the yin deficiency of the liver and kidney with deficiency-heat harassing the interior. Nourishing yin medicine such as *biē jiǎ*, *shēng dì*, *zhī mǔ* and clearing heat medicine like *qīng hāo*, *yín chái hú*, *dì gǔ pí* are used to treat these syndromes usually. There are typical formulas such as *Qīng Hāo Biē Jiǎ Tāng* (Sweet Wormwood and Turtle Shell Decoction, 青蒿鳖甲汤), *Qīng Gǔ Sǎn* (Bone-Clearing Powder, 清骨散).

Qīng Hāo Biē Jiǎ Tāng (Sweet Wormwood and Soft-shelled Turtle Shell Decoction, 青蒿鳖甲汤)

Systematic Differentiation of Warm Diseases (*Wēn Bìng Tiáo Biàn*, 温病条辨)

[Ingredient]

Qīng Hāo (Herba Artemisiae Annuae)　2 *qian* (6 g)

Biē Jiǎ (Carapax Trionycis)　5 *qian* (15 g)

Shēng Dì (Radix Rehmanniae)　4 *qian* (12 g)

Zhī Mǔ (Rhizoma Anemarrhenae)　2 *qian* (6 g)

Mǔ Dān Pí (Cortex Moutan)　3 *qian* (9 g)

[Usage]　5 cups of water in the original formula boiled into 2 cups, two times a day.

Modern Usage: Decocted with water.

[Action]　Nourish yin and vents heat.

[Indication]　Patients in the late period of warm disease and yin is readily damaged. Heat pathogen penetrates deeply into the *yin fen* which has symptoms such as feeling hot at night but [hot feeling] disappearing in the morning, with no sweating as the fever reduces, normal appetite but with emaciation, red tongue with less coating, thready and rapid pulse.

[Formula Analysis]　The qi of *wei* yang moves on the exterior during the day and enters the interior at night. During the late period of the warm-febrile disease, yin fluid is consumed, heat pathogen lurking in the *yin fen* deeply, yang qi moves into yin [area] and enhances the heat pathogen. In this formula, salty, cold *biē jiǎ* is used to nourish yin and clear heat, which can enter the *yin fen* straightly and *qīng hāo*, which vents the clear heat and cool the blood, which is both used as chief medicines. The deputies, *shēng dì* and *zhī mǔ* assist *biē jiǎ* in nourishing yin and clearing heat, while *mǔ dān pí* can help *qīng hāo* venting and clearing the hiding heat, which is both used as assistant medicines. Wu Ju-Tong[50] thinks that: "this formula has the advantages of entering [into the interior]firstly and then getting out [through the exterior]. *Qīng hāo* which is unable to enter into the yin fen straightly unless under the guidance of *biē jiǎ*; While *biē jiǎ* fails to go to the yang fen separately unless the *qīng hāo* lead

it." so *qīng hāo* and *biē jiǎ* can act as channel conductor herbs. These five ingredients combined with the effect of nourishing yin without lingering pathogen and dispel pathogen without damaging healthy qi, this formula is designed for patients with less excessive manifestation but severe deficiency symptoms. It is an effective formula to nourish yin, vent heat and clear the pathogen of *yin fen*.

[Clinical Application]   This formula is used to treat the late period of warm diseases. The critical point of differentiation is that the hot feeling at night but [burning sensation] disappears in the morning, with no sweating as the fever reduces, but the fever returns at night. As for the one who has manifested with yin deficiency and night fever, *shí hú*, *dì gǔ pí*, *tiān huā fěn* can be used to nourish yin and clear heat.

Qīng Gǔ Sǎn (Bone-Clearing Powder, 清骨散)
Standards for Diagnosis and Treatment (*Zhèng Zhì Zhǔn Shéng*, 证治准绳)

[Ingredient]

Yín Chái Hú (Radix Stellariae)   1.5 *qian* (4.5 g)

Hú Huáng Lián (Rhizoma Picrorhizae)   1 *qian* (3 g)

Qín Jiāo (Radix Gentianae Macrophyllae)   1 *qian* (3 g)

Biē Jiǎ (Carapax Trionycis)   dry-fried drugs with rice vinegar 1 *qian* (3 g)

Dì Gǔ Pí (Cortex Lycii)   1 *qian* (3 g)

Qīng Hāo (Herba Artemisiae Annuae)   1 *qian* (3 g)

Zhī Mǔ (Rhizoma Anemarrhenae)   1 *qian* (3 g)

Gān Cǎo (Radix Et Rhizoma Glycyrrhizae)   5 *fen* (1.5g)

[Usage]   2 *zhong* of water from the original formula decocted into 8 *fen* and taken a long time after the meal.

Modern Usage: Decocted with water.

[Action]   Clear deficiency-heat and alleviates steaming bone fever.

[Indication]   Patients with yin deficiency, steaming bone fever, red lips and flushed cheeks, thin and night sweat, red tongue and little coating, thready and rapid pulse.

[Formula Analysis]   This syndrome is caused by liver and kidney yin

deficiency, with deficiency-heat harassing the interior. The chief ingredient, sweet and slightly cold *yín chái hú*, is good at clearing the deficiency-heat and venting steaming bone fever without the disadvantage of draining, ascent and dissipating, in *Summarized Dissemination of the Classic of Materia Medica* (*Běn Căo Jīng Shū*, 本草经疏[51]) says: "it [*yín chái hú*] can treat taxation fever and steaming bone." There are three deputies: *dì gŭ pí*, *hú huáng lián*, *zhī mŭ* can clear heat in yin fen which removes heat interior; two assistant herbs support these three herbs: *qín jiāo* can clear heat of the liver and gallbladder and conduct the heat outward to the exterior, while *biē jiǎ* can nourish yin and clear heat, guide other medicine into the interior. *Gān cǎo* is used as an envoy medicine to harmonize all the medicines and avoid the bitter and cold medicine damaging the stomach qi. This formula gathers clearing heat and venting steaming fever medicine which focuses on clearing, so it is called: "*Qīng Gŭ Săn*".

[Clinical Application]   This formula is used to treat steaming bone fever and exhausting heat, usually has a good effect on patients with yin deficiency resulting in vigorous fire, steaming bone fever and tidal fever. If the patient with yin deficiency than tidal fever, this formula can be modified with subtracting *hú huáng lián*, *yín chái hú*, *qín jiāo* and adding *shēng dì*, *mŭ dān pí*, *mŭ dān pí* to nourish yin and clear heat.

Chapter 7

Resuscitative Formulas

The formulas in this chapter are formed by opening the orifices (resuscitate) with aromatics medicine with the effect of opening the orifices and unblocking to treat the syndromes of orifices blocking and unconsciousness is called as the formula for resuscitation or opening the orifices formula.

Section 1   Formulas that opens the orifices (resuscitate) with cool

The formula of opening the orifices (resuscitate) with cool medicines applies to the syndromes of warm-heat pathogen sinking into pericardium, and heat-phlegm veiling the heart orifice of the heart [*xīn qiào*] which leads to hyperpyrexia, unconsciousness, delirious speech or even convulsive syncope or attacked by filthy qi, sudden fall into a swoon without consciousness or stroke and the orifices blocking with heat symptoms.

The core medicine of these formulas are *niú huáng*, *xī jiǎo*, *huáng lián* and *shí gāo*, which can clear heat, resolve toxins and drain fire with *shè xiāng*, *bīng piàn* and *ān xī xiāng* which can open the orifices (resuscitate). If the patients have exuberant heat stirring wind and convulsion, medicines like *líng yáng jiǎo* and *dài mào* should be used to cool the liver and extinguish wind. Clearing heat and resolving toxins aim to determine the warm and heat pathogens, and also prevent these pathogens from sinking into the pericardium; opening the orifices (resuscitate) with aromatics aims to treat the main syndrome of blocking orifices and unconsciousness.There are typical formulas such as *Ān Gōng Niú Huáng Wán* (Peaceful Palace Bovine Bezoar Pill, 安

宫牛黄丸), *Zǐ Xuě Dān* (Purple Snow Elixir, 紫雪丹), *Zhì Bǎo Dān* (Supreme Jewel Elixir, 至宝丹).

Ān Gōng Niú Huáng Wán (Peaceful Palace Bovine Bezoar Pill, 安宫牛黄丸)
Systematic Differentiation of Warm Diseases (*Wēn Bìng Tiáo Biàn*, 温病条辨)

[Ingredient]

Niú Huáng (Calculus Bovis)

Yù Jīn (Radix Curcumae)

Xī Jiǎo (Cornu Rhinocerotis)

Huáng Lián (Rhizoma Coptidis)

Zhū Shā (Cinnabaris)

Shān Zhī (Fructus Gardeniae)

Xióng Huáng (Realgar)

Huáng Qín (Radix Scutellariae)

Each of them uses 1 *liang* (30 g)

Tiān Rán Bīng Piàn (Borneolum)　2 *qian* and 5 *fen* (7.5 g)

Shè Xiāng (Moschus)　2 *qian* and 5 *fen* (7.5 g)

Zhēn Zhū (Margarita)　5 *qian* (15 g)

Jīn Bó (Gold Foil)

[Usage]　In the original formula, grind all the medicines into a powder and form them into pills with honey; each pill is 1 *qian* (3 g), coating it with *jīn bó* (Gold Foil) and wrapping with wax for protection. Patients with deficient pulse need to take a pill with *Rén Shēn Tāng* (Ginseng Decoction, 人参汤); patients with excess pulse need to take a pill with *Yín Huā Bò Hé Tāng* (honeysuckle flower and peppermint Decoction, 银花薄荷汤). This formula can also treat sudden fainting, five epilepsies, malignity stroke, and convulsive caused by heat. The original text advised that if the adults were seriously ill, however, the constitution was strong then they can take the pills twice per day even three-time. While children can take a one-half pill at a time. If not recover, take the other half.

　　Modern Usage: Grind the medicine into a powder and form them into pills with

honey; each pill is 1 g with *jīn bó* clothing (some without gold foil). 1 pill a time, 1 or 2 times a day with water. Children take it depending on their age.

[Action]   Clear heat and resolve toxins, eliminate phlegm to open the orifices.

[Indication]   Warm-heat disease, the pathogen heat inward sinking into the pericardium, and heat-phlegm clouding the heart orifice, which causes high fever, irritability, restlessness, unconsciousness, incoherent speech or even convulsive syncope, red tongue with yellow turbidity in the middle and bad breath. For the patient with a stroke and orifices blocking. Children's convulsion were mainly caused by the heat-phlegm blocking interior.

[Formula Analysis]   Ye Tian-shi said in *Externally-Contracted Warm-Heat Diseases* (*Wài Gǎn Wēn Rè Piān*, 外感温热篇) that, "warm pathogen goes upward, attacks the lung first, then reversely transmit to the pericardium". So clearing heat and resolving toxicity in the pericardium are the foremost step. However, the phlegm and heat are combined together. Without draining the phlegm, the heat pathogen is hard to be cleared. In this formula, one of the chief ingredients, bitter, cool, and aromatic, *niú huáng* is very effective in clearing heat from the heart and resolving toxins, extinguishing wind and stopping the spasms, tremors, or convulsions, eliminating phlegm to open the orifices, which gets three effective results from one medicine. The second chief medicine, *xī jiǎo* [using *shuǐ niú jiǎo* (buffalo horn) instead] is used to calm the spirit, cool the blood, and resolve toxicity. Its cool, aromatic properties quickly vent pathogenic heat from the pericardium. *Zhēn zhū* and *zhū shā* are used to help *xī jiǎo* clear heart heat and settle [down] convulsion. *Yù jīn* is used to clear heat and cool blood. *Tiān rán bīng piàn* is used to open the orifices (resuscitate) because of its aromatics properties. *Xióng huáng* dislodges phlegm and resolves toxicity, thus helping to open the orifices by draining the turbid phlegm. *Shè xiāng* is used to open the orifices and dispel filth. Those medicines with aromatics that can lead the warm pathogen and toxins out of the interior and eliminate phlegm. *Huáng Lián*, *shān zhī* and *huáng qín* are used to clear heat and resolve toxins. All of these medicines are assistant medicine. *Jīn bó* serves as an envoy by calming the spirit with *honey* which can harmonize the actions of all medicines, both used as envoy medicine. Combined

with these medicines, this formula has the effect of clearing heat and resolving toxins and eliminating phlegm to open the orifices. The pericardium is the imperial palace of heart. In *The Spiritual Pivot-Invasion of Xie* (*Líng Shū-Xié Kè*, 灵枢·邪客), it says, "The heart is the emperor of the five *zang*-organs and the six *fu*-organs, and the residence of the essence and the spirit. [When] the heart is firm and cannot be invaded by *xie* (evil). If a pathogenic factor enters the inside [heart], the heart will be damaged. [If] the heart is damaged, the spirit will be lost. [If] the spirit is lost, [it will] lead to death. All the pathogenic influences that [appear to be] in the heart are the heart's wrap [i.e., the pericardium]. The collateral of the pericardium is the channel controlled by the heart." This formula can clear the heat of the pericardium and it uses *niú huáng* as chief medicine which is made into pills, so it is called *Ān Gōng Niú Huáng Wán*.

[Clinical Application] This formula is the model formula for clearing heat and resolving toxins, eliminating phlegm and opening the orifices which treats heat-phlegm veiling the heart orifice and leads to hyperpyrexia, unconsciousness and delirious speech. If the patient has a stroke or child convulsion which belongs to blocking with heat-phlegm, this formula can clear heat and drain phlegm medicine.

Zǐ Xuě Dān **(Purple Snow Elixir, 紫雪丹)**
Arcane Essentials from the Imperial Library **(*Wài Tái Mì Yào*, 外台秘要)**
Quote From Su Gong Formula, 苏恭方[52]

[Ingredient]
Shí Gāo (Gypsum Fibrosum)
Hán Shuǐ Shí (Glauberitum)
Cí Shí (Magnetitum)
Huá Shí (Talcum)
Each of them use 3 *jin* (1500 g)
Xī Jiǎo (Cornu Rhinocerotis)
Líng Yáng Jiǎo (Cornu Saigae Tataricae)
Qīng Mù Xiāng (Radix Aristolochiae)
Chén Xiāng (Lignum Aquilariae Resinatum)

Each of them use 5 *liang* (150 g)

Xuán Shēn (Radix Scrophulariae)

Shēng Má (Rhizoma Cimicifugae)

Each of them use 1 *jin* (500 g)

Zhì gān Cǎo (Radix Et Rhizoma Glycyrrhizae Praeparata Cum Melle)

8 *liang* (250 g)

Dīng Xiāng (Flos Caryophylli)   1 *liang* (30 g)

Huáng Jīng (Rhizoma Polygonati)   100 *liang* (3000 g)

Pò Xiāo (Mirabilitum)   high quality, 10 *jin* (5000 g)

Xiāo Shí (Saltpēteris)   4 *sheng* (1500 g)

Zhū Shā (Cinnabaris)   grind, 3 *liang* (90 g)

Shè Xiāng (Moschus)   grind, 5 *fen* (1.5 g)

[Usage]   In the original formula, the mineral medicines are crushed into small pieces and with 1 *hu* water boiled into 4 *dou*, then add the other 8 medicines with this decoction and boil into 1 *dou* and 5 *sheng*, take without sediment. Put *xiāo shí* (4 *sheng*) and *pò xiāo* (10 *jin*) into the decoction and boil it on the charcoal, stirring it incessantly with a willow comb and get 7 *sheng* decoction. Put it in a wooden basin and wait until it is half curdled, add *zhū shā* (3 *liang*), *shè xiāng* (5 *fen*) and continue stirring it; after two days of cooling, it turns purple with cream. A patient with a muscular body constitution takes 2 *fen*, the heat toxins can be drained, while an old or weak patient takes 1 fen.

Modern Usage: Made into powder and takes 1.5–3 g each time, 1–2 times a day with cold water. Children's dosage depends on themselves.

[Action]   Clear heat and resolve toxins, control convulsion and open the orifices.

[Indication]   Warm febrile disease caused by warm-heat pathogens sinking into the pericardium, and leads to high fever, irritability and restlessness, unconsciousness, delirious speech, thirsty and anxious lips, red urine and stool retention, or even convulsive, red tongue without coating. Children with hyperpyrexia and convulsive.

[Formula Analysis]   These syndromes are caused by intense pathogenic heat

sinking into the pericardium, heat stirring the *ying* [*fen*] and generating wind. In this formula, *shí gāo* and *hán shuǐ shí* are used to clear heat and drain fire, dispel vexation and stop thirst with *huá shí* which can clear heat, lubricate the orifices and guide the heat pathogen out through urine. These three medicines can reduce hyperpyrexia and dispel vexation and thirst. *Xī jiǎo* is used to clear heat, cool blood and resolve toxins for its fragrance which is cold and can get into the heat of pericardium. *Líng yáng jiǎo* is particularly useful for draining liver fire and cooling the liver and extinguish wind, clearing heat and resolving toxins. The combination of *xī jiǎo* and *líng yáng jiǎo*, makes the great formula to treat exuberant heat in heart *ying* [*fen*] and the wind stirred by heat. The intensely aromatic properties of *shè xiāng* can open the orifices (resuscitate). All these medicines are an essential part of this formula. *Xuán shēn*, *shēng má* and *zhì gān cǎo* are used to drain fire and resolve toxins, and *xuán shēn* can nourish yin and promote fluid production, *zhì gān cǎo* can calm the center and harmonize the stomach. *Cí shí*, *huáng jīng* and *zhū shā* can calm the mind with heavy sedatives. *Qīng mù xiāng*, *chén xiāng* and *dīng xiāng* can motivate qi and dispel turbid which can help *shè xiāng* open the orifices (resuscitate) with aromatics. *Pò xiāo* and *xiāo shí* are used to drain heat and nourish the dryness, drain fire and promote defecation. These medicines are an assistant part of this formula. This formula clears heat, resolves toxins, extinguishes wind, and suppresses convulsion, calms the mind and opening the orifices. And this pill has a color purple of frost and snow and has cold[nature], so it is called "*Zǐ Xuě Dān* (Purple Snow Elixir)".

[Clinical Application] This is a very commonly used formula for clearing heat and resolving toxins, controlling convulsion and opening the orifices, which is used to treat intense heat pathogen sinking into pericardium. Heart *ying* with intense heat and stirring liver wind causes hyperpyrexia, unconsciousness, delirious speech and convulsive, Children with intense heat and convulsive which belong to the wind caused by heat. This formula can also treat children with measles, intense heat toxins, purple and red measles or hyperpyrexia, short breath, coma with purple and red figer venae.

Zhì Bǎo Dān (Supreme Jewel Elixir, 至宝丹)
Formulary of the Pharmacy Service for Benefiting the People in the Taiping Era
(*Tài Píng Huì Mín Hé Jì Jú Fāng,* 太平惠民和剂局方)

[Ingredient]

Xī Jiǎo (Cornu Rhinocerotis)   grind and purify

Zhū Shā (Cinnabaris)   grind and purify

Xióng Huáng (Fel Ursi)   grind and purify

Sheng Dài Mào Xiè (Carapax Eretmochelydis)   grind

Hǔ Pò (Succinum)   grind

Each of them use 1 *liang* (30 g)

Shè Xiāng (Moschus)   grind

Hé Chéng Lóng Nǎo (Borneolum Syntheticum)   grind

Each of them use 1 *fen* (0.3 g)

Jīn Bó (Zelta folija)   half used as medicine, half used as cloth

Yín Bó (Sudraba folija)   grind, 50 slices

Niú Huáng (Calculus Bovis)   grind, 0.5 *liang* (15 g)

Ān Xī Xiāng (Benzoinum)   1.5 *liang*, made into a powder, purifying drug by water grinding, filter sediment and get 1 *liang*, decocted into paste (45 g)

[Usage]   In the original formula, grain the *xī jiǎo, sheng dài mào xiè* into powder, and add with other medicines. Boiled *ān xī xiāng* solidify and put other medicines together. Roll them into pills like Tung seed size, and swallow 3 or 5 pills with *Rén Shēn Tāng* (Ginseng Decoction). It can treat children who have epilepsy and heart heat, stroke, insomnia, vexation, wind drooling and tetanus. 1 pill for kid under the age of two, and melts the pill with *Rén Shēn Tāng*.

Modern Usage: Each time one pill (3 g), grind it and takes it with warm water. Children take 0.5 pills.

[Action]   Remove turbidity, open the orifices, clear heat and resolve toxins.

[Indication]   Patients with heatstroke, stroke and attacked by filthy [qi], (manifested with fainting suddenly, short of breath and warm disease which the heat-phlegm block the orifices, unconsciousness without speaking), exuberant phlegm and

heavily breathing, fever and vexation, red and crimson tongue with yellow greasy and thick coating, slippery and rapid pulse, and children convulsive syncope which belongs to the heat-phlegm blocking.

[**Formula Analysis**] These syndromes are caused by warm pathogen attacking the interior and phlegm veiling the pericardium. In this formula, *xī jiǎo* clears *ying*, cools blood and resolves toxins, vents the heat pathogen of the pericardium, and *niú huáng* can clear heat and resolve toxins, eliminate phlegm to open the orifices. They are both chief medicines. *Sheng dài mào xiè* can help *xī jiǎo* clear heat and resolve toxins. *Lóng nǎo* can open the orifices (resuscitate) with aromatics which can move and flee. S*hè xiāng* can move and flee with aromatics, open the orifices and dispel filth. *Ān xī xiāng* is highly aromatics without dryness, and good at scurrying but not too fierce. It opens the orifices (resuscitate), dispels filth, which can help *niú huáng to* eliminate phlegm and open the orifices used as deputy medicine. *Xióng huáng* can drain phlegm and resolve phlegm. *Hǔ pò* and *zhū shā* can tranquilize the heart and calm the mind, which are assistant medicines. *Jīn bó* and *yín bó* belong to the heart meridian which can tranquilize the heart and calm the mind, used as envoy medicines. Combined with all of these medicines, this formula has the effect of dispelling filth and opening the orifices, clearing heat and resolving toxins. Because of the valuable medicine and its striking effect, this formula is named "*Zhì Bǎo Dān* (Supreme Jewel Elixir)".

[**Clinical Application**] This formula, by dispelling filth and opening the orifices, clearing heat, and resolving toxins, is prescribed for treating disorders due to heat-phlegm veiling the pericardium, unconsciousness and blocking in the interior. The original book records that this formula needs to take with *Rén Shēn Tāng* (Ginseng Decoction). When the patient has a complicated situation and serious deficiency of healthy qi, it needs the *rén shēn*'s power of reinforcing qi and nourishing the heart, combined with opening the orifices (resuscitate) with aromatics and acrid medicine, which has a great effect on recovering conscious, reinforcing healthy qi and dispelling pathogen. It is also suitable for patients who have a deficient pulse, sweating and cold limbs which belong to [qi] blocking in the interior and desertion exterior. In the

original book, it can take with children's urine and *shēng jiāng zhī* (Ginger Juice), which can promote the effect of clearing heat and opening the orifices; it is suitable for patients with excess, slippery and rapid pulse, which has a reference value in the clinical application.

Section 2　Formulas that opens the orifices (resuscitate) with warm

The formula of opening the orifices (resuscitate) with warm medicine applies to cold-type block disorders manifested as cold-stroke, syncope due to the accumulation of phlegm, sudden collapse by attacking of noxious factor, clenched jaw, loss of consciousness, white tongue coating and slow pulse which belong to the pattern of pathogenic cold and phlegm and dampness blocking qi. These formulas are formed by the opening the orifices (resuscitate) with aromatics medicine like *sū hé xiāng*, *bīng piàn*, *shè xiāng*, combined with moving qi and dispel filth acrid warmherbs. The typical formula is *Sū Hé Xiāng Wán* (Storax Pill, 苏合香丸). The formula of opening the orifices (resuscitate) can rectify qi and relieve pain, dispel filth and resolve toxins to treat chest and abdominal pain, cholera, vomiting and diarrhea despite warming, and unblocking the orifices to treat a cold block.

Sū Hé Xiāng Wán (**Storax Pill,** 苏合香丸)
Arcane Essentials from the Imperial Library (***Wài Tái Mì Yào,*** 外台秘要)
Quote From Extensive Aiding Formula Collection (***Guang Ji Fang,*** 广济方)[53]

[Ingredient]
Chī Li Jiā[Bái Zhú] (Rhizoma Atractylodis Macrocephalae)
Qīng Mù Xiāng (Radix Aristolochiae)
Wū Xī Xuè [Shuǐ Niú Jiǎo] (Cornu Bubali)
Xiāng Fù (Rhizoma Cyperi)　remove the furing by dry-fried
Zhū Shā (Cinnabaris)　grind and purifying drug by water grinding
Hē Zǐ (Fructus Chebulae)　remove the coating by roasting
Tán Xiāng (Lignum Santali Albi)

Ān Xī Xiāng (Benzoinum)   made into powder and decocted into paste with wine

Chén Xiāng (Lignum Aquilariae Resinatum)

Shè Xiāng (Moschus)   grind

Dīng Xiāng (Flos Caryophylli)

Bì Bá (Fructus Piperis Longi)

Each of them use 2 *liang* (60 g)

Hé Chéng Lóng Nǎo (Borneolum Syntheticum)   grind

Sū Hé Xiāng oil (Styrax)   mix with the *ān xī xiāng* paste

Xūn Lù Xiāng (Boswellia Thurifera)   grind

Each of them use 1 *liang* (30 g)

[Usage]   Grind the 15 medicines into a powder and form the sieved powder into pills with white honey. Take 4 pills like *tung seed* with fresh well water in the morning, and the pills should be crushed in a clean pot first. The aged or children take 1 pill.

[Action]   Warming and aromatic properties open the orifices, promote the qi and remove turbidity.

[Indication]   Patients with a stroke, phlegm syncope, sudden collapse, clenched jaw, white face and cyan lips with a short but intense of breath, unconsciousness with a white greasy and glossy coating and deep and slippery pulse. The patient who was attacked by filthy qi, appeared with chest and abdominal pain, even a coma.

Patients, attacked by cold-damp and filthy qi, manifest with vomiting and diarrhea, miasmic malaria with white, glossy and greasy tongue coating.

[Formula Analysis]   This formula represents the typical method of warming to open the acute closed disorders. In this formula, *sū hé xiāng* is used to open the orifices and dispel filth. It is mentioned in *Encountering the Sources of the 'Classic of Materia Medica'* (*Běn Jīng Féng Yuán*, 本经逢原[54]) that, "it is gathered all incenses which can vent the various orifices and organs and clear away all abnormal qi. Whenever there is qi collapse (气厥) from phlegm accumulation, one must firstly use this to open and guide out. Regulating qi is the foundation for treating phlegm. *Ān*

xī xiāng can open the orifices (resuscitate) and dispel filth which is aromatics without dryness, can flee but mild. *Lóng nǎo* and *shè xiāng* can dispel filth and open the orifices, which is good at scurrying but not too fierce. These four medicines are the main part of this formula. *Qīng mù xiāng, xiāng fù, ān xī xiāng, bái tán xiāng, chén xiāng, dīng xiāng* and *xūn lù xiāng* can move qi and resolve constraint, dispel cold and remove turbidity to resolve the heat and constraint of *zang fu* organs and qi and blood. *Bì bá* can help those herbs to strengthen the effect of dispelling cold and warming the middle. *Shuǐ niú jiǎo* is used to clear heat and resolve toxins for its taste of salty and cold without inhibition, a fragrance which can vent, and *zhū shā* can tranquilize the heart and calm the mind because the heart is the fire organ which is unable to stand the acrid and warm medicine, used as paradoxical assistant medicine. *Bái zhú* can strengthen the spleen to consolidate qi for the taste of sweet and warm and help other medicine circulate around the body. *Hē zǐ* combined with other incense is used to avoid that too much acrid and aromatic medicines consume the healthy qi for its taste of warm, astringent which can restrain qi. These medicine are the assistant part of this formula. This formula has all the incense in one pill. However, it can ascend and descend, dissipate and restrain, which has the effect of warming and unblocking, opening the orifices, moving qi and removing turbidity.

[Clinical Application] This formula is quite a typical representative warm formula for opening the orifices. Patients with a stroke, qi stroke, attack of noxious factor and loss of consciousness suddenly, clenched jaw, or unconsciousness with white, glossy, and greasy tongue coating can take this formula.

Chapter 8

Tonifying and Replenishing Formulas

The formulas in this chapter are formed by tonifying, nourishing, enriching and replenishing medicine which has the effect of tonifying human bodies qi and blood, yin and yang are used to treat various deficiency syndromes. It belongs to the "tonifying method" of the "eight methods".

There are lots of tonifying and replenishing formulas. As for the deficiency of qi, blood, yin and yang, they can be divided into five types: supplement qi, supplement blood, supplement qi and blood, supplement yin and supplement yang.

Section 1   Formulas that tonify qi

Tonifying qi formulas apply to the syndromes of qi deficiency of the lung and spleen, such as exhaustion-fatigue and lack of strength, weak breathing with no desire to speak, weak voice, sallow yellow or white complexion, hasty breath when doing some acts, reduced appetite and thin, loose stool, deficiency weak or large pulse, pale tongue and thin and white coating with teeth-marked. There are usual tonifying qi medicines like *rén shēn, dǎng shēn, huáng qí, bái zhú, shān yào*. But because the qi prefers moving, so some regulating qi medicines like *chén pí, mù xiāng, shā rén* should be combined with tonifying-qi medicnals to avoid qi blocking which is possibly caused by sweet medicines. There are typical formulas like *Sì Jūn Zǐ Tāng* (Four Gentlemen Decoction, 四君子汤), *Shēn Líng Bái Zhú Sǎn* (Ginseng, Poria and Atractylodes Macrocephalae Powder, 参苓白术散), *Bǔ Zhōng Yì Qì Tāng* (Center-Tonifying and Qi-Boosting Decoction, 补中益气汤), *Shēng Mài Sǎn* (Pulse-Engendering Powder, 生脉散).

Sì Jūn Zǐ Tāng (Four Gentlemen Decoction, 四君子汤)
Ji Feng Formulas of Universal Benefit (Jī FēngPǔ Jì Fāng, 鸡峰普济方)[55]

[Ingredient]

Rén Shēn (Radix Et Rhizoma Ginseng)　1 *liang* (30 g)

Bái Zhú (Rhizoma Atractylodis Macrocephalae)　1 *liang* (30 g)

Fú Líng (Poria)　1 *liang* (30 g)

Gān Cǎo (Radix Et Rhizoma Glycyrrhizae)　1 *liang* (30 g)

[Usage]　In the original text, it advises grinding the ingredients into a thready powder and taking 2 *qian* with 1 *zhan* water, 3 pieces of *shēng jiāng*, 1 piece *dà zǎo* and decocted into 6 *fen* without sediment.

Modern Usage: Decoct with water, the dosage depends on the original formula, or it can be made into pills and taken 6–12 g pills, twice a day.

[Action]　Nourish qi and tonify the middle, strengthen the spleen and stomach.

[Indication]　Patients who have deficient qi of spleen and stomach, sallow yellow or pale face, weak voice, lassitude, reduced appetite, thin and loose stool, pale tongue and thin and white coating, weak pulse.

[Formula Analysis]　The spleen governs transportation and transformation, and the stomach governs intake (of food and drinks), which are the source of qi and blood production. In this formula, *rén shēn* has powerful supplementation of original qi, strengthens the spleen and nourishes the stomach, which is the chief medicine. The spleen is averse to dampness but prefers dryness, so *bái zhú* is the deputy medicine to strengthen the spleen and nourish qi, dry dampness and harmonize the center for its taste of bitter sweet and warm once the spleen gets dampness; *fú líng* is used to strengthen spleen, tonify the center and drain dampness for the taste sweet, bland, neutral, as Huang Xiu-gong[56] said, "*fú líng* in this formula can help *rén shēn* and *bái zhú* to drain the dampness of spleen." While Zhang Bing-cheng[57] said, "it can drain the dampness of lung and spleen downward and then the effect of *rén shēn* and *bái zhú* can be manifested." Thus, it is used as an assistant medicine. *Gān cǎo* is used as an envoy medicine to nourish qi, calm the stomach and harmonize the center for a

sweet and warm taste. This formula has the effect of nourishing qi and tonifing the middle, strengthening the spleen, and nourishing the stomach. These four flavors in this formula are all neutral medicine which have the quality of harmonious, so this formula is called "*Sì Jūn Zǐ Tāng* (Four Gentlemen Decoction)".

[Clinical Application] This formula is quite a basic formula for treating spleen and stomach qi deficiency. Many tonifying qi and strengthening spleen formulas are derived from this formula. For the spleen and stomach qi deficiency caused by various reasons, it can be used in addition and subtraction of this formula.

Shēn Líng Bái Zhú Sǎn (Ginseng, Poria and Atractylodes Macrocephalae Powder, 参苓白术散)

Formulary of the Pharmacy Service for Benefiting the People in the Taiping Era (Tài Píng Huì Mín Hé Jì Jú Fāng, 太平惠民和剂局方)

[Ingredient]

Lián Zǐ Xīn (Plumula Nelumbinis)

Yì Yi Ren (Semen Coicis)

Shā Rén (Fructus Amomi)

Jié Gěng (Radix Platycodonis)　　dry-fried ito deep yellow

Each of them use 1 *jin* (500 g)

Bái Biǎn Dòu (Semen Lablab Album)　　soak by ginger ale,1.5 *jin* (750 g)

Bái Fú Líng (Poria)

Rén Shēn (Radix Et Rhizoma Ginseng)　　remove the sediment of rhizome

Gān Cǎo (Radix Et Rhizoma Glycyrrhizae)　　dry-fried

Bái Zhú (Rhizoma Atractylodis Macrocephalae)

Shān Yào (Rhizoma Dioscoreae)

Each of them use 2 *jin* (1000 g)

[Usage] The original book advises grinding the herbs into thready powder and taking 2 *qian* with *dà zǎo* soup. The dosage for children depends on their ages.

Modern Usage: Each 6 g thready powder with *dà zǎo* soup, twice a day. It can make into pills. Alternatively, decocted with water, the dosage should be reduced

proportionally according to the original formula.

[Action] Strengthen the spleen and nourish qi, harmonize the stomach and eliminate dampness.

[Indication] Patients with weakness of the spleen and stomach, which lead to dampness produced in the interior, poor appetite, vomit or diarrhea, sallow yellow face and lassitude, distention feeling in the chest and epigastrium, white and pale tongue but with greasy coating, deficiency and slow pulse.

[Formula Analysis] Those with a strong spleen and stomach can restrain the dampness normally. While the spleen and stomach are weak thus cannot guide transportation and transformation, the fluids are accumulated and transform into dampness. This formula is formed by *Sì Jūn Zǐ Tāng* (Four Gentlemen Decoction) with *lián zǐ xīn, yì yǐ rén, shā rén, bái biǎn dòu, shān yào, jié gěng*. In this formula, *bái fú líng, rén shēn* and *bái zhú* can nourish qi and strengthen the spleen, which is used as chief medicines; *lián zǐ xīn, yì yǐ rén, bái biǎn dòu, shān yào* are used as deputy medicines to strengthen the effect of chief medicine, and *yì yǐ rén, bái biǎn dòu, bái fú líng* and *bái zhú* can strengthen the spleen and eliminate dampness; *gān cǎo* is used to nourish qi and harmonize the center, *shā rén* serves as the assistant medicine, used to remove dampness with intensely aromatic, harmonize the stomach and regulate qi; the envoy, *jié gěng* is used to guide other medicines upward and to disseminating [lung-qi], also directs the turbid downward, drain the dampness in order to strengthen the spleen. With all these medicines, deficiency can be tonified, dampness can be drained, stasis can be moved, qi can be regulated. When the spleen is strong and the dampness go away, the body will recover by itself.

[Clinical Application] This formula is quite a typical applicator in the clinic for its mild nature and taste, warm but not dry, which can strengthen the spleen and nourish qi, harmonize the stomach and eliminate dampness. And this formula can treat the lung [qi] deficiency and consumption, for it can tonify the lung-qi deficiency, regulate qi and dissolve phlegm, stimulate one's appetite, which is the method of backing up earth to generate metal.

Bŭ Zhōng Yì Qì Tāng (Center-Tonifying and Qi-Boosting Decoction, 补中益气汤)

Treatise on the Spleen and Stomach (Pí Wèi Lùn, 脾胃论)[58]

[Ingredient]

Huáng Qí (Radix Astragali)   patient with high feveruse 1 *qian* (18 g)

Zhì Gān Căo (Radix Et Rhizoma Glycyrrhizae Praeparata Cum Melle)   each of them use 5 *fen* (9 g)

Rén Shēn (Radix Et Rhizoma Ginseng)   remove the sediment of rhizome, 3 *fen* (9 g)

Dāng Guī (Radix Angelicae Sinensis)   bake or bask, 2 *fen* (6 g)

Jú Pí (Pericarpium Citri Reticulatae)   don't remove the white inner surface of exocarp, 2 or 3 *fen* (6 g)

Shēng Má (Rhizoma Cimicifugae)   2 or 3 *fen* (6 g)

Chái Hú (Radix Bupleuri)   2 or 3 *fen* (6 g)

Bái Zhú (Rhizoma Atractylodis Macrocephalae)   3 *fen* (9 g)

[Usage]   In the original book, chew it coarsely, boil it with 2 *zhan* water into 1 *zhan*, then remove the sediment and take it warmly after the meal.

Modern Usage: Decocted with water. It can make into pills, 6–9 g a time, 2–3 times a day with warm water.

[Action]   Tonify the center and reinforce qi, raises the yang and lifts what has sunken.

[Indication]   Patients with fever caused by the qi deficiency, sweating, thirst but prefer warm beverages, headache and aversion to cold, the laziness of speech, with surging and large but forceless pulse. Or the one with deficiency qi of spleen and stomach, lassitude, cannot tolerate manual labor, rapid panting on exertion, pale tongue and thin and white coating.

The qi deficiency causes the sinking manifested as rectal or uterine prolapse, chronic diarrhea or dysentery, bloody stool, flooding and spotting, diarrhea and dribbling urination, and other syndromes of the sinking of clearing yang.

[Formula Analysis]

Treatise on the Spleen and Stomach (*Pí Wèi Lùn,* 脾胃论) says: "true qi or original qi is the essential qi of human body which can be nourished by stomach qi"; "[if]the spleen and stomach qi have been damaged, then the original qi can not be nourished as well, all the diseases come out." and "improper diet causes the stomach disease...overexertion causes the spleen disease." This formula is created by Li Gao[59], based on the "warm to treat overexertion", "boost to treat consumption" in *Basic Questions-Comprehensive Discourse on the Essentials of the Most Reliable* (*Sù Wèn-Zhì Zhēn Yào Dà Lùn,* 素问·至真要大论). In this formula, *huáng qí* is in an critical position and used as the chief medicine which can augment the lung qi to consolidate the exterior, boost the center to raise yang for the sweet and little warm taste, belonging to the spleen and lung meridian. *Zhì gān cǎo* and *rén shēn* are used as deputy medicines to tonify spleen and reinforce qi, helping *huáng qí* to tonify the center for its sweet and warm taste, which said by Li Gao that, "*huáng qí, zhì gān cǎo* and *rén shēn* are holy medicines to drain fire" Because that vexation and overexertion lead to deficiency and are manifested as pyrexia, while the sweet and warm medicine can nourish original qi which makes the deficient fever reduced by itself. *Bái zhú* can strengthen the spleen, *dāng guī* can nourish the blood, *jú pí* can regulate qi, they are used as assistant medicines; *shēng má* and *chái hú* can raise clear yang, combined with chief medicines, [it] can raise the sinking yang qi, *The Grand Compendium of Materia Medica* (*Běn Cǎo Gāng Mù,* 本草纲目) says: "*shēng má* guides the *yangming* clear qi upwards while *chái hú* leads the *shaoyang* clear qi upward, which are the important medicines to treat congenital deficiency, weak original qi, overexertion, irregular eating, interior damage by raw or cold food." The combination of these medicines has the effect of tonifying the center and boosting qi, raising yang and lifting the sunken.

[Clinical Application]

1. This formula is a famous representative formula that is good at tonfiying the center and augmenting the qi, raising the yang, It has indeed effective to treat insufficiency of middle qi or sinking of deficiency qi in clinical treatment.

2. Combining upraising medicine and tonifying qi medicine are the characteristic

of this formula. Without upraising medicine, the effect of raising yang and lifting the sunken cannot work; without tonifying qi medicine, the upraising medicine will not be noticeable. Qi deficiency causes the sinking of clear yang, so the tonifying qi medicine should be put in an important position. If qi is insufficient, the sinking will rise by itself. [but]A small amount raising medicine can be used, but not too much.

Shēng Mài Sǎn (Pulse-Engendering Powder, 生脉散)
Clarifying Doubts about Damage from Internal and External Causes (*Nèi Wài Shāng Biàn Huò Lùn*, 内外伤辨惑论)[60]

[Ingredient]

Rén Shēn (Radix et Rhizoma Ginseng)　(10 g)

Mài Dōng (Radix Ophiopogonis)　(15 g)

Wǔ Wèi Zǐ (Fructus Schisandrae Chinensis)　(6 g)

The original book does not record the dosage.

[Usage]　The original book does not record the administration.

Modern Usage: Decocted with water.

[Action]　Boost qi and engender fluid, maintains yin and check excessive sweating.

[Indication]

1. The patient's original qi been damaged by heat, [leads to]deficiency of qi and yin, shortness of breath and lassitude, thirst and sweating, deficient thready or rapid pulse, even profuse sweating, panting and coughing, large without its roots pulse, dry and red tongue without coating.

2. Patients with chronic cough and lung deficiency, cough with sparse phlegm, shortness of breath and spontaneous sweating, dry mouth, deficient pulse.

[Formula Analysis]　Heat damages the original qi and causes a deficiency of qi and yin. In this formula, as the chief medicine, *rén shēn* is used to powerfully tonify the original qi, release thirst and promote fluid production for its sweet and warm taste; *mài dōng* is used as the deputy medicine to nourish yin and clear heat, moisten the lung and promote fluid production for its taste sweet and cold; the assistant, *wǔ*

wèi zǐ can consolidate the kidney qi and restrain heart qi. Together with these three medicines, one for tonifying, one for clearing, and one for restraining, which ensures this formula is good at boosting the qi and engendering fluid, preserving the yin and checking excessive sweating. Wang Ang said, "people have a thready and faint pulse which is nearly going to stop, taking this [formula] can be revived [normal]. What a great achievement". This formula can enrich qi and recover the pulse, so it is called as "*Shēng Mài Sǎn* (Pulse-Engendering Powder)."

[Clinical Application] This formula is usually used to treat original qi damaged by heat, deficiency of qi and yin, which can be used to treat fluid and qi desertion caused by warm and heat diseases damaging fluid and consuming qi and has the effect of boosting the qi and engendering fluid, preserving the yin and checking excessive sweating. Patients attacked by summer heat result in yin and qi consuming, profuse sweating, exhaustion and thirst, this formula is fit.

Section 2　Formulas that tonifies lood

Tonifying blood formula applies to the syndromes of blood deficiency which includes dizziness, vertigo, pale and lusterless complexion, dry and cracked nails without shine, palpitations, insomnia and dreaminess, muscular spasms or cramp, dry and itchy skin, dry hair, thready weak or choppy pulse, pale tongue with thin and white coating. Women have abnormal menstruation, prolonged menstrual cycles with scanty or even amenorrhoea. There are some tonifying blood medicines such as *dāng guī*, *bái sháo yào*, *shú dì huáng*, *lóng yǎn ròu*. However, visible blood cannot be produced by itself; only invisible qi can do this. Qi is the commander of blood while blood is the mother of qi, so too much blood loss will cause the failure of the qi. Therefore, tonifying blood formula is usually combined with *huáng qí*, *rén shēn* to boost qi and nourish the blood. Representative formulas like *Sì Wù Tāng* (Four Substances Decoction, 四物汤), *Dāng Guī Bǔ Xuè Tāng* (Chinese Angelica Blood-Tonifying Decoction, 当归补血汤), *Guī Pí Tāng* (Spleen-Restoring Decoction, 归脾汤) and *etc*.

Sì Wù Tāng (Four Substances Decoction, 四物汤)
Formulary of the Pharmacy Service for Benefiting the People in the Taiping Era
(*Tài Píng Huì Mín Hé Jì Jú Fāng*, 太平惠民和剂局方)

[Ingredient]

Dāng Guī (Radix Angelicae Sinensis)　removes the sediment of rhizome from the root, soaking in rice wine and dry-fried slightly

Chuān Xiōng (Rhizoma Chuanxiong)

Bái Sháo Yào (Radix Paeoniae)

Shú Dì Huáng (Radix Rehmanniae Praeparata)　steaming drugs with rice wine, equal dose

[Usage]　In the original formula, grind the ingredients into a thick powder, take 3 *qian* with 1.5 *zhan* water, decoct into 8 *fen*, remove the sediment and take it before a meal. If the patient has threatened abortion, 10 leafs *ài yè*, *ē jiāo* 1 slice needs to be added and decocted like the former way; if the patient has a deficiency cold of blood and organs who lost too much blood, this formula needs more *Jiāo Ài Tāng* (Donkey-Hide Gelatin and Mugwort Decoction).

Modern Usage: Decocted with water, modified the dosage according to the original formula.

[Action]　Tonify and harmonize blood and regulate menstruation.

[Indication]　Patients with deficient stasis of *ying* blood manifested as frighted, dizziness, dizzy vision, nails without shiny, abnormal menstruation or scant menstrual flow, or amenorrhoea, umbilical and abdominal pain, pale tongue with white coating, thready weak or choppy pulse.

[Formula Analysis]　The heart governs the blood and the liver stores the blood. In this formula, *Shú dì huáng* is the chief medicine to nourish yin and tonify blood, it tastes sweet and a little warm; *dāng guī* acts as deputy medicine to tonify blood and nourish the liver, harmonize blood and regulate the menstruation for its taste of sweet, acrid, bitter, warm; *bái sháo yào* is used as assistant medicine to nourish blood and soft liver, harmonize *ying* and stop the pain; *chuān xiōng* is used as

envoy medicine to invigorate blood and regulate qi for its tastes of acrid and warm. *Bái sháo yào* and *shú dì huáng* are the yin medicines of blood while *chuān xiōng* and *dāng guī* are the yang medicines of blood. Combined with these four medicines, it has the effect of tonifying without stasis, harmonizing the *ying* and blood. So, not only can the blood deficiency pattern use this formula to tonify blood, but also the blood stagnation can use this formula to harmonize blood which has relieving in tonifying, astringency within dissipation, which is the basic formula to treat blood disease.

[Clinical Application]

1. This formula is fundamental to tonify and harmonize blood, regulate the menstruation. Such syndromes like blood deficiency, blood stagnation, abnormal menstruation, Pre-fetal postpartum can use this formula with a ddition and subtraction to treat.

2. If it mainly needs tonifying blood, this formula can add the dosage of *bái sháo yào* and *shú dì huáng*, change *dāng guī* into *dāng guī shēn* [trunk part], use less *chuān xiōng* or don't use it; if it mainly needs harmonizing blood, this formula can add the dosage of *chuān xiōng* and *dāng guī*, and change *bái sháo yào* into chì sháo. If the patient has blood deficiency with fever, *shú dì huáng* need to change into *xiān dì huáng* [fresh].

Dāng Guī Bǔ Xuè Tāng (Chinese Angelica Blood-Tonifying Decoction, 当归补血汤)

Clarifying Doubts about Damage from Internal and External Causes (*Nèi Wài Shāng Biàn Huò Lùn*, 内外伤辨惑论)

[Ingredient]

Huáng Qí (Radix Astragali)   1 *liang* (30 g)

Dāng Guī   washing with rice wine, 2 *qian* (6 g)

[Usage]   In the original formula, it is chewed[ground] into coarse pieces and decocted with 2 *zhan* water into 1 *zhan*, remove the sediment and take it warmly before a meal.

Modern Usage: Decocted with water.

[Action]   Tonify qi and generate blood.

[Indication]   Overexertion and internal exhaustion-fatigue, deficient blood and qi, yang floating to the superficial, hot sensation in the muscle and red face, vexation and thirst with desire for warm beverages, surging, large but deficient pulse when pressed deeply, or women who have menorrhagia, flooding and spotting, deficient blood, and fever after delivery; or with ulcerating skin and external diseases who can not recover by himself.

[Formula Analysis]   Exhaustion-fatigue damages the interior, original qi is deficient and the yin blood is also deficient. The visible blood is produced by the invisible qi, so in this formula, *huáng qí*, sweet and warm, plays a important role in nourishing the origin of blood production by tonifying qi. *Essentials of Materia Medica (Běn Cǎo Bèi Yào*, 本草备要[61]) says: "[it can] drain yin fire, clear the heat in muscle". *Dāng guī* is an important medicine of nourishing blood and the holy medicine of tonifying ying for its taste of sweat, acrid, bitter, warm. The dosage of *huáng qí* is five times of *dāng guī* in terms of the meaning that when yang arises, yin grows when qi is in excess, blood can be produced by itself.

[Clinical Application]   This formula is typical for tonifying qi and producing blood to treat deficient blood and fever. The key point of differentiation is that the patient has a large but deficient pulse that is faint when pressed deeply.

Guī Pí Tāng (Spleen-Restoring Decoction, 归脾汤)
Formulas to Aid the Living (Jì Shēng Fāng, 济生方)[62]

[Ingredient]

Bái Zhú (Rhizoma Atractylodis Macrocephalae)   (9 g)

Fú Shén (Sclerotium Poriae Pararadicis)   remove the woody   (12 g)

Huáng Qí (Radix Astragali)   remove the sediment of basal leaf from the root (12 g)

Lóng Yǎn Ròu (Arillus Longan)   (12 g)

Suān Zǎo Rén (Semen Ziziphi Spinosae)   remove the peel by dry-fried, each of them uses 1 *liang* (12 g)

Rén Shēn (Radix Et Rhizoma Ginseng)　　(9 g)

Mù Xiāng (Radix Aucklandiae)　　invisible fire, 0.5 *liang* (6 g)

Zhì gān Cǎo (Radix Et Rhizoma Glycyrrhizae Praeparata Cum Melle)
2.5 *qian* (4.5 g)

Dāng Guī (Radix Angelicae Sinensis)　　(9 g)

Yuǎn Zhì (Radix Polygalae)

Each of them uses 1 *qian* (3 g) [the last two medicines are from *Corrections and Annotations to Fine Formulas for Women* (*Jiào Zhù Fù Rén Liáng Fāng*, 校注妇人良方)]

[Usage]　　In the original book, [it] advised to chewed and decocted 4 *qian* with 1.5 *zhan* water, 5 slices of *shēng jiāng*, and 1 *mei dà zǎo* into 7 *fen*, remove the sediment and take it warmly anytime.

Modern Usage: Add 3 slices *shēng jiāng* and 5 *mei dà zǎo* decocted with water. Or made into pills, each time take 6–9 g, 2–3 times a day with warm water.

[Action]　　Augment the qi and tonify the blood, strengthen the spleen and nourishes the heart.

[Indication]　　Excessive contemplation damage the heart and spleen and leads to severe palpitations, forgetfulness, palpitations due to phobia and night sweating, bad appetite, and insomnia; or the deficient spleen which fails to contain blood and occur with vomiting blood, nosebleed, bloody stool; or women with abnormal menstruation, metrorrhagia, with pale tongue and thin and white coating, thready and weak pulse.

[Formula Analysis]　　The heart stores the spirit and governs the blood; the spleen governs thoughts and controls the blood. Excessive deliberation will damage the heart and spleen. In this formula, *huáng qí* and *rén shēn* are sweet and a little warm, invigorating the spleen and nourishing qi, and *lóng yǎn ròu* is sweet and neutral, nourishing the heart and calming the mind, nourishing the spleen and blood, those three medicines are used as chief medicines; *bái zhú* is bitter, sweet and warm, and helps *huáng qí* and *rén shēn* tonify the spleen and boost qi, *fú shén* and *suān zǎo rén* are used to help *lóng yǎn ròu* are sweet and neutral, nourish the heart and calm

the mind, *dāng guī* is acrid, bitter and warm, used to nourish *ying* and blood, and is compatible with *huáng qí* and *rén shēn* which strengthen the power of tonifying blood, used as deputy medicine. *yuǎn zhì* is bitter, acrid and warm, can restore communication between the heart and kidney, calm the heart and mind, *mù xiāng* can regulate qi and awaken the spleen which can promote the effect of tonifying qi and blood medicine without stagnation for the taste acrid, bitter and warm, which are used as assistant medicine. *Zhì gān cǎo* is sweet and warm, can boost qi and harmonize all the medicines, *shēng jiāng* and *dà zǎo* can harmonize *ying* and *wei* levels, which are all used as envoy medicine. This formula combines nourishing heart and strengthening spleen, nourishing the heart with tonifying blood, strengthening the spleen with tonifying qi so that excessive qi and blood will calm the heart and mind promote the spleen qi transportation. This formula uses lots of augmenting and strengthening spleen medicines because the heart blood is produced by the essence which transported and transforms from the spleen, *The Spiritual Pivot-Discourse on Qi* (*Líng Shū-Jué Qì*, 灵枢·决气) says: "Middle *jiao* (Middle Energizer) receives qi (nutrients of food), absorbs the juice and changes [transforms] it into red. That is what *xue* (blood) means". Thus, it can nourish the heart by tonifying the spleen qi. The spleen controls the blood and when it is strong, it can controls and contains blood, and restore blood, hence the name *Guī Pí Tāng* (Spleen-Restoring Decoction).

[Clinical Application]   This formula is appropriate for treating any disorder due to the deficiency of the heart and spleen, qi and blood. The key points of its differentiation are that the patients have severe palpitations, forgetfulness, palpitations, night sweating, lassitude, poor appetite and insomnia with pale tongue, thin and white coating, thready and weak pulse.

Section 3   Formulas that tonifies qi and blood

These formulas apply to the syndromes of qi and blood deficiency, such as lusterless complexion, dizziness and dizzy vision, palpitations and shortness of breath, lack of appetite and exhaustion-fatigue, pale tongue with thin and white coating,

thready and weak pulse. There are some usual qi-tonifying medicines *like rén shēn*, *huáng qí*, *gān cǎo*, *dà zǎo* and some usual blood-tonifying medicines like dì huáng, *dāng guī*, *bái sháo yào*, *ē jiāo* and so on. There are typical formulas such as *Bā Zhēn Tāng* (Eight-Gem Decoction, 八珍汤), *Shǔ Yù Wán* (Deltoideae Root Pills, 薯蓣丸), *Zhì Gān Cǎo Tāng* (Honey-Fried Licorice Decoction, 炙甘草汤).

Bā Zhēn Tāng (Eight-Gem Decoction, 八珍汤)
Categorized Essentials for Normalizing the Structure (Zhèng Tǐ Lèi Yào, 正体类要)[63]

[Ingredient]

Rén Shēn (Radix Et Rhizoma Ginseng)   1 *qian* (9 g)

Bái Zhú (Rhizoma Atractylodis Macrocephalae)   1 *qian* (9 g)

Bái Fú Líng (Poria)   1 *qian* (9 g)

Dāng Guī (Radix Angelicae Sinensis)   1 *qian* (9 g)

Chuān Xiōng (Rhizoma Chuanxiong)   1 *qian* (9 g)

Bái Sháo Yào (Radix Paeoniae)   1 *qian* (9 g)

Shú Dì Huáng (Radix Rehmanniae Praeparata)   1 *qian* (9 g)

Gān Cǎo (Radix Et Rhizoma Glycyrrhizae)   dry-fried with liquid adjuvant, 5 *fen* (4.5 g)

[Usage]   In the original book, it is decocted with *shēng jiāng* and *dà zǎo*.

Modern Usage: Add 3 slices s*hēng jiāng* and 5 pieces *dà zǎo*, decocted with water.

[Action]   Tonify qi and blood.

[Indication]   Patients with deficiency of qi and blood, sallow yellow or pale complexion, dizziness and blur vision, lassitude, palpitation, shortness of breath, poor appetite, pale tongue with thin and white coating, thready and weak or deficient and large without power pulse. Or treats excessive blood loss, fever with aversion to cold, vexation but thirst; or patients with chronic skin and external diseases which is cannot heal for a long time.

[Formula Analysis]   This formula is composed by *Sì Jūn Zǐ Tāng* (Four

Gentlemen Decoction, 四君子汤) and *Sì Wù Tāng* (Four Substances Decoction, 四物汤). In the formula, *rén shēn*, *bái zhú*, *bái fú líng* and *gān cǎo* are used to boost qi, *dāng guī*, *chuān xiōng*, *bái sháo yào* and *shú dì huáng* are used to nourish the blood, *shēng jiāng* and *dà zǎo* are used to harmonize *ying* and *wei* levels. These medicines form the tonifying qi and blood formula, which has the effect of rising yang and growing yin.

[Clinical Application] This formula often used for chronic disease and weakness, for women with abnormal menstruation, metrorrhagia, stillborn fetus, uterine atrophy, postpartum depletion and persistent sores and external diseases for a long time.

Shǔ Yù Wán (deltoideae root pills, 薯蓣丸)
Essentials from the Golden Cabinet (*Jīn Guì Yào Lüè,* 金匮要略)

[Ingredient]

Shǔ Yù (Rhizoma Dioscoreae Deltoideae)   *30 fen* (22.5 g)

Dāng Guī (Radix Angelicae Sinensis)

Guì Zhī (Ramulus Cinnamomi)

Shén Qǔ (Massa Medicata Fermentata)

Gān Dì Huáng (Radix Rehmanniae Recens)

Dà Dòu Juǎn (Semen Sojae Germinatum)

Each of them uses 10 *fen* (7.5g)

Gān Cǎo (Radix Et Rhizoma Glycyrrhizae)   *28 fen* (21 g)

Rén Shēn (Radix Et Rhizoma Ginseng)   *7 fen* (5.3 g)

Chuān Xiōng (Rhizoma Chuanxiong)

Sháo Yào (Radix Paeoniae)

Bái Zhú (Rhizoma Atractylodis Macrocephalae)

Mài Mén Dōng (Radix Ophiopogonis)

Xìng Rén (Semen Armeniacae Amarum)

Each of them uses 6 *fen* (5.3 g)

Chái Hú (Radix Bupleuri)

Jié Gĕng (Radix Platycodonis)

Fú Líng (Poria)

Each of them use 5 *fen* (3.8 g)

Ē Jiāo (Colla Corii Asini)　7 *fen* (5.3 g)

Gān Jiāng (Rhizoma Zingiberis)　3 *fen* (2.3 g)

Bái Liăn (Radix Ampelopsis)　2 *fen* (1.5 g)

Fáng Fēng (Radix Saposhnikoviae)　6 *fen* (4.5 g)

Dà Zăo (Fructus Jujubae)　100 *mei* made into cream (30 *mei*)

[Usage]　In the original book, grind those medicines into a powder and rolls them into pills with honey; take 1 pill with alcohol before a meal, 100 pills a period.

Modern Usage: Grind into powder, make it into pills, and take 6–9 g, twice a day with warm water or yellow rice wine.

[Action]　Tonify deficiency and dispel wind.

[Indication]　Patients who have deficiency consumption, dizziness and blurred vision, poor appetite, loss of weight, heavy body and shortness of breath, numbness and pain in the limbs.

[Formula Analysis]　Patients with deficiency and weak body situations can easily be attacked by the external wind. In this formula, the chief medicial, *shŭ yù*, with a sweet and neutral taste, is good at tonifying the spleen and stomach, which is recorded in *Shen Nong's Classic of the Materia Medica* (*Shén Nóng Bĕn Căo Jīng*, 神农本草经) says: "it can treat center damage, tonify deficiency, dispel the heat and cold pathogenic qi, tonify qi and strengthen the power and regenerate the muscle, strengthen yin." and is good at tonifying deficiency and dispelling wind, *rén shēn, bái zhú, gān căo* and *fú líng, gān jiāng* and *dà zăo* are used to boost qi and warm yang, *dāng guī, gān dì huáng, chuān xiōng, sháo yào, mài mén dōng* and *ē jiāo* are used to nourish blood and yin and help *shŭ yù* tonify its deficiency which is used as deputy medicines; *chái hú, bái liăn, fáng fēng, guì zhī* are used to dissipate and dispel wind and clear heat, *xìng rén* and *jié gĕng* can ascend and descend qi movement, *dà dòu juăn* can drain dampness, *shén qǔ* can promote digestion and harmonize the center, which is the assistant medicines. *gān căo* and *dà zăo* can harmonize all the medicines

which are the envoy medicines. This formula has dissipated in tonifying; with a small number of pills, it can recover the deficiency and dispel the wind slowly.

[Clinical Application] In *Important Formulas Worth a Thousand Gold Pieces* (*Qiān Jīn Fāng*, 千金方), this formula belongs to the treating wind and dizziness group, which adds *huáng qín* and changes *ē jiāo* into *lù jiǎo jiāo* to treat deficiency-consumption wind and dizziness.

According to professor Yue Mei-zhong's experience, this formula is suitable for elderly people with a deficiency of qi and blood, who feels uncomfortable, dizziness, pain and numbness of limbs, so-called "wind dizziness", "wind *bi*" or "five taxations and seven injuries". This formula has an effect of enriching, nourishing and strengthening which can be used to treat poor sleep, low-spirited and deficient yin and yang, qi and blood.

Zhì Gān Cǎo Tāng (Honey-Fried Licorice Decoction, 炙甘草汤) *Fù Mài Tāng* (Pulse-Restoring Decoction, 复脉汤)
Revised Popular Guide to 'Treatise on Cold Damage' (*Chóng Dìng Tōng Sú Shāng Hán Lùn,* 重订通俗伤寒论)

[Ingredient]

Gān Cǎo (Radix Et Rhizoma Glycyrrhizae)   4 *liang*, dry-fried with liquid adjuvant (12 g)

Shēng Jiāng (Rhizoma Zingiberis Recens)   3 *liang*, cut (9 g)

Guì Zhī (Ramulus Cinnamomi)   3 *liang*, remove the outer bark (9 g)

Rén Shēn (Radix Et Rhizoma Ginseng)   2 *liang* (6 g)

Xiān Dì Huáng (Radix Rehmanniae Recens)   1 *jin* (30 g)

Ē Jiāo (Colla Corii Asini)   2 *liang* (6 g)

Mài Mén Dōng (Radix Ophiopogonis)   0.5 *sheng*, remove the plumule from lotus seed (12 g)

Má Rén (Fructus Cannabis)   0.5 *sheng* (12 g)

Dà Zǎo (Fructus Jujubae)   30 *mei*, breaking off with hands (10 *mei*)

[Usage]   In the original formula, 8 medicines are decocted with 7 *sheng* sake

and 8 *sheng* water, take 3 *sheng* of them, remove the sediment and add *ē jiāo* to melt, drink 1 *sheng* warmly, three times a day.

Modern Usage: Decocted with water and 60 g alcohol, then added *ē jiāo* to melt and drink it.

[Action] Nourish yin and blood, boost qi and unblock yang.

[Indication]

1. The main pattern for this formula is knotted and intermittent pulse, palpitation, weak and shortness of breath, light red tongue with little coating or tenellous and dry tongue caused by deficient yin and yang, qi and blood of the heart.

2. Patients with lung *wěi* (肺痿), cough, profuse saliva and spittle, weakness and shortness of breath, palpitation, sweating, throat and tongue dryness, dry stool with deficient rapid or slow pulse.

[Formula Analysis] *Basic Questions-Discourse on the Essentials of Vessels and the Subtleties of the Essence* (*Sù Wèn-Zāng Qì Fǎ Shí Lùn*, 素问·脉要精微论) says: "Intermittent pulse means qi failure." and Chen Wu-ji also said that: "knotted and intermittent pulse is that the slow pulse with an occasional dropped beat. The beats dropped at regular intervals, caused by deficiency and failure of yang qi and blood that can't continue living. That points to the inner deficiency of true qi.", it means that the knotted and intermittent pulse and palpitation are caused by the deficiency of yin and yang, qi and blood. The deficiency of yin blood causes the heart fail to be nourished, and the debilitation of yang qi causes a forceless beating. This formula is called *Zhì Gān Cǎo Tāng* (Honey-Fried Licorice Decoction) by Zhang Zhong-jing, because *gān cǎo* is used as the chief medicine which can boost qi that is said in *Miscellaneous Records of Materia Medica* (*Běn Cǎo Bié Lù*, 名医别录). "It can unblock the vessels and promote qi and blood, so it can be used to treat the knotted and intermittent pulse and palpitation"; *xiān dì huáng*, *ē jiāo*, *mài mén dōng* and *má rén* can nourish blood and reinforce yin, *rén shēn* and *dà zǎo* can boost qi and promote the production of fluid, which as deputy medicines. *Shēng jiāng* and *guì zhī* are assistant medicines, combined with tonifying medicines which can nourish yin and blood without cloying, boost qi and promote the production of fluid without

blocking, so that tonifying medicines can play a better role. Alcohol is used as an envoy medicine to invigorate blood to unblock the meridians, blood circulation and pulse become regular. The dosage of *xiān dì huáng* decocted with rice wine is quite large for a greater effect of nourishing yin and blood and avoiding too greasy to damage the spleen and stomach. Combined with all of the medicines, it nourishes the heart yin, reinforces the heart blood, warming the heart yang which makes the qi and blood sufficient, harmonizes the yin and yang to calm the palpitation and restores the pulse. That is why this formula is called *Fù Mài Tāng* (Pulse-Restoring Decoction)

[Clinical Application] This formula is quite effective for treating of both deficiency of heart yin and yang, qi and blood of the heart, with knotted and intermittent pulse and palpitation. In Tonify to *'Supplement to Important Formulas Worth a Thousand Gold Pieces' (Qiān Jīn Yì Fāng*, 千金翼方)[64], this formula is used to "treat deficiency-consumption syndrome, sweating but with distention feeling, knotted and palpitation who can act as usual but the situation will turns worse within 100 days, even [will] dead after 21 days.". *Arcane Essentials from the Imperial Library (Wài Tái Mì Yào*, 外台秘要) uses this formula to "treat lung wilting with lots of saliva and palpitation[manifestation]". In *Medical Formulas Collected and Analyzed (Yī Fāng Jí Jiě*, 医方集解), Yu Jia-yan once said, "in *the Arcane Essentials from the Imperial Library*, this formula can boost the deficiency of lung qi, and nourish the dryness of lung, as for the *guì zhī* which seems inappropriate for its taste of acrid and warm can dredge *ying* and *wei* qi to promote the production of fluid and then transport the lung qi, get the saliva downflow gradually,which is quite important and is the reason why it can treat palpitation.".

Section 4　Formulas that tonifies yin

The tonifying yin formulas, are suitable for the syndrome of yin deficiency, symptoms as thin with dry mouth and throat, deficient vexation and insomnia, dryness in the large intestine and constipation, dizziness and tinnitus, lumbago and weakness of the legs, even bone steaming fever and night sweating, cough with blood, red

checks, *xiāo kě*, seminal emission, red tongue with few coating, thready and rapid pulse. Yin deficiency will cause internal heat which has the symptoms that deficiency-fire flaming upward which can't be cleared only by the bitter and cold medicine. *Basic Questions-Comprehensive Discourse on the Essentials of the Most Reliable* (*Sù Wèn-Zhì Zhēn Yào Dà Lùn*, 素问·至真要大论) says, "heat disease, showing more heat after being treated by cold medicine, should be treated by nourishing yin (*zhū hán zhī ér rè zhě, qǔ zhī yīn*)". Wang Bing said, "strengthen the kidney yin to suppress yang hyperactivity" which all refers to the method of nourishing yin and subduing fire. This kind of formula is mainly com posed of yin-tonifying medicines, such as *dì huáng*, *guī bǎn*, *běi shā shēn*, *mài dōng* and *gǒu qǐ zǐ*, *shān zhū yú*, *shān yào* and so on. The representative formulas are *Liù Wèi Dì Huáng Wán* (Six-Ingredient Rehmannia Pill, 六味地黄丸), *Zuǒ Guī Yǐn* (Left-Restoring Beverage, 左归饮), *Dà Bǔ Yīn Wán* (Major Yin-Tonifying Pill, 大补阴丸), *Yī Guàn Jiān* (Effective Integration Decoction, 一贯煎), and so on.

Liù Wèi Dì Huáng Wán (Six-Ingredient Rehmannia Pill, 六味地黄丸)
Craft of Medicines and Patterns for Children (*Xiǎo Ér Yào Zhèng Zhí Jué*, 小儿药证直诀)

[Ingredient]

Shú Dì Huáng (Radix Rehmanniae Praeparata)   8 *qian* (24 g)

Shān Zhū Yú (Fructus Corni)

Shān Yào (Rhizoma Dioscoreae)

Each of them uses 4 *qian* (12 g)

Zé Xiè (Rhizoma Alismatis)

Mǔ Dān Pí (Cortex Moutan)

Bái Fú Líng (Poria)   remove the skin

Each of them use 3 *qian* (9 g)

[Usage]   Ground the medicine into a powder and roll it into pills with honey like *tung* seed size, take 3 pills with warm water before taking food.

Modern Usage: Grind it into a fine powder and refine honey into pills, take 6–9 g

a time, 2–3 times a day, take it on an empty stomach with warm water or light salt water, or just decocted with water.

[Action]　Reinforce yin and tonify kidney.

[Indication]　Patients with kidney yin deficiency, lumbago, sourness and weakness of the legs, dizziness and dizzy vision, tinnitus and deafness, night sweating, nocturnal emissions, *xiāo kě*, steaming bone fever, feverish feeling in palms and soles, continuous, dribbling urination, gomphiasis, dryness tongue and throat pain, heel pain, as well as the non-closure of the fontanels in the child, red tongue with less tongue coating, feeble and empty in *chǐ* area.

[Formula Analysis]　The kidney stores the essence, which is the foundation of the congenital (prenatal) constitution, and [if] yin [essence] deficiency will cause lots of syndromes. In the formula, *shú dì huáng*, sweet and light warm, which belongs to the liver and kidney meridian, is the chief medicine to nourish yin and tonify blood, tonify essence and generates the marrow, the powerful tonification of true yin which makes it become the important medicine of strengthening kidney. The *shān zhū yú* is sour and sweet, astringent and light warm, it belongs to the liver and kidney meridian, which can tonify the liver and kidney, generate essential qi, the kidney qi can be boosted to store essence moderately, and the liver yin can be nourished to free flow unimpededly; *shān yào* belongs to the lung, spleen and kidney meridian which can strengthen the spleen and tonify lung, consolidate kidney and generates essence for its taste of sweet and neutral which is in terms of earth excess can produce metal and metal excess can produce water, they two are both used as deputy medicines. The above three medicines mainly tonifying the kidney, the liver and the spleen, called "three tonifying".

Zé xiè is sweet and salt, enters the kidney and bladder meridians which can drains water and eliminates dampness, relieves fire, and dispels the pathogenic water in the kidney. *Mǔ dān pí is* acrid, bitter and slightly cold, enters the heart, liver and kidney meridians, which can clear heat and cool the blood, harmonize the blood and disperse stasis, drain the latent fire in yin to treat deficiency-fire flaming upward; *bái fú líng* with a sweet and bland taste, enters the heart, spleen and lung meridians which

can tonify heart and spleen, percolate and drain dampness, help *shān yào to* boost the spleen, combine with *zé xiè* to drain water. They are all used as assistant and envoy medicines. The above three medicines are called "three draining".

This is "not only the formula can treat the deficiency of liver and kidney, but also can treat three yins which has the *shú dì huáng* to tonify kidney water with *zé xiè*'s diffusing and draining kidney turbidity to coordinate with it, has the warming and astringing liver meridian of *shān zhū yú* with the clearing and draining liver fire of *mǔ dān pí* to assistant it, has the restraining spleen meridian of *shān yào* with the percolating and draining spleen dampness with the bland taste of *bái fú líng* to harmonize it. And it has six medicines which have the broad effect of treating three yins [spleen, liver, kidney] together, like shooting a bull's eye, it is the representative formula for tonifying." (*Treatise on Medical Formulas Yī Fāng Lùn*, 医方论). All in all, this formula can nourish but without pathogenic retention, drain without damaging the healthy qi which is quite better than the formula which only can tonifying.

[Clinical Application]   By deducting *ròu guì* and *fù zǐ*, Qian Yi[65] evolved *shèn qì wán* (kidney qi pill, 肾气丸) of *essentials from the golden cabinet (Jīn Guì Yào Lüè*, 金匮要略), which treats children kidney deficiency and other diseases in the original recording.

The kidney mainly stores the essence and water, so the "three tonifying" are used to supplement the essence, *zé xiè* and *bái fú líng* are used to disinhibit water; yin deficiency resulting in effulgent fire, so the *mǔ dān pí* is used to drain ministerial fire. In this formula, "three tonifying" supplements the healthy qi, "three draining" eliminates the pathogenic qi which has the benefit of tonifying health qi. The dosage of "three tonifying" is heavier than that of "three draining". This formula can be used to treat the syndromes of deficiency of kidney yin in the clinical.

Zuǒ Guī Yǐn (Restore the left[kidney] Beverage, 左归饮)
The Complete Works of [Zhang] Jing-yue (Jǐng Yuè Quán Shū, 景岳全书)

[Ingredient]
Shú Dì Huáng (Radix Rehmanniae Praeparata)   2,3 *qian* or 1,2 *liang* (6–60 g)

Shān Yào (Rhizoma Dioscoreae)   2 *qian* (6 g)

Gǒu Qǐ Zǐ (Fructus Lycii)   2 *qian* (6 g)

Fú Líng (Poria)   1 *qian* and 5 *fen* (4.5 g)

Shān Zhū Yú (Fructus Corni)   1, 2 *qian*, people who are afraid of sourness use less (3–6 g)

Zhì Gān Cǎo (Radix Et Rhizoma Glycyrrhizae Praeparata Cum Melle) 1 *qian* (3 g)

[Usage]   In the original formula, it is decocted with 2 *zhong* water into 7 *fen*, and then take it after meals.

Modern Usage: Decocted with water.

[Action]   Tonify kidney and nourish yin.

[Indication]   True yin deficiency, soreness and weakness in the lower back, spontaneous and nocturnal emission, night sweating, thirsty and dry mouth and throat, red tongue, thready and bit rapid pulse.

[Formula Analysis]   True yin, which is also called original yin, true essence, is stored in the kidney. This formula strongly reinforces the water [true yin] with sweet herbs. *Basic Questions-Discourse on the True [Qi Endowed by] Heaven in High Antiquity (Sù Wèn-Shàng Gǔ Tián Zhēn Lùn,* 素问·上古天真论) says, "The kidney controls water, which receives and stores *jing* (essence) from five *zang*-organs and the six *fu*-organs." In this formula, *shú dì huáng* is used as chief medicine to boost kidney water and tonify true [yin]; *gǒu qǐ zǐ* and *shān zhū yú* are used as deputy medicines to tonify and boost liver[blood] and kidney, help chief medicine tonify kidney and nourish yin; *shān yào* is used to nourish kidney yin, reinforcing stomach yin and *fú líng* is used to tonifies the spleen as the source of the postnatal constitution, which are both used as assistant medicine; *zhì gān cǎo* is used to harmonize all the medicines and nourish the yin of spleen and stomach which is because that the reinforcing spleen can nourish kidney and the congenital essence relies on acquired essence to produce. With all the medicines, it can reinforce the kidney, tonify the congenital essence and acquired essence which has the effect of tonifying and replenishing kidney water, nourishing true yin. This formula can supplement the true water of the left kidney to make the yin

essence go back to its origin, so it is called *Zuǒ Guī Yǐn* (Left-Restoring Beverage).

[Clinical Application] This formula derives from *Liù Wèi Dì Huáng Wán* (Six-Ingredient Rehmannia Pill, 六味地黄丸) which is combined by six medicines but is different from *Liù Wèi Dì Huáng Wán*. *Liù Wèi Dì Huáng Wán* is a mixture of tonifying and draining herbs that are used to clear signs of fire from deficiency; this formula is the pure sweet and tonifying kidney formula that applies to the syndrome of deficiency and doesn't need *Zé Xiè*'s draining [function] or *Mǔ dān pí*'s cooling [function].

Dà Bǔ Yīn Wán (Great Yin-Tonifying Pill, 大补阴丸)
Essential Teachings of [Zhu] Dan-xi (*Dān Xī Xīn Fǎ*, 丹溪心法)

[Ingredient]

Huáng Bǎi (Cortex Phellodendri Chinensis)   stir-heat till (the drugs) become dark yellow 4 *liang* (120 g)

Zhī Mǔ (Rhizoma Anemarrhenae)   soaking in rice wine, dry-fried, each of them uses 4 *liang* (120 g)

Shú Dì Huáng (Radix Rehmanniae Praeparata)   steaming drugs with rice wine 6 *liang* (180 g)

Guī Bǎn (Plastrum Testudinis)   dry-fried with butter each of them use 6 *liang* (180 g)

[Usage] Grind the ingredients into a powder and make them into pills with honey and the marrow from pigs' vertebrae. Take 70 pills with salt soup before taking food.

Modern Usage: Thready powder, make it into pills with steamed marrow from pigs'vertebrae and honey, roll into a pill like *Tung* seed size. The normal dosage is 6–9 g twice a day with salty water. Or make it decocted with water. And the dosage depends on the original formula to plus or minus.

[Action] Enrich yin and direct fire [downward].

[Indication] Patients with flourishing fire due to yin deficiency, manifests as steaming bone disorder with afternoon tidal fever, night sweating and seminal

emission, cough and hemoptysis, vexation and irritability, heat and pain in the feet and knees, with red tongue and less coating, *chǐ* pulse is rapid and powerful.

[Formula Analysis] The true yin is deficient and the ministerial fire is rising up. In this formula, *huáng bǎi* is used to consolidate the true yin to defeat the ministerial fire for its taste of bitter and cold, *zhī mǔ* is used to enrich yin and subdue the fire, moisten the lung and clear the lung fire for its taste of bitterness and coldness. *The Grand Compendium of Materia Medica* (*Běn Cǎo Gāng Mù*, 本草纲目) says, "It can moisten the kidney dryness to enrich yin in the lower part, clear the lung metal to drain fire in the upper part". *Huáng bǎi* and *zhī mǔ* are mutual reinforcements between each other and can drain the ministerial fire to protect the true yin, which has the advantage of mutual generation between metal and water that is the method of clearing the source. *Shú dì huáng* can enrich the kidney and nourish yin, supplement essence and boost marrow for its taste of sweet and light warm, *guī bǎn* can enrich yin and subdue yang, strengthen the water to defeat the fire for its taste of sweet and neutral, which is the important medicine of the kidney meridian. *Zhū jǐ suǐ* is flesh and blood medicine that uses marrow from pigs' vertebrae to tonify the essence and enrich the kidney water to reduce the deficient fire that is the method of cultivating the root. This enriching yin and subduing fire formula formed by these medicines can clear the ministerial fire and tonify the true yin, so it is called "*Dà Bǔ Yīn Wán* (Major Yin-Tonifying Pill)".

[Clinical Application] Enrich yin and subdue fire, as known as "cultivating the root and clearing the source". Zhu Dan-xi[66] said, "yin is often insufficient, while yang is often in excess. We should always enrich the yin to balance the yin and yang and let the water control the fire, and then there are few diseases". This formula is based on this theory. Especially for the deficiency-consumption disease of yin deficiency resulting in flourishing fire, [Zhu] Dan xi thought, "eighty or ninety percent of this disease is caused by flourishing fire [caused by yin deficiency]; less than twenty thirty percent of this disease is caused by fire [yang] deficiency." Thus, before enriching yin, the fire should be subdued first for it can protect true yin and display the effect of nourishing yin medicines.

Yī Guàn Jiān (Effective Integration Decoction, 一贯煎)
Supplement to 'Classified Case Records of Famous Physicians' (Xù Míng Yī Lèi Àn, 续名医类案) [67]

[Ingredient]

Běi Shā Shēn (Radix Glehniae)   (9 g)

Mài Dōng (Radix Ophiopogonis)   (9 g)

Xiān Dì Huáng (Radix Rehmanniae Recens)   (15 g)

Dāng Guī (Radix Angelicae Sinensis)   (9 g)

Gǒu Qǐ Zǐ (Fructus Lycii)   (9 g)

Chuān Liàn Zǐ (Fructus Toosendan)   (4.5 g)

[the original formula doesn't record the dosage]

[Usage]   The original book does not record the usage.

Modern Usage: Decoct with water.

[Action]   Nourish yin and soothe the liver.

[Indication]   Patients with the liver and kidney yin deficiency, [while] liver qi failing to flow smoothly, manifested as rib-side distending pain, acid reflux and bitterness vomiting, dry mouth and throat, thready and weak or deficient and wiry pulse, with red tongue and few salivae. Or the hernia and mass.

[Formula Analysis]   The liver is yin in the body [essence] but manifests through its yang shape [functions], prefers activity and is averse to constraint. In this formula, *xiān dì huáng* is used as chief medicine to enrich yin and nourish the blood, supplement the liver and kidney; *dāng guī* and *gǒu qǐ zǐ* can nourish blood and soften the liver, *běi shā shēn* and *mài dōng* can enrich yin and promote the production of fluid, which all are good at enriching the yin of lung and stomach because the wood can over restrict the earth, so should promote the earth to generate metal, clear metal to control the wood, the above all are used as deputy medicines. *Chuān liàn zǐ* can soothe the liver, rectify qi and drain fire, but the bitter nature would tend to damage the yin, but the sweet, moistening nature of the other herbs in this formula mitigates this property. Nourish the liver, free activity of liver qi, clear all the syndromes. This formula is excellent for treating yin deficiency and hypochondriac pain.

[Clinical Application]

1. Wei Yu-heng[68] used this formula frequently and has many modifications. If the patient has a bitter and dry mouth, it should add *huáng lián* 3 to 5 *fen*; if the patient has constipation, *guā lóu rén* should be added, if the patient has deficient fever or sweating, it should add *dì gǔ pí*; if the patient has lots of phlegm, *bèi mǔ* can be applied; if the patient has red and dry tongue with severe yin deficiency, *shí hú* are suitable; if the patient has rib-side distending pain and hard feeling when pressed, *biē jiǎ* can be used; if the patient has abdominal pain, it should add *sháo yào*, *gān cǎo*; if the patient has vexation heat and thirsty, *zhī mǔ*, *shí gāo* are fit to add; if the patient has feet weakness, *niú xī*, *yì yǐ rén* should be used; if the patient has insomnia, *dà zǎo* can release it.

2. Regulating qi medicines are mainly used to treat rib-side distending pain; however, most are aromatic and dry [in nature], for treating the liver and kidney yin deficiency, those medicines will easily consume the fluid and exacerbate the disease. So when the rib-side distending pain is caused by yin deficiency, blood can not nourish the liver and leds to the binding constraint of liver qi, the editor always uses this formula as the basic one. With bái *sháo*, *gān cǎo*, it will strengthen the effect of soothing the liver and stop the pain; adding *fó shǒu*, *mài yá*, *lù è méi* will have a better effect on soothing the liver and rectifying qi and the gentle medicine can regulate qi without damaging yin.

Section 5 Formulas that tonifies yang

The tonifying yang formula can treat yang deficiencies. However, the yang deficienies include heart yang deficiency, spleen yang deficiency, kidney yang deficiency and so on. The formula for treating the heart and spleen yang deficiency has been introduced in the warming the interior formula chapter. This section mainly introduces the formula for treating kidney yang deficiency. All the exhaustion and lacking strength, waist and knees sourness and pain, cold feeling under of waist, weakness of lower limbs, frequent clear and white urine, continuous urination,

impotence and premature ejaculation, deep and thready pulse, especially in the *chǐ* pulse, pale tongue with white coating all belong to the kidney yang deficiency and lower origin losing warming. In *Basic Questions-Comprehensive Discourse on the Essentials of the Most Reliable (Sù Wèn-Zhì Zhēn Yào Dà Lùn,* 素问·至真要大论), it says: "Hot or warm [nature] medicine to treat the cold syndrome, but the cold getting serious, this is not a cold syndrome of external cold evil, but the deficiency of kidney yang (true yang), should using the tonify yang [method]." Wang Bing said, "boost the origin of fire to disperse the shroud of yin.", it all refers to the method of warming and tonifying the kidney yang. Commonly used *ròu guì, fù zǐ, lù jiāo jiāo, dù zhòng, tù sī zǐ, Shú Dì Huáng, shān zhū yú, xiān máo, xiān líng pí, etc.* If the yang deficiency can not warm, [leads to] qi transformation fails to move and the pathogenic water lingers, the draining water medicines should be added, which can tonifying the yang to clear the pathogenic water and recover the kidney's control of water. The representative formulas are *Shèn Qì Wán* (Kidney Qi Pill, 肾气丸) and *Yòu Guī Yǐn* (Right-Restoring Beverage, 右归饮).

Shèn Qì Wán (Kidney Qi Pill, 肾气丸)
Essentials from the Golden Cabinet (Jīn Guì Yào Lüè, 金匮要略)

[Ingredient]

Gān Dì Huáng (Radix Rehmanniae Recens)   8 *liang* (250 g)

Shān Zhū Yú (Fructus Corni)   4 *liang* (125 g)

Sān Jiǎo Yè Shǔ Yù (Rhizoma Dioscoreae Deltoideae)   4 *liang* (125 g)

Zé Xiè (Rhizoma Alismatis)   3 *liang* (90 g)

Fú Líng (Poria)   3 *liang* (90 g)

Mǔ Dān Pí (Cortex Moutan)   3 *liang* (90 g)

Guì Zhī (Ramulus Cinnamomi)   1 *liang* (30 g)

Fù Zǐ (Radix Aconiti Lateralis Praeparata)   process of roasting or dry-fried, 1 *liang* (30 g)

[Usage]   In the original book, grind the eight medicines into a powder and form into pills with honey like *tung* seeds size, take 15 pills with wine twice a day.

Modern Usage: Grind into a powder, form them into pills with honey, take 6–9 g a time, twice a day with warm water or salty water. Or decocted with water, and the dosage should be reduced in proportion to the original formula.

[Action] Warm the kidney and transform qi.

[Indication] [Patients with] kidney yang deficiency, lumbago and feet weakness, cold sensation in the lower part of the body, the tenseness of the lower abdomen, urinary retention or excessive urination, especially at night, pale and swollen tongue, deep and thready *chǐ* pulse. Phlegm and fluid retention, *xiāo kě* [consumptive thirst], beriber, bladder colic and pregnant dysuria.

[Formula Analysis] The kidney is the foundation of the congenital (prenatal) constitution which has the *mìng mén* fire. If the kidney yang is deficient, it can not warm the lower *jiao*. In this formula, *gān dì huáng*, enriches the yin and generates fluids, with a large dosage, as the chief medicine of this formula. The deputy medicines, *shǔ yù*, can consolidate kidney and supplement essence, *shān zhū yú* can tonify the liver and kidney, astringe the essence and qi, *fù zǐ* and *guì zhī* can warm the kidney and reinforce yang. *Mǔ dān pí* can cool the liver, *zé xiè* and *fú líng* can drain water and direct the turbid downward, they are the assistant medicines. *Fù zǐ, guì zhī* and *shān zhū yú* combined with *mǔ dān pí* can warm without dryness, *gān dì huáng*, *shǔ yù* and *shān zhū yú* combined with *zé xiè* and *fú líng* can supplement without stagnation. In this formula, a small amount of *fù zǐ* and *guì zhī* are added to the yin-nourishing medicines to lightly ignite a fire to inspire the kidney qi, which is the method of "mild fire generates qi", so it is called "*Shèn Qì Wán* (Kidney Qi Pill)". Yin and yang are rooted in each other; without yang, the yin can not be produced; without yin, the yang can not be generated. This formula tonifies water and fire, nourishes yin to help yang which can clear the pathogen and recover the healthy qi, enrich the kidney qi. Just like Zhang Jing-Yue said, "people who are good at supplement yang, must seek yang based on yin [medicine], the yin can help yang and promotes the transformation", and the effect of "boosting the origin of fire to clear the shadow." This formula is the original formula of treating kidney.

[Clinical Application] This formula is usually used to treat kidney yang

deficiency. Later generations always use *shú dì huáng* instead of *gān dì huáng* use *ròu guì* instead of *guì zhī* which can use as a reference.

Yòu Guī Yǐn (Right-Restoring Beverage, 右归饮)
The Complete Works of [Zhang] Jing-yue (Jǐng Yuè Quán Shū, 景岳全书)

[Ingredient]

Shú Dì Huáng (Radix Rehmanniae Praeparata)   2, 3 *qian* or 1, 2 *liang* (6–60 g)

Shān Yào (Rhizoma Dioscoreae)   dry-fried, 2 *qian* (6 g)

Shān Zhū Yú (Fructus Corni)   1 *qian* (3 g)

Gǒu Qǐ Zǐ (Fructus Lycii)   2 *qian* (6 g)

Zhì Gān Cǎo (Radix Et Rhizoma Glycyrrhizae Praeparata Cum Melle)   1, 2 *qian* (3–6 g)

Ròu Guì (Cortex Cinnamomi)   1, 2 *qian* (3–6 g)

Dù Zhòng (Cortex Eucommiae)   processed with ginger, 2 *qian* (6 g)

Zhì Fù Zǐ (Radix Aconiti Lateralis Praeparata)   1, 2, 3 *qian* (3–9 g)

[Usage]   In the original book, decocted it with 2 zhong water into 7 fen, take it warmly long time after a meal.

Modern Usage: Decocted with water.

[Action]   Warm the kidney and tonify the essence.

[Indication]   Patients with kidney yang deficiency even [yang] failure, exhaustion and timidity, abdominal pain and waist sourness, cold limbs and thready pulse, pale tongue and white coating or exuberant yin repelling yang, true cold with false heat.

[Formula Analysis]   *Basic Questions-Discourse from the Secret Classic of the Miraculous Orchid (Sù Wèn-Líng Lán Mì Diǎn Lùn,* 素问·灵兰秘典论) says, "The kidney is the official functioning as operator with great power, technical skills and expertise originate from it." This formula is a variation of *Shèn Qì Wán* (Kidney Qi Pill) which is also formed by eight medicines. *Shú dì huáng,* taste sweet and light warm, is good at nourishing kidney and tonifying essence; as the chief medicine, *shān yào* is sweet and neutral, good at strengtheing the spleen, consolidating the kidney

and boosting essence, *shān zhū yú* can tonify the liver and kidney, astringe essence and qi for its taste of sourness and light warm, *ròu guì* can tonify the deficiency of *mìng mén*, boost fire to clear yin, *zhì fù zǐ* can drastically tonify the original yang and boost the origin of fire for its taste of large acrid and heat. They are all used as deputy medicines; *gǒu qǐ zǐ* is sweet and neutral, which can nourish the liver and kidney, tonify deficiency and boost essence, *dù zhòng* can tonify liver and kidney, strengthen tendon and bone, boost essence and qi for its sweet and warm taste, they are both used as assistant medicines; *zhì gān cǎo* can warm the center [middle *jiao*] and strengthen the spleen, harmonize all the medicines which is used as envoy medicine. The combination of this formula is wonderful in seeking yang from yin [medicine], warming kidney and replenishing essence, which can tonify *Mìng Mén* fire of the right kidney and let the original yang go back to its origin place, so it is called "*Yòu Guī Yǐn* (Right-Restoring Beverage)".

[Clinical Application] This formula belongs to the "boost the source of fire" formula. The original book said, "if [the syndrome changes into]exuberant yin repelling yang, [manifested as] true cold with fake heat, 2 *qian* of *zé xiè* should be added and decocted, taking it after soaking to cold by cool water is better." This is the usage of *Basic Questions-Discourse on the Five Regular Policies* (*Sù Wèn-Wǔ Cháng Zhèng Dà Lùn*, 素问·五常政大论) that "treating cold use heat medicine and use cool medicine to move it."

Chapter 9

Astringent Formulas

According to "treating dispersion with astringent", in *Basic Questions-Comprehensive Discourse on the Essentials of the Most Reliable* (*Sù Wèn-Zhì Zhēn Yào Dà Lùn*, 素问·至真要大论), all the formula are mainly composed of astringing and consolidating essence medicines which are used to treat qi, blood, essence and fluid dissipation and slippery syndrome, so called as consolidating essence formula. It belongs to the "astringent relieving collapse" of "ten formula types (*shí jì*)".

Section 1　Formulas that consolidates exterior and stops sweating

Consolidating exterior and stopping sweating formula are suitable for the syndromes of weakness and insecurity of the *wei* [qi] exterior can not keep the yin fluid inside, which can cause spontaneous sweating or night sweating. The representative medicines are *huáng qí, mǔ lì, má huáng gēn, fú xiǎo mài*, and the representative formula is *Mǔ Lì Sǎn* (Oyster Shell Powder, 牡蛎散). In this section, some formulas are used to consolidate the exterior, which can dispel the cause of sweating as well, like *Yù Píng Fēng Sǎn* (Jade Wind-Barrier Powder, 玉屏风散), which uses tonifying [method] as consolidating, *Dāng Guī Liù Huáng Tāng* (Chinese Angelica Six Yellow Decoction, 当归六黄汤) can enrich yin and drain fire to treat the exterior deficiency with night sweating which is caused by yin deficiency and fire disturbing. They both reflect the spirit of this compatibility.

Mǔ Lì Sǎn (Oyster Shell Powder, 牡蛎散)
Formulary of the Pharmacy Service for Benefiting the People in the Taiping Era
(*Tài Píng Huì Mín Hé Jì Jú Fāng,* 太平惠民和剂局方)

[Ingredient]

Huáng Qí (Radix Astragali)   remove the sediment of basal leaf and soil 1 *liang* (30 g)

Má Huáng Gēn (Radix Et Rhizoma Ephedrae)   wash 1 *liang* (30 g)

Mǔ Lì (Concha Ostreae)   soaking in rice-washed water, wash the soil, scorching on fire until turning red, 1 *liang* (30 g)

[Usage]   The original book mentioned that all medicines are ground into a coarse powder, take 3 *qian* with 1.5 *zhan* water, hundreds of grains of *xiǎo mài* and decoct into 8 *fen*, remove the sediment, drink it warmly, twice a day.

Modern Usage: Coarse powder, take 9 g of them, decocted with 30 grams of *fú xiǎo mài*. Or decocted *fú xiǎo mài* with those medicines, the dosage should be modified based on the original formula.

[Action]   Replenish qi and consolidate exterior, restrain yin and inhibit sweating.

[Indication]   Deficiency leads to the insecurity of a defensive exterior, spontaneous sweating that worsens at night, palpitations, susceptibility to fright, shortness of breath, irritability, fatigue, a pale-red tongue, and a thin, frail pulse.

[Formula Analysis]   *Basic Questions-The Great Treatise on Yin Yang Correspondence in phenomena* (*Sù Wèn-Yīn Yáng Yīng Xiàng Dà Lùn,* 素问·阴阳应象大论) says, "yin maintains inside to preserve yang while yang stays outside to protect yin." In this formula, *mǔ lì* is salty astringent and light cold, as the chief medicine to constrain yin and subdue yang, consolidate the exterior and inhibit sweating; *huáng qí* is sweet and light warm [nature], used as deputy medicine to boost qi, consolidate exterior and inhibit sweating; *má huáng gēn* is sweet and neutral, used as assistant medicine to inhibit sweating especially; *fú xiǎo mài* is sweet and cool, which belongs to the heart channel used as envoy medicine to nourish heart qi, reduce deficient fever, inhibits sweating. This formula can boost qi and consolidate the exterior, constrain yin and stop sweating, [when] the qi and yin recover, spontaneous

sweating will stop.

[Clinical Application]　This formula is designed for the sweating syndrome of insecurity of the *wei* exterior and [cause] yin fluid leaking, which can also treat night sweating as well. If it is yang deficiency, *bái zhú*, *fù zǐ* can be added to help yang consolidate the exterior; if it is qi deficiency, it needs to add *rén shēn* and *bái zhú* to strengthen the spleen and boost qi; if it is yin deficiency, *shēng dì*, *bái sháo* can be added to nourish yin and stop sweating. The severe sweating, should use a high dosage of *huáng qí*; for night sweating, *jī dòu yī* and *nuò dào gēn xū* will have significant effect.

Yù Píng Fēng Sǎn (Jade Wind-Barrier Powder, 玉屏风散)
Analogous Medical Prescriptions Collection (*Yī Fāng Lèi Jù*, 医方类聚) [69]
Quote From The Original Prescription Collection (*Jiū Yuán Fāng*, 究原方)[70]

[Ingredient]

Fáng Fēng (Radix Saposhnikoviae)　1 *liang* (30 g)

Huáng Qí (Radix Astragali)　dry-fried drugs with water-diluted honey 2 *liang* (60 g)

Bái Zhú (Rhizoma Atractylodis Macrocephalae)　2 *liang* (60 g)

[Usage]　Chew the original medicines, each 3 *qian* of them, decocted with 0.5 *zhan* water, 1 *dà zǎo*, boiling into seven-tenths, remove the sediment, take it warmly after a meal.

Modern Usage: Grind into a coarse powder, take 6–9 g, twice a day, decoct with water.

[Action]　Replenish qi, consolidat exterior and inhibit sweating.

[Indication]　Exterior deficiency and spontaneous sweating or the one with deficiency inside who is easily attacked by wind or aversion to wind, manifested as a sallow white face, pale tongue and white coating, floating, deficient and weak pulse.

[Formula Analysis]　Qi deficiency fails to defend the exterior, [when] *wei* qi is insecurity, *ying* yin is leaking easily. In the formula, *huáng qí* is sweet and warm, which can consolidate the exterior and inhibit sweating, replenishing qi; *bái zhú* is

used as deputy medicine to strengthen the spleen and reinforce qi, consolidate the exterior and inhibit sweating. *Huáng qí* combined with *bái zhú* powerfully tonifies the lung and spleen qi, which respectively tonifies skin and muscle. Thus, sweating will be inhibited, the pathogen will be eliminated. *Fáng fēng* is used as assistant medicine to expel wind pathogens, enhance the spleen and clear yang, help *huáng qí* replenish qi and defense wind. *The Grand Compendium of Materia Medica* (*Běn Cǎo Gāng Mù*, 本草纲目) quoted Li Gao says: "*fáng fēng* can control *huáng qí*, while *huáng qí* been assisted by *fáng fēng* will have a greater effect, which is assistance and restraint." Futhermore, *huáng qí* supported by *fáng fēng* can consolidate the exterior without lingering the pathogen, *fáng fēng* combined with *huáng qí* can dispel the pathogen without damaging the healthy qi. The compatibility of the three medicines can strengthen the *wei* qi to consolidate striae and interstices so the pathogen will not re-attack. Strengthen the spleen to recover the healthy qi, strengthen the interior to dispel the pathogen to recover all the symptoms. This formula is the maintain internal security and repel foreign invasion formula. Its effect is like the protective screen (*píng fēng*, 屏风) of resisting wind and which is as precious as jade, so it is called *Yù Píng Fēng Sǎn* (Jade Wind-Barrier Powder).

[Clinical Application] This formula is excellent for replenishing qi, consolidating exterior and restraining sweating which can treat qi deficiency with spontaneous sweating and vacuity patients who are easily to be attacked by the wind pathogen mainly. Alternatively, it can treat patients with qi deficiency attacked by the wind pathogen, spontaneous sweating, and cannot bearing the exterior-releasing medicines.

Dāng Guī Liù Huáng Tāng (**Chinese Angelica Six Yellow Decoction,** 当归六黄汤)
Secrets from the Orchid Chamber (*Lán Shì Mì Cáng*, 兰室秘藏)

[Ingredient]
Dāng Guī (Radix Angelicae Sinensis)   (6 g)
Xiān Dì Huáng (Radix Rehmanniae Recens)   (6 g)
Shú Dì Huáng (Radix Rehmanniae Praeparata)   (6 g)

Huáng Bǎi (Cortex Phellodendri Chinensis)　　(6 g)

Huáng Qín (Radix Scutellariae)　　(6 g)

Huáng Lián (Rhizoma Coptidis)　　(6 g)

Huáng Qí (Radix Astragali)　　(12 g)

[Usage]　The original formula is cut into a coarse powder, each 5 *qian* of them with 2 *zhan* water and decocted into 1 *zhan*, take it before the meal. Children take it in half dosage.

Modern Usage: Decoct with water, the dosage should be increased or decreased according to the original formula.

[Action]　Enrich yin and drain fire, consolidate the exterior and restrain sweating.

[Indication]　The yin deficiency with stirring fire, aversion to cold with fever, red facial complexion with vexation, dry mouth and lips, constipation and red urine, red tongue, rapid pulse.

[Formula Analysis]　Patients with yin deficiency and internal heat. In this formula, *dāng guī*, *xiān dì huáng* and *shú dì huáng* are used as chief medicines to nourish yin and blood, which can subdue fire; *huáng lián*, *huáng bǎi* and *huáng qín* are used as deputy medicines to clear heat and drain fire to consolidate yin. Profuse sweating not only consumes yin blood but also damages yang qi, which causes insecurity of the *wei* exterior. So double the dosage of *huáng qí* to boost qi and consolidate the exterior. The combination of these medicines in this formula can recover yin, reduce heat, strengthen *wei* qi and restrain sweating.

[Clinical Application]

1. This formula is suitable for treating night sweating caused by the yin deficiency and fire disturbance. If the patient has the deficiency without fire, the bitter and cold, descending and floating medicines like *huáng lián*, *huáng bǎi* and *huáng qín* should not be used. However, it should use the nourishing yin and promoting the fluid production formula like *Shēng Mài Sǎn* (Pulse-Engendering Powder) and *Liù Wèi Dì Huáng Wán* (Six-Ingredient Rehmannia Pill).

2. This formula has the insufficient effect of consolidating essence, so the patient

with severe night sweating can add *má huáng gēn*, *mǔ lì* and *fú xiǎo mài* into this formula which will have a better effect.

Section 2 Formulas that restrains enuresis and emission with astringents

The formula of restraining enuresis and emission with astringents is suitable for the syndromes of kidney deficiency. It cannot store essence causing spontaneous seminal emission, kidney qi deficiency, bladder losing control, causing enuresis and frequent urination. There are restrain enuresis and emission with astringent medicines like *sāng piāo xiāo*, *lóng gǔ*, *qiàn shí*, *lián xū*, *mǔ lì* and *jīn yīng zǐ* and so on. The representative formula are *Sāng Piāo Xiāo Sǎn* (Mantis Egg Shell Powder, 桑螵蛸散), *Jīn Suǒ Gù Jīng Wán* (Golden Lock Essence-Securing Pill, 金锁固精丸).

Sāng Piāo Xiāo Sǎn (Mantis Egg Shell Powder, 桑螵蛸散)
Extension of the Materia Medica (Běn Cǎo Yǎn Yì, 本草衍义)*[71]

[Ingredient]

Sāng Piāo Xiāo (Oötheca Mantidis)　1 *liang* (30 g)

Yuǎn Zhì (Radix Polygalae)　1 *liang* (30 g)

Shí Chāng Pú (Rhizoma Acori Tatarinowii)　1 *liang* (30 g)

Lóng Gǔ (Os Draconis; Fossilia Ossis Mastodi)　1 *liang* (30 g)

Rén Shēn (Radix Et Rhizoma Ginseng)　1 *liang* (30 g)

Fú Shén (Sclerotium Poriae Pararadicis)　1 *liang* (30 g)

Dāng Guī (Radix Angelicae Sinensis)　1 *liang* (30 g)

Guī Bǎn Jiāo (Colla Testudinis Plastri)　processing with rice vinegar, 1 *liang* (30 g)

[Usage]　Grind all the ingredients into a powder, take 2 *qian* with *Rén Shēn Tāng* (Ginseng Decoction) before bedtime.

Modern Usage: Grind into powder, take 6 g before bedtime every day with *Rén Shēn Tāng* (Ginseng Decoction), or make into a decoction, boiled with water, the dosage depends on the original formula.

[Action]　Regulate and tonify the heart and kidney, stabilize the essence and restrain seminal emission.

[Indication]　Deficiency in the heart and kidney manifested as frequent urination, or enuresis and spermatorrhea, pale tongue and white coating, thready and weak pulse.

[Formula Analysis]　The syndrome of this formula is caused by insufficient heart qi and kidney deficiency, which fail to control the essence. The chief medicine, *sāng piāo xiāo* is used to tonify the kidney and stabilize the essence, restrain seminal emission. *Miscellaneous Records of Materia Medica (Běn Cǎo Bié Lù*, 本草别录) says, "it can treat male deficiency, five viscera qi failure, seminal emission while dreaming and enuresis". The deputy medicine, *lóng gǔ* is good at astringing and consolidating the essence. Recorded in *Miscellaneous Records of Materia Medica (Běn Cǎo Bié Lù*, 本草别录) says: "it can concentrate urine, nourish the spirit and calm the soul"; *sāng piāo xiāo* combined with *lóng gǔ* can strengthen its effect of consolidating essence, restrain the frequent urine, enuresis and spontaneous seminal emission; among the assistant medicines, *rén shēn* can powerfully tonify, the original qi, *fú shén* can boost qi and calm the spirit and descend the heart qi to the kidney, *shí chāng pú* can open the heart orifice, *yuǎn zhì* can calm the mind and steady the will, which can ascend the kidney qi to heart and promote heart-kidney interaction. In contrast, *dāng guī* can tonify heart and blood, *guī bǎn jiāo* can nourish kidney yin and *dāng guī* combined with *rén shēn* will tonify qi and blood in pair. This formula coordinates the heart and the kidney, tonifies and boosting qi and blood, stabilizes the essence, and restrains seminal emission.

[Clinical Application]　This formula is used to treat the patient with the heart and kidney deficiency which causes frequent urine, enuresis and spermatorrhea, especially for children who have bed-wetting or can not control their urination.

Jīn Suǒ Gù Jīng Wán (Golden Lock Essence-Securing Pill, 金锁固精丸)
Medical Formulas Collected and Analyzed (*Yī Fāng Jí Jiě*, 医方集解)

[Ingredient]

Shā Yuàn Jí Lí (Semen Astragali Complanati)   dry-fried 2 *liang* (60 g)

Qiàn Shí (Semen Euryales)   steaming 2 *liang* (60 g)

Lián Xū (Stamen Nelumbinis)   2 *liang* (60 g)

Lóng Gǔ (Os Draconis; Fossilia Ossis Mastodi)   processing with butter 1 *liang* (30 g)

Mǔ Lì (Concha Ostreae)   boiling in salty water a day and night, calcining into powder, 1 *liang* (30 g)

[Usage]   Mixed the ingredients with lotus seed powder and make them into pills, take it with salty water.

Modern Usage: Grind the ingredients into a fine powder, coated with lotus seed powder, and form them into pills, 6–9 g, twice a day, take with salty water on an empty stomach.

[Action]   Nourish the kidney and receive the semen.

[Indication]   The patients with kidney deficiency and lost control of essence, spontaneous seminal emission, mental fatigue and lacking of strength, lumbago and tinnitus, pale tongue and white coating, thready and weak pulse.

[Formula Analysis]   *Basic Questions-Discourse on the Sexagenary cycles and Organ Manifestation* (*Sù Wèn-Liù Jié Zàng Xiàng Lùn*, 素问·六节藏象论) says, "The kidney governs dormancy, it is the root of sealing up and storing as well as the location of the *jing* (essence)". In this formula, *shā yuàn jí lí* is sweet and warm, used as chief medicine to tonify the kidney and consolidate essence. In *The Grand Compendium of Materia Medica* (*Běn Cǎo Gāng Mù*, 本草纲目) says: "it can tonify kidney and treat lumbago, and seminal emission and deficiency-consumption", and in *Encountering the Sources of the 'Classic of Materia Medica'* (*Běn Jīng Féng Yuán*, 本经逢原) says, "It is the important medicine of treating seminal emission and deficiency-consumption which is most able to consolidate essence" *Qiàn shí* and *lián zǐ*, taste sweet, astringent and neutral, both used as deputy medicines to harmonize the

heart and the kidney, nourish the kidney and consolidate the essence, tonify the spleen qi; The assistants, *duàn lóng gǔ* and *duàn mǔ lì* are powerful restraining substances to bind the semen and prevent it from leaking. This formula is quite a great one to treat the root and branch simultaneously by tonifying the kidney and consolidateing the essence. Because this formula can boost kidney qi and consolidate the essence which is specially designed for patients who have kidney deficiency and spontaneous seminal emission, it is called *Jīn Suǒ Gù Jīng Wán* (Golden Lock Essence-Securing Pill).

[Clinical Application]   This formula can tonify the kidney and consolidate the essence mainly with the function of restore interaction between the heart and the kidney, which is used to treat kidney deficiency and insecurity of essence. If the female has leukorrhea which belongs to kidney deficiency, this formula can also be used.

Section 3   Formulas that astringes intestines and arrests proptosis

The formulas in this section are indicated for the syndrome of long-lasting diarrhea.The drug usually used are *ròu dòu kòu, hē zǐ, chì shí zhǐ* and *yǔ yú liáng*. The typical formulas are *táo huā tāng* (Peach Blossom Decoction, 桃花汤) and *sì shén wán* (Four-Miracle Pill, 四神丸).

Táo Huā Tāng (Peach Blossom Decoction, 桃花汤)
Treatise on Cold Damage (*Shāng Hán Lùn*, 伤寒论)

[Ingredient]

Chì Shí Zhǐ (Halloysitum rubrum)   1 *jin*, half keep in raw, half screen out the powder, (24 g, half keep in raw, half screen out the powder)

Gān Jiāng (Zingiberis Rhizoma)   1 *liang* (6 g)

Jīng Mǐ (Nonglutinous rice)   1 *jin* (24 g)

[Usage]   In the original text, half of the *chì shí zhǐ* is decocted with the other two herbs with 7 *sheng* water; using this liquid for cooking the rice, and discard the rice, drink 7 *he* (150 ml) warmed strained decoction, then add the small powder

tablespoon [方寸匕 *fāng cùn bǐ*] (2.5–5 g), drink it 3 times per day. The medicine is no longer needed, if the symptoms disappear after the first taken.

Modern usage: Decocting the three herbs, take the strained decoction after the rice is cooked, and add the *chì shí zhǐ* powders (6 g), twice per day.

[Action] Warm the middle, dispel cold, bind up the bowels, and stop dysenteric.

[Indication] Chronic dysenteric disorders with dark blood and pus in the stool, abdominal pain that prefer local pressure or warmth, pale tongue with thin and white tongue coating, slow and frail or faint and thin pulse.

[Formula Analysis] The *shaoyin* [spleen and stomach have injured] yang deficiency, Causes the cold generated and led to internal obstruction of damp-cold, which disrupts the lower *jiao* and injures the collaterals of the intestines and brings about dark blood and pus in the stool. The *chì shí zhǐ* is good at binding up the bowels, and governing dysenteric. In *Ben Jing*, it was mentioned to "govern dysenteries, intestinal afflux, blood and pus", *Bie Lu* says "treating the abdomen pain and diarrhea, dysenteries with blood and white pus", it is the first choice of chronic dysentery and diarrhea.

The ingenious method of making *chì shí zhǐ* into a powder and drinking it with decoction, which easily remains in the intestine and induces astringency, so it can be the chief medicine; *gān jiāng* is acrid and hot, good at warming the middle [spleen and stomach] for dispelling cold, stanching blood and diarrhea. *Ben Jing* describes it can "warming middle and stanching blood", governs "dysenteric and diarrhea.". It works as the minster, *jīng mǐ*, sweat and neutral, nourishing the stomach and spleen, which can assistant the *chì shí zhǐ* and *gān jiāng* to firm the intestine and stomach. All the herbs altogether play the bind up the bowels and stop dysenteric. For the name "*Táo Huā Tāng* [Peach Blossom Decoction], Zhang Zhi-Cong refers to "the *chì shí zhǐ*'s color is like the peach flower's color, so the decoction was named after it.", Ke Yun-Bo said "peach flower also refers to the spring, which is gentle and warm, not only because of the color", Wang Jin-San[72] also mentioned, "*Táo Huā Tāng* was not named after the color, it can be used in the Kidney Yang deficiency situation, like the

warm and gentle [spring] comes to the cold valley". All sayings are reasonable and can be accepted.

[Application]

With a warming and astringent nature, this formula is frequently used to treat dysenteric diarrhea with pus and blood in the stools, and efflux desertion caused by *shaoyin* yang deficiency. If [patients] accompany with reversal cold of hands and feet, sinking and faint pulse, that belongs to the *shao-yin* yang debilitation, *fù zǐ*, those[warm and hot nature] herbs can be added. *Emergency Formulas to Keep Up One's Sleeve* (*Zhǒu Hòu Bèi Jí Fāng*, 肘后备急方) records, "*chì shí zhǐ tang fang* can heal dysenteric diarrhea with pus and blood in the stools which caused by cold damage, (ingredients: *chì shí zhǐ* two *liang*, *gān jiāng* two *liang*, *fù zǐ* one *liang* [cracked], with five *sheng* water decocted into three *sheng* [volume], drink it warmly; if complain painful feeling below the umbilicus, one *liang dāng guī* and two *liang sháo yào* should be applied".

Sì Shén Wán (Four-Miracle Pill, 四神丸)
Summary of Internal Medicine (*Nèi Kē Zhāi Yào*, 内科摘要)[73]

[Ingredient]

Ròu Dòu Kòu (Myristicae Semen)　2 *liang* (60 g)

Bǔ Gǔ Zhǐ (Psoraleae Fructus)　4 *liang* (120 g)

Wǔ Wèi Zǐ (Schisandrae Fructus)　2 *liang* (60 g)

Wú Zhū Yú (Evodiae Fructus)　2 *liang* (60 g)

[Usage]　Grind the ingredients into a powder and decocted with *shēng jiāng* 4 *liang*, and 50 pieces of *dà zǎo*. When all the materials are thoroughly cooked, take the *dà zǎo* and remove the pit and rub it into tiny pills (dia.0.5cm), take 50–10 pills before three meals.

Modern usage: Grind the ingredients into a powder and mix with water, then boil with *shēng jiāng* (125 g) and *dà zǎo* (50 pieces). After cooking, remove the ginger and *dà zǎo* pit, roll the remaining ingredients into pills (dia.0.5 cm). Take 6–9 g before meals and bedtime with boiled water, twice daily. It can also be prepared as a

decoction with an appropriate reduction in the dosage of the ingredients.

[Action]　Warm and tonify the spleen and kidneys, bind up the intestines, and stop diarrhea.

[Indication]　Spleen and kidney deficiency-cold lead to diarrhea that occurs daily just before sunrise, lack of interest in food, and inability to digest what is eaten, there may also be abdominal pain, fatigue and lethargy, a pale tongue with a thin, white coating, and a submerged, slow, and forceless pulse.

[Formula Analysis]　*Wu Geng Xie* (五更泄, daybreak diarrhea), also known as "*Ji Ming Xie*" (rooster-crow diarrhea), "*shen xie*". *Basic Questions-True Words from the Golden Cabinet* (*Sù Wèn-Jīn Kuì Zhēn Yán Lùn*, 素问·金匮真言论) says, "from the crowing of the rooster to dawn, this is the yin of heaven; it is the yang in the yin, the fact is, man, too, corresponds to this". The bitter and acrid, *bǔ gǔ zhī* is used in a large dosages, which directly tonifies the gate of vitality and benefits the earth (spleen) by fortifying this aspect of fire. It also has an astringent nature that acts on the kidney to secure the primal yang, and on the spleen to stop diarrhea, *The Grand Compendium of Materia Medica* (*Běn Cǎo Gāng Mù*, 本草纲目) describes that it is good at "treating *shen xie* (肾泄)", it is the chief medicine; *ròu dòu kòu* is acrid and warm, is good at warming the spleen and stomach, which works as a minister and interacts with the chief to restraining intestine and stop diarrhea. The other assistant, *wǔ wèi zǐ*, is a strong, warm, and astringent herb that strengthens the deputy's ability to bind up the intestines, warming the spleen and stomach, relieving yin-cold. Ginger is good at removing cold in the stomach and cooperating with *dà zǎo* which is good at nourishing, they are all envoys. All the four ingredients allied together make the formula named "*si shen* (四神)" [four miracle pill]. Wang Jin-Shan says "four types of herbs which have the magic power of treating daybreak diarrhea [spleen-kidney cold deficiency diarrhea]".

[Application]　This formula is adopted in treating diarrhea caused by spleen-kidney cold deficiency; if companied with cold and sour sensation in lumber and limbs, *Yòu Guī Wán* (Right-Restoring Pill) can come to use together for tonifying the kidney-yang.

Section 4   Formulas that arrests leucorrhea and metrorrhagia

This section's formulas indicate chronic, un-remitting uterine bleeding and vaginal discharge. Accompanying signs and symptoms include palpitations, shortness of breath, weakness, lower back soreness, a pallid complexion, pale tongue, and a deficient, thin, and frail pulse. The common medicine like *lóng gǔ, mǔ lì, hǎi piāo xiāo, wǔ bèi zǐ,* etc, the representative formulas are *Gù Chōng Tāng* (Stabilize Gushing Decoction, 固冲汤), *Wán Dài Tāng* (End Discharge Decoction, 完带汤)

Gù Chōng Tāng (Stabilize Gushing Decoction, 固冲汤)
Source Essays on Medicine Esteeming the Chinese and Respecting the Western
Yī Xué Zhōng Zhōng Cān Xī Lù, 医学衷中参西录[74]

[Ingredient]

Baí Zhú (Dry-Fried Atractylodis Macrocephalae Rhizoma)   1 *liang* fried (30 g)

Shēng Huáng Qí (Astragali Radix)   6 *qian* (18 g)

Shān Zhū Yǔ (Corni Fructus)   8 *qian* (24 g)

Shēng Háng Sháo[Sheng Bai Shao] (Paeoniae Radix Alba)   4 *qian* (12 g)

Duàn Lóng Gǔ (Calcined Fossilia Ossis Mastodi)   8 *qian* (24 g)

Duàn Mǔ lì (Calcined Ostreae Concha)   8 *qian* (24 g)

Haǐ Pīao Xiāo (Cuttlefish Bone)   4 *qian* (12 g)

Zōng Biǎn Tàn [Zōng Lǔ Tàn] (Charred Palm)   2 *qian* (6 g)

Wǔ Beì Zǐ (Galla Chinensis)   5 *fen* (1.5 g)

Qiàn Cǎo (Rubiae Radix)   3 *qian* (9 g)

[Usage]   In the original book, the decoction method was not mentioned.

Modern usage: Boiled, *wǔ bèi zǐ* is ground into a powder, and taken with the strained decoction.

[Action]   Augment the qi, strengthen the spleen, stabilize the *Chong* vessel, and stop bleeding.

[Indication]   The spleen deficiency and instability of the *Chong* vessel lead to Uterine bleeding or profuse menstrual bleeding in which the blood is thin and pale

and either gushes out or continuously trickles out. Accompanying signs and symptoms include palpitations, shortness of breath, a pale tongue, and a deficient, big, thin and weak pulse.

[Formula Analysis]　A person's sea of blood is called the *Chong* [meridian]. While the spleen is the post-heaven which produces qi and blood, and governs blood. The high dosage of *bái zhú* and *shēng huáng qí* are good at invigorating qi and strengthening the spleen; hence, spleen-qi becomes strong that can control the blood and solidified *Chong* vessel, as the chief medicines. The uterine bleeding [metrorrhagia and metrostaxis] will lead to blood deficiency, *shān zhū yú*, *shēng bái sháo* as the minster medicines can nourish the liver and kidney and produce blood. The synergistic combination of *duàn lóng gǔ* and *duàn mǔ lì* is frequently used to secure leakage. However, there is an attendant risk that blood stasis will form because of the large dosage of these ingredients mentioned above. The final assistant, *hǎi piāo xiāo*, *qiàn cǎo gēn*, not only stop bleeding, but also invigorate the blood, therefore they are able to prevent the formation of blood stasis. It is precise because of this formula is good at stopping and binding the gushing blood from the uterus, and firms the *Chong* vessel, hence the name [*Gù Chōng Tāng*].

[Application]　With the appropriate presentation, this formula may treat metrorrhagia and metrostaxishy, hypermenorrhea, excessive bleeding which cause by *spleen-qi* deficiency, and frailish *Chong* vessel. But if companie with cold limbs and sweating, a faint pulse that is the yang depletions, should quickly increase the dosage of *huáng qí* and co-use with the "*Shēn Fù Tāng*" to save yang qi.

Wán Dài Tāng (End Discharge Decoction, 完带汤)
Fu Qing-Zhu's Women's Disorders (*Fù Qīng Zhǔ Nǚ Kē*, 傅青主女科)[75]

[Ingredient]

Tǔ Chǎo Bǎi Zhú (Earth-Fried Atractylodis Macrocephalae Rhizoma) 1 *liang* (30 g)

　Chǎo Shān Yào (Dry-Fried Rhizoma Dioscoreae)　1 *liang* (30 g)

　Rén Shēn (Ginseng Radix)　2 *qian* (6 g)

Jiŭ Chăo Baí Sháo (Wine-Fried Paeonia Lactiflora Pall)   *5 qian* (15 g)

Jiŭ Chăo Chē Qián Zĭ (Wine-Fried Plantaginis Semen)   *3 qian* (9 g)

Zhì Cāng Zhú (Prepared Atractylodis Rhizoma)   *3 qian* (9 g)

Gān Căo (Glycyrrhizae Radix)   *1 qian* (3 g)

Chén Pí (Citri Reticulatae Pericarpium)   *5 fen* (1.5g)

Heī Jìe Suì (Charred Schizonepetae Spica)   *5 fen* (4.5g)

Chaí Hú (Bupleuri Radix)   *6 fen* (1.8 g)

[Usage]   Original usage: boiling into a decoction, modern usage is the same.

[Action]   Tonify the spleen and soothe the liver, transform dampness, and stop vaginal discharge.

[Indication]   Liver depression and spleen deficiency, turbid dampness streaming down, the vaginal discharge that is white or pale yellow in color, thin in consistency, the worse situation have particularly foul-smelling and usually continuous. Accompanying signs and symptoms include fatigue, lethargy, a shiny, pale complexion, a pale tongue with a white tongue coating, and a soggy and frail or moderate pulse.

[Formula Analysis]   Profuse vaginal discharge [*dài xià*, 带下]. The *bái dài* (vaginal discharge) is mainly associated with the actions of *Dài Mài* (带脉),which wraps around the lower trunk like a belt, securing all the channels that traverse the area. The [earth-fried] *tŭ chăo bái zhú* is good at nourishing qi and eliminating dampness. *Chăo shān yào* is adept in tonifying qi and spleen, arresting seminal emission. These two co-act as the chief medicines which assist the spleen (earth) in curbing the food nutrients; the minister: *rén shēn*, prepared *cāng zhú* not only nourishes the spleen-qi but is also are very effective against drying dampness. The cooperative work of the four herbs guarantees that the spleen works normally and avoiding from dampness. The assistants are meant to regulate the liver, in concert with chief medicine to balance the liver with the spleen, *chē qián zĭ*, it eliminates dampness downward. The inventive using little dosage of *chái hú* for promoting liver-qi, corresponds to *jiu chăo bái sháo, chén pí* work with *bái zhú, shān yào* which can regulate qi-flowing for strengthening the spleen but without jammed, *jīng jiè*

suì which enters the blood-level [*xuè fēn*, 血分], eliminating dampness and binding the vaginal discharge, also soothing liver, relieving wind. Meanwhile, *gān cǎo* can harmonize all the medicines. This is a liver-spleen co-treating formula, and it contains tonification within dispersion, and places elimination in [a generally] ascending. This purposive method can tonify the spleen and soothe the liver concurrently, eliminating dampness and binding vaginal discharge (*bái dài*, 白带). That's the name "End Discharge Decoction" (*wán dài*) comes.

[Application] This is a commonly-used formula for turbid and profuse virginal discharge due to spleen deficiency and liver-qi stagnation.

Chapter 10

Tranquilizing Formulas

It is composed mainly of tranquilizing or nourishing medicines, which have a tranquilizing effects and can be used to treat mental disturbances, collectively referred to as tranquilizing formulas.

Section 1   Formulas that tranquilizes the mind with heavy sedatives

According to the principle of the *Basic Questions-Comprehensive Discourse on the Essentials of the Most Reliable* (*Sù Wèn-Zhì Zhēn Yào Dà Lùn*, 素问·至真要大论) "treating fright by calming", all the formulas that are mainly composed of heavy minerals or crustaceans, with the effect of sedating and calming the mind, belong to tranquilizing mind with heavy sedatives group. In the "ten formula types", it belongs to the category of "heavy [medicines] eliminating timidity".

In this section, the medicines are mostly used to treat panic, epilepsy, palpitation, insomnia, restlessness and other symptoms such as *zhū shā*, *cí shí*, and *lóng gǔ, etc.* The representative formula is *Zhū Shā Ān Shén Wán* (Cinnabar Pill to Calm the Spirit, 朱砂安神丸).

Zhū Shā Ān Shén Wán (Cinnabar Pill to Calm the Spirit, 朱砂安神丸)
Clarifying Doubts about Injury from Internal and External Causes (*Nèi Wài Shāng Biàn Huò Lùn,* 内外伤辨惑论)

[Ingredient]
Shuǐ Feī Zhū Shā (Aqueous Trituration Of Cinnabaris)   *5 qian* (15 g)

Huáng Lián (Coptidis Rhizoma)　remove the fibril, wash them with alcohol 6 *qian* (18 g)

Dāng Guī (Angelicae Sinensis Radix)　*2 qian 5 fen* (7.5 g)

Shēng Dì Huáng (Radix Rehmanniae)　*2 qian 5 fen* (7.5 g)

Gān Cǎo (Glycyrrhizae)　*5 qian 5 fen* (17 g)

[Usage]　Grind the four ingredients (without *zhū shā*) together into a fine powder, using water knead and form them into pills, which are as big as millet, clothing with *zhū shā*. Each serving is 15–20 pills per time, swallowed with saliva, or a little warm or cold water, either once before bedtime or twice daily.

Modern usage: Grind the fours (without *zhū shā*) together into a powder that is covered with *zhū shā*. Take in 4.5–9 g per time with warm water, either once before bedtime. It can also be used as a decoction, and all the dosage is reduced according to the original formula; the *zhū shā* is originally taken with the strained decoction.

[Action]　Sedat the Heart, calm the mind, clear heat, and nourish the blood.

[Indication]　Hyperactivity of heart-fire which consumes the blood, manifested as insomnia, continuous palpitations, irritability and heat in the chest, a desire to vomit without result, dream-disturbed sleep, a tongue that is red at the tip, and a thready and, rapid pulse.

[Formula Analysis]　*Basic Questions-Discourse from the Secret Classic of the Miraculous Orchid (Sù Wèn-Líng Lán Mì Diǎn Lùn*, 素问·灵兰秘典论) says, "the heart, the emperor [of organs], housing the *shen*"; *Basic Questions-Discourse on the Sexagenary cycles and Organ Manifestation (Sù Wèn-Liù Jié Zàng Xiàng Lùn* 素问·六节藏象论) says, "the heart is the origin of life, and the place of god". When the fire of the heart rises, the fire should be cleared; if the yin of the heart is insufficient, the yin should be replenished, but if the replenishment without cleaning, the evil heat will still damage the yin; while clearing without replenishment, the yin blood will be difficult to recover. The chief ingredient, sweet and slightly cold *zhū shā*, in *Ben Jing*, is described as "nourish the essence-spint, calm the ethereal and corporeal soul"; The *Thoroughly Revised Materia Medica (Běn Cǎo Cóng Xīn*, 本草从新) [76], describes it can enter the heart channel and sedate excessive yang activity by way of its heavy

nature. It calms the mind and also clears fire from the heart. The deputy ingredient, bitter and cold *huáng lián*, strongly drains excess heat from the heart and works synergistically with the chief ingredient to reinforce its actions. They address both the branch and root of this disorder. The assistant ingredients are acrid, sweet, and warming *dāng guī*, which enters the heart, liver, and spleen channels, and sweet, bitter, and strongly cool *shēng dì huáng*, which enters the heart, liver, and kidney channels. Together they nourish the blood and replenish the yin to tonify those aspects that have been injured by the heart fire and prevent further injury. The latter ingredient also helps clear fire from the nutrional and blood aspects. The envoy, *gān cǎo*, harmonizes the actions of the other ingredients while protecting the stomach from the harsh effects of the chief and deputy ingredients.

[Application]   In clinical practice, this formula is thought to be particularly effective in treating the heart fire flaming up, burning yin-blood, causing insomnia and palpitations. The palpitations and insomnia, red tip of the tongue, thready and rapid pulse are the critial points of syndrome differentiation.

Cí Zhū Wán (Magnetite and Cinnabar Pill, 磁朱丸)
(*Primitive name: shén qū wán, "Valuable Prescriptions for Emergency"*)
(原名神曲丸, 备急千金要方)

[Ingredient]
Cí Shí (Magnetitum)   2 *liang* (60 g)

Zhū Shā (Cinnabaris)   1 *liang* (30 g)

Shén Qǔ (Massa Medicata Fermentata)   4 *liang* (120 g)

[Usage]   Grind the ingredients into a powder and form them into small pills (phoenix tree seed size) with honey. Take 3 pills, three times per day.

Modern usage: Grind the front two ingredients into a fine powders, mix it with the powder of *shén qǔ*, and form them into small pills (dia.0.5 cm), take 6 g with thin rice soup or warm water, twice daily.

[Action]   Heavily sedate and calm the spirit, weigh down the yang and tonfiy the yin.

[Indication] Disharmony of heart and kidney, dim and blurred vision, tinnitus, diminished hearing and vision acuity, palpitations and insomnia. Also used for seizures.

[Formula Analysis] This syndrome is caused by kidney yin (essence) insufficiency, partial heart fire hyperactivity, disharmony between the heart and kidney, and inbalance between water and fire. The chief ingredient, salty, cold and heavy *cí shí* enters the kidney, calms the mind, subdues the yang nourishing the yin. The deputy, *zhū shā*, is cold and sweet which enters the heart channel, sedates and calms the spirit, clearing the heat of the heart. The cooperation of these two can tranquilize the floating-yang [the fire flee out of the kidney], harmonize the water and fire which keep the essence transporting upward, heart-fire going downward. One assistant, *shén qǔ* strengthens the spleen and stomach and aids digestion. It prevent injury to the stomach qi from the heavy metals and helps disseminate their actions throughout the body. It also plays an active role in stabilizing the regular ascending and descending of the essence and fire. The other assistant, honey, serves as the filler for the pills. In a word, this formula tranquils the floating-yang [the fire flees out of the kidney], sedate and calm the spirit and help the movement in the middle palace [middle *jiao*], which balances the water and fire.

[Application] This formula focuses on treating dim and blur vision, tinnitus, diminished acuity of hearing and vision, palpitations, and insomnia caused by disharmony of heart and kidney, and it will work better together with *Liù Wèi Dì Huáng Wán*.

Section 2   Formulas that nourishes and calms the spirit

Formulas that nourish and calm the spirit are appropriate for the disturbances of the spirit due to deficiency of the qi, blood, and yin, usually manifested as palpitations, irritability and insomnia. The typical medicines, like *suān zǎo rén*, *bǎi zǐ rén*, and *fú líng*, *xiǎo mài* which are good at tonifying and regulating the qi, enriching the yin and nourishing the blood. The representative formula like: *Suān Zǎo Rén Tāng* (Sour Jujube Decoction, 酸枣仁汤), *Tiān Wáng Bǔ Xīn Dān* (Emperor of Heaven's Special

Pill to Tonify the Heart, 天王补心丹), *Gān Mài Dà Zǎo Tāng* (Licorice, Wheat, and Jujube Decoction, 甘草小麦大枣汤).

Suān Zǎo Rén Tāng (Sour Jujube Decoction, 酸枣仁汤)
Essentials from the Golden Cabinet (*Jīn Guì Yào Lüè*, 金匮要略)

[Ingredient]

Suān Zǎo Rén (Ziziphi Spinosae Semen)　2 *sheng* (12 g)

Gān Cǎo (Glycyrrhizae Radix)　1 *liang* (3 g)

Zhī Mǔ (Anemarrhenae Rhizoma)　2 *liang* (6 g)

Fú Líng (Poria)　2 *liang* (6 g)

Chuān Xiōng (Chuanxiong Rhizoma)　2 *liang* (6 g)

[Usage]　Decoct *suān zǎo rén* with 8 *sheng* water. with 6 *sheng eft*. Then, put the other five herbs into it, boil into 3 *sheng*, and drink it warmly. Three times per day.

Modern usage: Boiling all the ingredients together.

[Action]　Nourish the blood, calm the spirit, clear heat, and eliminate irritability.

[Indication]　Deficiency overwork (*xū láo*, 虚劳) and deficiency irritability (*xū fán*, 虚烦). Insomnia, a wiry or thready, rapid pulse.

[Formula Analysis]　The liver governs the blood and ethereal soul. When a person lies down [falls asleep], the blood returns back to the liver. In terms of people who are exhausted or overworked, their liver qi is not glorious and the liver blood is inadequate, which fails to store the soul.

Basic Questions-Discourse on the Sexagenary cycles and Organ Manifestation (*Sù Wèn-Liù Jié Zàng Xiàng Lùn*, 素问·六节藏象论) says, "the liver is the basis of exhaustion to the utmost. It is the location of the *hun* (soul)". *Basic Questions-The Generation and Completion of the Five Depots* (*Sù Wèn-Wǔ Zàng Shēng Chéng*, 素问·五脏生成) says, "the liver longs for sour[flavor]". Sweet, sour and bland *suān zǎo rén* nourishes the liver, and calm the *hun-soul*. According to *Miscellaneous Records of Famous Physicians* (*Míng Yī Bié Lù*, 名医别录), "it focuses on heart irritability with an inability to sleep", it act as the chief. *Basic Questions-Discourse on How the Qi in the Depots Follow the Pattern of the Seasons* (*Sù Wèn-Zāng Qì Fǎ Shí Lùn*, 素

问·藏气法时论) mentioned, "The liver [qi] longs for dispersion, [in case of a disease in the liver]quickly consume acrid [flavor]to disperse its[qi], use acrid[flavor] to supplement it, sour[flavor] to drain it". The deputy is acrid, warming and aromatic *chuān xiōng*, which regulates the liver blood by encouraging it to flow freely and calm the spirit by providing them with its natural abode. The assistant medicines are sweet and bland *fú líng*, which calms the spirit and tonifies the spleen and stomach. Along with bitter, sweet and cool *zhī mǔ*, clears heat to preserve the yin protects the stomach from dryness and indirectly enriches the fluids like most of the other medicines in this formula. Meanwhile, *Basic Questions-Discourse on How the Qi in the Depots Follow the Pattern of the Seasons* (*Sù Wèn-Zāng Qì Fǎ Shí Lùn*, 素问·藏气法时论) says, "when the liver suffers from tensions, quickly consume sweet [flavor] to relax [these tensions]", so the envoy, *gān cǎo*, tonifies the middle burner[spleen] and relaxes hypertonicity of the Liver.

[Clinical Application]　This formula is mainly used to treat liver blood deficiency and internal heat caused by blood deficiency syndrome, manifested as irritability and insomnia. According to the editor's clinical experience, blood deficiency can even be treated with *Si Wu Tang*, for better efficacy.

Tiān Wáng Bǔ Xīn Dān (Emperor of Heaven's Special Pill to Tonify the Heart, 天王补心丹)
Fine Formulas for Women with Annotations and Commentary (*Jiào Zhù Fù Rén Liáng Fāng*, 校注妇人良方)

[Ingredient]
Shēng Dì Huáng (Rehmanniae Radix)　4 *liang* (120 g)
Rén Shēn (Ginseng Radix))　5 *qian* (15 g)
Tiān Mén Dōng (Asparagi Radix)　1 *liang* (30 g)
Maì Mén Dōng (Ophiopogonis Radix)　1 *liang* (30 g)
Xuán Shēn (Scrophulariae Radix)　5 *qian* (15 g)
Dān Shēn (Salviae Miltiorrhizae Radix)　5 *qian* (15 g)
Fú Líng (Poria)　5 *qian* (15 g)

Yuǎn Zhì (Polygalae Radix) 5 *qian* (15 g)

Dāng Guī (Angelicae Sinensis Radix) 1 *liang* (30 g)

Wǔ Weì Zǐ (Schisandrae Fructus) 1 *liang* (30 g)

Baǐ Zǐ Rén (Platycladi Semen) 1 *liang* (30 g)

Chǎo Suān Zǎo Rén (Dry-Fried Ziziphi Spinosae Semen) 1 *liang* (30 g)

Jié Gěng (Platycodi Radix) 5 *qian* (15 g)

[Usage] Grind the ingredients into a powder and form them into small pills (Phoenix Tree Seed size) with honey, coating with *zhū shā*. Take 20–30 pills before sleep, with *zhú yè tāng* [decocting bamboo leaf into soup].

Modern usage: Grind the ingredients into a powder and form into small pills (Phoenix Tree Seed size) with honey, coating with *zhū shā* take 6–9 g with warm water twice per day; or discretionary reduction, make it into a decoction.

[Action] Enrich the yin and clear heat, nourish the blood, and calm the spirit.

[Indication] Yin and blood deficiency lead to irritability, palpitations with anxiety, fatigue, insomnia with restless sleep, forgetfulness, dry stools, a red tongue with less coating, and a thready, rapid pulse.

[Formula Analysis] *Basic Questions-Discourse from the Secret Classic of the Miraculous Orchid (Sù Wèn-Líng Lán Mì Diǎn Lùn, 素问·灵兰秘典论)* says, "the heart is the organ [similar to] a monarch and is responsible for *shenming* (mental activity or thinking)". The large dosage of *shēng dì huáng* goes to the heart and kidney[meridian], tonfiying yin and clearing heat, and the adequate water [yin] can quell the fire, acting as the chief medicine. The three deputies, *xuán shēn*, *tiān dōng* and *mài dōng*, enrich the yin and clear the heat from deficiency, and the *xuán shēn* and *tiān dōng* go to the kidney channel controling the fire; with sweet and cold nature, *mài dōng* goes to the heart channel, which can nourish the heart-yin and clear the heart heat. There are four groups of assistants: *dāng guī* and *dān shēn* tonify the blood to nourish the heart, calming the heart-*shen*; as the relationship between blood and qi, the *rén shēn* and *fú líng* can assist the heart qi, and also tranquilize *shen*; *suān zǎo rén*, *yuǎn zhì*, *bǎi zǐ rén*, the *yuǎn zhì* also can connect the kidney with the heart, restoring coordination between the heart and kidney; the *wǔ wèi zǐ* can preserve the heart-qi.

The envoy is *jié gěng*, which conducts the other medicines, actions toward the upper burner, the abode of the spirit. *Zhū shā*, red goes into the heart, clears the heat and calms the wayward spirit. All those medicines work together, clearing heat, enriching yin, and calming the s*hen*. As "*Effective Use of Established Formulas* (*Chéng Fāng Qiè Yòng*, 成方切用)"[77] recorded, "the [religious discipline] interpreter in *Zhong Nan Shan* (Zhong Nan Mountain, 终南山) recited and explained [all day], consuming the heart-shen, and got this formula from the heavenly king in the dream".

[Clinical Application] This formula is good at enriching the yin and clearing heat, nourishing the blood and calming the spirit, which is appropriate for the syndromes, including palpitation, insomnia, fatigued spirit and lassitude, dry stool and ulcer in the mouth, *etc.*

Gān Cǎo Xiǎo Mài Dà Zǎo Tāng (Licorice, Wheat, and Jujube Decoction, 甘草小麦大枣汤)
Essentials from the Synopsis of Golden Chamber (*Jīn Guì Yào Lüè*, 金匮要略)

[Ingredient]

Gān Cǎo (Glycyrrhizae Radix)   3 *liang* (9 g)

Xiǎo Mài (Tritici Fructus)   1 *sheng* (30 g)

Dà Zǎo (Jujubae Fructus)   10 pieces

[Usage] Use 6 *sheng* water and boil the ingredients into 3 *sheng*, drinking it warmly.

Modern usage: Decocted with water.

[Action] Nourish the heart, calm the mind, harmonize the middle burner, and relax hypertonicity.

[Indication] Visceral agitation (*zàng zào*, 脏躁), disorientation, frequent attacks of melancholy and the desire to cry, inability to control oneself, frequent bouts of yawning, red tongue with less coating, thready and rapid pulse.

[Formula Analysis] Viscera here refers to the heart. Heart deficiency generates the blood deficiency which results in visceral agitation, manifested as deficiency-fire disturbed inside, heart-shen disquieted. However, this fire is a deficiency type that could

not be treated with the bitter descending method; meanwhile, this deficiency is not a total infirmity, and tonification is not suitable. In *Basic Questions-Discourse on How the Qi in the Depots Follow the Pattern of the Seasons* (*Sù Wèn-Zàng Qì Fǎ Shí Lùn*, 素问·藏气法时论), "when the liver suffers from tensions [rapid flow of qi], which can be relieved by sweet flavor", *The Spiritual Pivot-Discourse on Five Flavors* (*Líng Shū-Wǔ Wèi*, 灵枢·五味) says, "the wheat is good for the [person who has] heart disease". So the sweet and mild medicine can release the liver-qi and tonify the heart-qi. In this formula, the chief herb-*xiǎo mài* is good at reinforcing the heat-qi to tranquilize the heart-shen. According to the mother-son relationship between liver and heart, the wheat also can soothe the liver-qi and this thought can be found in *Miscellaneous Records of Famous Physicians* (*Míng Yī Bié Lù*, 名医别录); *gān cǎo*, as the deputy medicine, can tonify the heart-qi, harmonize the middle and relax tension; *dà zǎo*, which augments the qi and moistens internal dryness, act as the assistant and guide medicines. Only three simple medicines, but this formula achieves remarkable effects of nourishing the heart, calming the spirit, harmonizing the middle burner, and relaxing hypertonicity. In the original book referred, "[this formula] also tonify the spleen-qi", because they can invigorate spleen and replenish qi action. Because the fire is the mother of earth. It mother [fire] is nourished, thus the son [earth] will be reinforced. Additionally, see the liver disease [liver been attacked], know the liver passes [transforms to] spleen, [should] firstly solid [reinforce] the spleen, which is the treatment for liver-deficiency, being related in *Classic of Difficult Issues* (*Nàn Jīng*, 难经)[78], "liver been injured, the middle [burner] should be moderated [tonified] ".

[Clinical Application] This formula acts appropriately to the visceral agitation (*zàng zào*, 脏躁), caused by excessive thought, preoccupation and yin deficiency. This syndrome not only appears in females but also males. However, this symptom commonly happens in women. In the early stage, it is mentally disoriented, sensitive, and suffering from unquiet sleep, attacks, [they] often the feeling of upset or depressed, uncontrollable crying, yawning, manic behavior or severe disorientation, and this formula is very effective for these syndromes.

Chapter 11

Wind-Relieving Formulas

The formulas expeling wind are composed of medicines that can scatter wind or enrich yin and subdue yang. These formulas have the impact of dredging and dispersing external wind or pacifying and extinguishing interior wind, to treat the disease caused by pathogenic wind.

Section 1   Formulas that dredges and disperses external wind

These formulas are suitable for all kinds of diseases caused by the external wind. As described in *The Spiritual Pivot-five Changes* (*Líng Shū-Wǔ Biàn*, 灵枢·五变), "When the flesh is not firm qi deficiency and the interstices and pores are sparse, one is prone to [have] wind disorders", which shows that if healthy qi of human body is weak and interstices are loose, he will be easily to be attacked by the external wind which leads to wind disease. The external wind is invading from outside, thus medicines must be used to disperse wind through the interstices, that is called external wind should be treated with the dispersing method. Because the wind attacks the channel which influences the fluid circulation and condenses it into phlegm. The phlegm-resolving medicines are often used tooperatively to dispers the exterior wind. The formula is mainly composed of *chuān xiōng, qiāng huó, fáng fēng, bái zhǐ, jīng jiè, jiāng cán, etc.*, and often combined with *bái fù zǐ, nán xīng* and other phlegm-resolving drugs.

"Dispelling the wind and regulating the blood first, [then] the wind is self-destructive", the pathogenic qi attacks the body and obstructs the channels, thus some

herbs like *rǔ xiāng, mò yào, dì lóng, dāng guī*, should be used to invigorate blood and dissolve stasis. If the average circulation of qi and blood becomes harmonious, the obstructive wind will be dispersed. Because wind is the pathogen of yang, it often causes constraint-heat that over-consumes the blood. Medicines that drain heat and nourish the blood, such as *shēng dì, chì sháo, mǔ dān pí* can be combined.

The representative formulas used for this syndrome include *Chuān Xiōng Chá Tiáo Sǎn* (Tea-Mix and Chuanxiong Powder, 川芎茶调散), *Qiān Zhèng Sǎn* (Symmetry-Correcting Powder, 牵正散) and *Huó Luò Dān* (Channel-Activating Elixir, 活络丹). The medicines in this section are warm and dry. Therefore one should be cautious when they are applied to a patient with fluid depletion or yin deficiency with yang hyperactivity.

Chuān Xiōng Chá Tiáo Sǎn (Tea-Mix and Chuanxiong Powder, 川芎茶调散)
Formulary of the Pharmacy Service for Benefiting the People in the Taiping Era (*Tài Píng Huì Mín Hé Jì Jú Fāng*, 太平惠民和剂局方)

[Ingredient]

Bái zhǐ (Radix Angelicae Dahuricae)   2 *liang* (60 g)

Gān cǎo (Radix Et Rhizoma Glycyrrhizae)   2 *liang* (60 g)

Qiāng huó (Rhizoma Et Radix Notopterygii)   2 *liang* (60 g)

Jīng jiè (Herba Schizonepetae)   remove the stalk 4 *liang* (120 g)

Chuān xiōng (Rhizoma Chuanxiong)   without peduncle, 4 *liang* (120 g)

Xì xīn (Radix Et Rhizoma Asari)   without reed, 1 *liang* (30 g)

Fáng fēng (Radix Saposhnikoviae)   1.5 *liang* (45 g)

Bò he (Herba Menthae)   avoids fire, 8 *liang* (250 g)

[Usage]   Grinding the ingredients and dividing the average dosage to 2 *qian*. Drink with tea after meals.

Modern usage: Grind the ingredients into a fine powder and take 6 g twice daily after meals with green tea. It may also be prepared as a decoction by reducing the dosage of the ingredients.

[Action]   Disperse wind and alleviate pain.

[Indication] This formula is used to treat patients who are attacked by externally-contracted wind disease, manifested as migraine or headache, or aversion to cold with heat effusion, dizzy vision with nasal congestion, white and thin coating and floating pulse.

[Formula Analysis] *Basic Questions-Discourse on the Major Yin and on the Yang Brilliance [conduits]* (*Sù Wèn-Tài Yīn Yáng Míng Lùn*, 素问·太阴阳明论) says, "So when wind invades [the body], it attacks the upper [part of the body] first". In the formula, *chuān xiōng* is good at dispersing wind to alleviate pain in the *shao-yang*[lesser yang], and *jue yin* channels (temporal and vertex), *Herbal Classic* (*běn jīng*, 本经) says, "medicine [chuān xiōng] is to treat the headache caused by wind-stroke", as the chief medicine; *qiāng huó* is acrid, bitter and warm, entering into the *taiyang* channel (occipital), *bái zhǐ* is acrid and warm, entering in the *yangming* channel. Li Shizhen explains in *The Compendium of Materia Medica* (*Běn Cǎo Gāng Mù*, 本草纲目) as follows, "For headaches, one must employ *chuān xiōng*. To enhance the efficacy, add the herbs guiding medicines into channels. For instance, *qiāng huó* enters into the *taiyang* meridian, *bái zhǐ* enters into *yangming* meridian", as deputy medicine;" The wind is the swift and changeable pathogen of yang which often causes constraint-heat [after a long time], so use a large amount of *bò he* to disperse wind and clear heat, *jīng jiè*, acrid, warm, dispel wind, and clear the head. *Fáng fēng*, acrid, sweet and warm, is used to dispel wind. *Xì xīn*, acrid, and warm, is used to dispel wind to alleviate pain. Four deputies aid the chief by dispersing wind from the head and releasing the exterior. *Gān cǎo*, the envoy, supplements the center and boosts qi, ascending without harming the healthy qi and harmonizing the actions of the other herbs in the formula. Tea can clear head by its bitterness and coolness as a final envoy medicine. Besides, it can avoid the wind medicine rising fire and regulate ascending and descending. Taking medicine after meals to promote the medicine goes to the upside. This formula contains many warm and acrid substances that specialize in soothing the wind to relieve the headache. As the *Medical Formulas Gathered and Explained* (*Yī Fāng Jí Jiě*, 医方集解) says, "For headaches, one must employ wind herbs because only the wind can reach upward to the vertex of the head." As the chief

191

medicine is *chuān xiōng*, the dosage form is powder, taken with green tea, so it is named "*Chuān Xiōng Chá Tiáo Sǎn* (Tea-Mix and Chuanxiong Powder)*".

[Clinical Application] This formula is commonly used to disperse wind and pathogens, regarded as a famous formula for treating head-wind and headache. It is more suitable for headaches from external contraction and headaches due to external wind-cold.

Qiān Zhèng Sǎn (Symmetry-Correcting Powder, 牵正散)
Secret Formulas of the Yang Family (*Yáng Shì Jiā Cáng Fāng*, 杨氏家藏方) [79]

[Ingredient]

Bái Fù Zǐ (Rhizoma Typhonii)

Bái Jiāng Cán (Bombyx Batryticatus)

Quán Xiē (Scorpio)

Detoxify, Unprocessed, equal dose

[Usage] Grind equal amounts of the ingredients into a fine powder and take 1 *qian* dose with hot wine.

Modern usage: Grind equal amounts of the ingredients into a fine powder and take 3 g with hot wine or warm water. The decoction is also available when the dosage is reduced.

[Action] Expels wind and resolves phlegm.

[Indication] Wind-phlegm obstructing the collateral, deviation eyes and mouth and facial spasm.

[Formula Analysis] This type of syndrome is caused by wind-phlegm pathogens obstructing the head and face collaterals. The chief ingredient, bái fù zǐ acrid and warm, resolves wind-phlegm and expels wind over the head by ascending and dispersing. *Bái jiāng cán* salty, sweet and neutral transforms phlegm, together with *quán xiē* acrid and neutral extinguishs wind and arrest convulsion. These two are regarded as deputy medicines. The envoy, hot wine, assists the other ingredients upward to the head and face by diffusing the collaterals. The combination of all the ingredients has an intense action of expelling wind, resolving phlegm and unblocking

the collaterals. After that, the symptom of facial palsy can be "pulled back", so the formula is called *Qiān Zhèng Săn* (Symmetry-Correcting Powder)

[Clinical Application] This formula is usually used to treat the syndrome of wind-phlegm obstructing the collaterals and facial palsy. This formula contains toxic substances and should not be taken in large doses for long-term time, or during pregnancy.

Huó Luò Dān (Invigorate the collateral Special Pil, 活络丹)
Formulary of the Pharmacy Service for Benefiting the People in the Taiping Era (*Tài Píng Huì Mín Hé Jì Jú Fāng,* 太平惠民和剂局方)

[Ingredient]

Zhì Chuān Wū (Radix Aconiti Praeparata)   without peel, 6 *liang* (180 g)

Zhì Căo Wū (Radix Aconiti Kusnezoffii Praeparata)   without peel, 6 *liang* (180 g)

Dì Lóng (Pheretima)   without soil 6 *liang* (180 g)

Zhì Tiān Nán Xīng (Rhizoma Arisaematis praeparatum)   6 *liang* (180 g)

Rŭ Xiāng (Olibanum)   grinding, 2 *liang* 2 *qian* (66 g)

Mò Yào (Myrrha)   grinding, 2 *liang* 2 *qian* (66 g)

[Usage]   In the original formula: grind the ingredients into a fine powder and form into pills with wine and batter. Roll into *Tung* (phoenix tree seed) size. Take once a day in 20 pills doses on an empty stomach with cold wine or a decoction made of *jīng jiè* tea (Herba Schizonepetae).

Modern usage: Grind the ingredients into a fine powder and form them into pills with wine and panada. Take once or twice a day in 3g doses on an empty stomach with wine or warm water.

[Action]   Warm the channels, unblock the collateral, dispel wind and eliminate dampness, resolve phlegm and expell stasis.

[Indication]   Wind, dampness and phlegm [pathogens] obstruct the channels and collaterals, which leads to persistent spasms and inflexible in the extremities. In severe cases, the obstruction causes wandering pain. It can also treat numbness of the

extremities after wind stroke, which lasts for a long time, while there is wet and stable stasis in the meridians pain between the legs and arms.

[Formula Analysis] Wind-cold-damp pathogens obstruct the channels and collaterals, stagnant qi and blood, disturb the circulation of *ying-wei* as well. The chief ingredients, *zhì chuān wū* and *zhì cǎo wū*, acrid, hot and toxic, have the action of warming the channels, dispersing cold, searching out wind, overcoming dampness and unblocking the channels. The deputy, *zhì tiān nán xīng*, bitter, acrid, warm and toxic, can overcome phlegm and dry dampness. Two of the assistants, *rǔ xiāng*, acid, bitter, warm, and *mò yào*, bitter, neutral, invigorate the blood and increase the flow in the channels to stop the pain. *Dì lóng*, cold in nature, is good at dredging channels, removing stasis and alleviating the toxicity of *zhì cǎo wū*. In *Materia Medica of Sichuan* (*Shǔ Běn Cǎo*, 蜀本草[80]), it is said that "it alleviates the toxicity of *shè wǎng* (射罔)" (according to *The Compendium of Materia Medica* (*Běn Cǎo Gāng Mù*, 本草纲目) records, "juice *cǎo wū* and turn into a poison after sunburn. It can be used to shoot animals, so it is called *shè wǎng*"). The wine is good at moving and dispersing, which can guide medicines to arrive at the affected area as envoy medicine. The combination of these two medicines removes the wind-cold and damp pathogens, turbidity, blood stasis, and have the actions of invigorate blood and unblock channels, the so-called "*Huó Luò Dān* (Channel-Activating Elixir)". *Basic Questions-Comprehensive Discourse on the Essentials of the Most Reliable* (*Sù Wèn-Zhì Zhēn Yào Dà Lùn*, 素问·至真要大论) says, "treating retention with purgation" and "treating stagnation by moving", reflected in this formula.

[Clinical Application] This formula is usually used to treat the *bì* syndrome manifested as pain or numbness of limbs after a wind-stroke. It is also suit for those who are impaired by wind-cold-damp or phlegm-damp pathogens or stable stasis; the premise is that the constitution is still strong.

Section 2 Formulas that calms down internal wind

The formulas in this section are used for treating conditions with internal

stirring of visceral lesions. Its clinical symptoms have sudden, swaying and variable characteristics like the wind's characteristics, so it is called the internal wind. It is typically characterized by a sudden loss of consciousness, facial palsy and hemiplegia, without any typical symptom of six-channel diseases such as wind-type stroke and the "liver wind" manifested as limbs fainting and convulsions which belongs to the category of internal wind. The pathogenesis of the disease varies. Disharmony of qi and blood due to extreme heat and liver wind stirring internally is characterized by dizziness, feverish sensation in the head, drunken complexion, even fainting, facial palsy and hemiplegia. Wind generated by blood deficiency is characterized by convulsion, mental fatigue, and weak pulse. Wind-turbid pathogens ascending due to kidney deficiency are characterized by aphasia and paralysis.

Further progression of these patterns may lead to coma, muscular tetany and sudden loss of consciousness. The internal wind is generally treated with herbs that calm, extinguish and sedate, and tonify the yin and regulate the liver. Avoid using any acrid herbs as the internally-generated wind arises inside. To treat these patterns, the formulas in this section tranquilizes the liver, enriches the yin or cools the liver to extinguish wind. Internally-generated wind arises when the internal organs, primarily the liver and kidney, lose the ability to exercise control over the yang qi, which their nature is wild and they readily transform into the pathogenic wind. Thus, nourishing yin is an vital measure to extinguish internal wind. There are some modifications in treatment. Moisturizing dryness, softening the liver, clearing the heat, subduing yang and extinguishing the wind can all be accomplished by enriching yin. In severe cases with heavy sedatives, those who are deficient both in yin and yang can be treated with the yang-tonifying medicines to return fire to its source. Avoid using bitter-cold medicines. Use the heat-clearing medicines if the yin deficiency leads to internal heat. External and internal wind can mutually produce or combine. "The *Feng qi* (wind-qi) communicates with the liver", as is said in *Basic Questions-Comprehensive Discourse on Phenomena Corresponding to Yin and Yang* (*Sù Wèn-Yīn Yáng Yīng Xiàng Dà Lùn*, 素问·阴阳应象大论). In some conditions, the external drives the internal wind,

in which case the treatment must deal with both aspects. Using a small amount of exterior wind-dispersing medicines among a large number of external wind-calming medicines, the curative action is better than the simple way.

To treat these patterns, the formulas in this section rely on medicines that can calm the liver and extinguish wind, such as *líng yáng jiǎo, tiān má, gōu téng, sāng yè, jú huā, shí jué míng, dài zhě shí, lóng gǔ* and *mǔ lì, etc.* and medicines of enriching yin and nourishing the fluid, such as *shēng dì, bái sháo, ē jiāo, jī zǐ huáng, guī bǎn, biē jiǎ* and *niú xī*. Representatives such as *Zhèn Gān Xī Fēng Tāng* (Liver-Sedating and Wind-Extinguishing Decoction, 镇肝熄风汤), *Dà Dìng Fēng Zhū* (Major Wind-Stabilizing Pill, 大定风珠), *Líng Jiǎo Gōu Téng Tāng* (Antelope Horn and Uncaria Decoction, 羚角钩藤汤) and *Dì Huáng Yǐn Zǐ* (Rehmannia Drink, 地黄饮子).

Zhèn Gān Xī Fēng Tāng (Liver-Sedating and Wind-Extinguishing Decoction, 镇肝熄风汤)

Essays on Medicine Esteeming the Chinese and Respecting the Western (*Yī Xué Zhōng Zhōng Cān Xī Lù,* 医学衷中参西录)

[Ingredient]

Huái Niú Xī (Radix Achyranthis Bidentatae)　1 *liang* (30 g)

Shēng Zhě Shí (Haematitum)　grind, 1 *liang* (30 g)

Shēng Lóng Gǔ (Os Draconis; Fossilia Ossis Mastodi)　pound to pieces, 5 *qian* (15 g)

Shēng Mǔ Lì (Concha Ostreae)　Pound, 5 *qian* (15 g)

Shēng Guī Bǎn (Plastrum Testudinis)　Pound to pieces, 5 *qian* (15 g)

Shēng Sháo Yào (Radix Paeoniae)　5 *qian* (15 g)

Xuán Shēn (Radix Scrophulariae)　5 *qian* (15 g)

Tiān Dōng (Radix Asparagi)　5 *qian* (15 g)

Chuān Liàn Zǐ (Fructus Toosendan)　pound to pieces, 2 *qian* (6 g)

Shēng Mài Yá (Fructus Hordei Germinatus)　2 *qian* (6 g)

Yīn Chén (Herba Artemisiae Scopariae)　2 *qian* (6 g)

Gān Cǎo (Radix Et Rhizoma Glycyrrhizae)　1.5 *qian* (4.5 g)

[Usage]   The original usage is not recorded in the book.

Modern usage: Decoction.

[Action]   Tranquilize the liver and extinguish the wind.

[Indication]   This internal wind-stroke mainly manifests as a strong long-wiry pulse which leads to dizziness and vertigo caused by upper excess and lower deficiency, feverish sensation in the head, eye swelling and tinnitus, vexing heat in the chest, frequent belching, unfavorable of extremities, face palsy gradually, drunk complexion, mental confusion with moments of clarity, and an inability to fully recover after a loss of consciousness, atrophy and withered.

[Formula Analysis]   The internal wind stroke, also known as a wind-like strike (stroke), [which] is impaired is caused by the endogenous wind. The relatively large dosage of *huai niú xī*, the chief ingredient, conducts the circulation of blood downward and subdues the ascendant yang, it also tonifies the liver-kidney yin for treating the root. *Dài zhě shí* has the heavy nature that enables it to direct the qi downward and control its rebelliousness, which calms the liver, directs the stomach qi downward, and pacifies the rebellious qi in the penetrating vessel. An aggregate action of *lóng gǔ*, *mǔ lì*, *guī bǎn* and *sháo yào* is subduing yang and directing counterflow downward, softening the liver and extinguishing wind. *Xuán shēn* and *tiān dōng* have the actions of tonifying water to moisten wood and clearing gold to restrict wood. In Zhang Xi-chun's opinion[81], "If the clearing and clarifying qi in the lung moves downward, it will naturally sedate and control liver wood", and the medicines mentioned aboved are especially suitable for helping the chief medicines to tranquilize the liver and extinguish wind as deputy medicines; liver, the organ of general, contains ministerial fire, prefers to free activity and dislikes depression. Thus, the property of the liver will be restrained, with ministerial fire ascending and liver yang being hyperactive if the setting method is used simply. Among the assistants, *yīn chén* can most handle the smoothing of liver wood's nature, excelling at draining liver heat. *Mài yá* has the function of smoothing liver wood's nature so that it does not become constrained. The other assistant medicine, *chuān liàn zǐ*, excels at guiding

the liver qi to spread downward, as well as turning back its contrary force. Processed *gān cǎo* is to soothe the liver and harmonize the actions of the other medicines. *mài yá*, as the envoy medicine, harmonizes the stomach and adjusts the middle burner, thereby preventing the metals and minerals in the formula from adversely affecting the stomach. This elegantly designed formula is an excellent example of simultaneously applying both the liver-tranquilizing and liver-soothing medicines to regulate descending-ascending circulation. So it is a promising agent for tranquilizing the liver and extinguishing wind.

[Clinical Application] This formula is commonly applied for treating wind stroke in any period due to hyperactivity of liver yang, which manifests as dizziness, vertigo, drunken complexion, string and powerful pulse.

Dà Dìng Fēng Zhū (Major Wind-Stabilizing Pill, 大定风珠)
Systematic Differentiation of Warm Pathogen Diseases (*Wēn Bìng Tiáo Biàn*, 温病条辨)

[Ingredient]

Shēng Bái Sháo (Radix Paeoniae Alba)　6 *qian* (18 g)

Ē Jiāo (Colla Corii Asini)　3 *qian* (9 g)

Shēng Guī Bǎn (Plastrum Testudinis)　4 *qian* (12 g)

Gān Dì Huáng (Radix Rehmanniae Recens)　6 *qian* (18 g)

Má Rén (Fructus Cannabis)　2 *qian* (6 g)

Wǔ Wèi Zǐ (Fructus Schisandrae Chinensis)　2 *qian* (6 g)

Shēng Mǔ Lì (Concha Ostreae)　4 *qian* (12 g)

Mài Dōng (Radix Ophiopogonis)　6 *qian* (18 g)

Zhì Gān Cǎo (Radix Et Rhizoma Glycyrrhizae Praeparata Cum Melle)
4 *qian* (12 g)

Jī Zǐ Huáng (Egg yolk)　raw, 2

Biē Jiǎ (Carapax Trionycis)　raw, 4 *qiaǐn* (12 g)

[Usage] The original formula uses eight cups of water to decoct the herbs into

3 cups, remove the sediment. After that, add *jī zǐ huáng* and mix it. Take it three times.

Modern usage: Blend the *ē jiāo* and *jī zǐ huáng* into the strained decoction and take warmly.

[Action]   Nourish yin, extinguish wind and rescue from desertion.

[Indication]   Weariness, muscle spasms with alternating flexion, an extension of the extremities, convulsion, a deficient pulse pertain to the internal stirring of wind due to yin deficiency, which may be caused by the long-standing retention of pathogenic heat from a warm pathogen disease, crimson tongue with less tongue coating; Constantly, the patient will appear as if about to go into shock.

[Formula Analysis]   This is an internal stirring of wind due to yin deficiency, which may be caused by the long-standing retention of pathogenic heat from a warm pathogen disease or improper treatment involving excessive sweating or purging. The chief medicines, *jī zǐ huáng,* and *ē jiāo*, nourish yin to extinguish wind. The deputy medicines, *bái sháo*, *wǔ wèi zǐ* and *zhì gān cǎo*, are a mix of sweet and sour substances that work in concert to nourish the yin and soften the liver. Taken with *gān dì huáng*, *má rén* and *mài dōng* to enrich yin and moisten dryness. The remaining ingredients serve as an assistant, *guī bǎn, biē jiǎ,* and *mǔ lì,* to enrich the yin to anchor the yang and extinguish the wind. *Mǔ lì* is especially good at calming the liver and sedating the liver yang. *Zhì gān cǎo* harmonizes the actions of all medicines, and acts as the envoy. The primary focus of this formula is to enrich and nourish the yin, extinguish wind and rescue from desertion which strongly treats the internal stirring of wind due to yin deficiency. This formula consists of plenty of yin-nourishing medicines. Instead, the chief medicine *jī zǐ huáng* looks like a ball and can extinguish wind, the so-called *Dà Dìng Fēng Zhū* (Major Wind-Stabilizing Pill).

[Clinical Application]   This formula impacts enriching yin and extinguishing wind, so it can treat the symptoms such as yin impairment, water failing to nourish the wood, convulsion caused by disturbance of internal stirring of wind due to yin deficiency. Convulsion, mental fatigue, weak pulse and crimson tongue with less coating are the dialectical points.

Líng Jiǎo Gōu Téng Tāng (**Antelope Horn and Uncaria Decoction,** 羚角钩藤汤)
Revised Popular Guide to the Discussion of Cold Damage (*Chóng dìng tōng sú*
shāng hán lùn, 重订通俗伤寒论)

[Ingredient]

Líng Yáng Jiǎo (Cornu Saigae Tataricae)   decocted first,1.5 *qian* (4.5 g)

Sāng Yè (Folium Mori)   2 *qian* (6 g)

Chuān Bèi Mǔ (Bulbus Fritillariae Cirrhosae)   without core, 4 *qian* (12 g)

Shēng Dì (Radix Rehmanniae)   fresh 5 *qian* (15 g)

Gōu Téng (Ramulus Uncariae Cum Uncis)   added later, 3 *qian* (9 g)

Jú Huā (Flos Chrysanthemi)   3 *qian* (9 g)

Fú Shén (Sclerotium Poriae Pararadicis)   3 *qian* (9 g)

Bái Sháo (Radix Paeoniae Alba)   3 *qian* (9 g)

Gān Cǎo (Radix Et Rhizoma Glycyrrhizae)   8 *fen* (2.4 g)

Zhú Rú (Caulis Bambusae In Taenia)   freshly scraped, decocted first with *líng yáng jiǎo* 5 *qian* (15 g)

[Usage]   The original usage is not recorded in the book.

Modern usage: Decoction.

[Action]   Cool the liver and extinguish wind, increase body fluids to eliminate phlegm, relax the sinews and unblock the collateral.

[Indication]   Excessive heat in the liver channel stirring up internal wind causes persistent high fever, restlessness, dizziness, vertigo, twitching, spasms of the extremities, deep-red, dry, or burnt tongue with prickles, and a wiry, rapid pulse.

[Formula Analysis]   This is heat excess in the liver channel stirring up internal wind. When pathogenic heat enters *jueyin*, it generates vigorous heat in the liver channel that causes the internal stirring of wind. *Líng yáng jiǎo*, one of the chief ingredients, enters the liver meridian to sedate the liver heat and extinguish wind. The other chief ingredients, *gōu téng*, clears heat, calms the liver, extinguishes wind, and suppresses convulsion. The deputies are *sāng yè* and *jú huā*, calming the liver and extinguishing wind to help the chief medicine clear heat and sedate the liver.

Wind and fire readily provoke one another, which exhausts the yin and scorches the fluids. Therefore, three of the assistant ingredients, *shēng dì*, *bái sháo* and *gān cǎo*, nourish yin and relieve the sinews. Excessive heat will scorch fluid into phlegm, so add *chuān bèi mǔ* and *zhú rú*, two other assistants, to clear heat and dissolve phlegm. The internal wind and fire will harm the heart, so apply *fú shén* to sedate the liver and extinguish the wind, relax the sinews, unblock the collateral, nourish the heart and calm the mind. *Gān cǎo*, regarded as envoy medicine, can harmonize the actions of all medicines in the formula. This is the representative formula for promoting the function of sedating the liver, extinguishing wind, increasing body fluids to dissolve phlegm, relaxing the sinews and unblocking the collateral.

[Clinical Application] This is the representative formula for treating the overabundance of heat causing the stirring of internal wind. When pathogenic heat enters *jueyin*, it generates vigorous heat in the liver channel that causes the internal stirring of wind. For heat trapped in the interior with impaired or loss of consciousness, *Zǐ Xuě Dān* can be combined to resuscitate. If the disease are combined with constipation, add *Xī Lián Chéng Qì Tāng* (*xī jiǎo*, *huáng lián*, *zhǐ shí*, *xiān dì huáng*, *dà huáng*, *jīn zhī*) to clear heat, drain fire, unblock the bowels and discharge the heat.

Dì Huáng Yǐn Zǐ (**Rehmannia Drink,** 地黄饮子)
Formulas from the Discussion Illuminating the Yellow Emperor's Basic Questions (*Huáng Dì Sù Wèn Xuān Míng Lùn Fāng,* 黄帝素问宣明论方) [82]

[Ingredient]
Shú Dì Huáng (Radix Rehmanniae Praeparata)

Bā Jǐ Tiān (Radix Morindae Officinalis)   without core

Shān Zhū Yú (Fructus Corni)

Shí Hú (Caulis Dendrobii)

Ròu Cōng Róng (Herba Cistanches)   wine-fried, baked

Zhì Fù Zǐ (Radix Aconiti Lateralis Praeparata)

Wǔ Wèi Zǐ (Fructus Schisandrae Chinensis)

Ròu Guì (Cortex Cinnamomi)

Fú Líng (Poria)

Mài Dōng (Radix Ophiopogonis)　without core

Shí Chāng Pú (Rhizoma Acori Tatarinowii)

Yuǎn Zhì (Radix Polygalae)

without core, equally divide

[Usage]　The original formula is fine-grinding equal amounts of the ingredients into a powder. A dose of 3 *qian* of the powder decocts with 5 slices of *shēng jiāng*, 1 piece of *dà zǎo*, 5 to 7 pieces of *bò he* and decocted with water.

Modern usage: Decoct with *shēng jiāng*, *dà zǎo* and *bò hé*. Adjust the dosage when necessary.

[Action]　Enriches the kidney yin, tonifies the kidney yang, dissolves phlegm to open the orifices.

[Indication]　Mute paraplegia (*yīn féi*, 喑痱), stiffness of the tongue with an inability to speak, disability or paralysis of the lower extremities, a greasy, yellow tongue coating, and a submerged, slow, thready, and frail pulse.

[Formula Analysis]　Mute paraplegia (*yīn féi*), manifests as the stiffness of the tongue with an inability to speak and disability or paralysis of the lower extremities. The chief, *shú dì huáng*, nourishes the kidney and boosts yin. The deputy, *shān zhū yú*, warms the liver, consolidates essence and supports yin and yang. Another two deputy ingredients, *ròu cōng róng* and *bā jǐ tiān*, supplement the kidney to tonify yang. Take with *zhì fù zǐ* and *ròu guì* to warm the kidney, assist yang and return fire to its source. These four herbs take back the floating yang by warming and tonifying the deficiency of the lower source. The deputies, *shí hú*, *mài dōng* and *wǔ wèi zǐ*, enrich the yin fluids and cool the fire from deficiency, simultaneously moderating the drying actions of *fù zǐ* and *ròu guì*. Due to the exuberance of heart fire and kidney deficiency, [kidney deficiency leads to] flooded water transform into phlegm, which obstructs the orifices. Therefore, apply *shí chāng pú* and *fú líng*, the assistant ingredients, to restore interaction between the heart and the kidney, open the orifices and eliminate phlegm. Add less *bò he* to scatter the pathogenic qi, together with *shēng jiāng* and *dà zǎo* to

harmonize *ying* and *wei*, strengthening the body's resistance to eliminate pathogenic factors as the envoy. This formula treats the upper and lower side, simultaneously for the root and branches. Under this premise, this formula combines a core strategy of warming and tonifying the lower source with a secondary strategy of opening the orifices and transforming the phlegm. After that, the kidney will be warmed up and the floating yang is restrained. Moreover, the heart and kidney can be harmonized, orifices can be opened, phlegm can be dissolved and the mute paraplegia (*yīn fěi*) can be cured.

The thought of a lightly decocting method makes the properties and actions descend or ascend to reach sinews and extremities. Additionally, *shú dì huáng*, the chief medicine, harmonizes yin and yang, so-called *Dì Huáng Yǐn Zǐ* (Rehmannia Drink).

[Clinical Application]

1. This formula aims at treating mute paraplegia (*yīn fěi*). It mainly manifested as the stiffness of the tongue that is unable to speak and disability or paralysis of the lower extremities. For disability or paralysis of the lower extremities only, remove *shí chāng pú*, *yuǎn zhì* and *bò hé*. This formula is not suitable for the other symptoms.

2. For yin deficiency and vigorous phlegm-fire, remove *fù zǐ* and *ròu guì* and add *chuān bèi mǔ*, *dǎn nán xīng* and *tiān zhú huáng* to clear and dissolve heat-phlegm.

Chapter 12

Dryness-Relieving Formulas

According to the theory of "If dryness has encroached upon the interior, it should be treated with bitter [flavor] and warm [qi]. To assist using sweet and acrid [flavor]"; "[to treat disease due to] dryness [of qi] with moistening [therapy] the dryness." From *Basic Questions-Comprehensive Discourse on the Essentials of the Most Reliable* (*Sù Wèn-Zhì Zhēn Yào Dà Lùn*, 素问·至真要大论), those formulas are used to treat the dryness syndrome that are mainly made of dispersing and acrid-disperse or sweet-cold moistening medicines, which have the function of moistening external dryness by dispersing, enriching yin and moistening dryness are all called dryness-treating formulas.

Section 1   Formulas that relieves external dryness by dispersing

External dryness relieving formulas are for relieving syndromes caused by cold-dryness or warm-dryness. Cold-dryness is usually caused by the cool qi in autumn, strong wind and wind-cold fettering the lung's function, manifested as the failure of the lung qi to diffuse, impairment of body fluids distribution which can cause the accumulation of phlegm, along with symptoms such as headache, aversion to cold, cough, clear phlegm, nasal congestion, throat discomfort that lead to blockage feeling during swallowing or breathing, thin and white tongue coating. The bitter, acrid, warm and moistening formulas, should be use to lightly diffuse the cold-dryness and the medicines such as *xìng rén*, *sū yè*, *qián hú*, and *jié gěng*, are commonly used the representative formula is *Xìng Sū Sǎn* (Apricot Kernel and Perilla Powder, 杏苏散).

Though cold-dryness is inferior to cold, it is easy to get fire transformation. Thus, while using those medicines to treat clod-dryness, we must pay attention to whether the dryness has transformed into a fire in case of overdosing on the formulas. Warm-dryness is more common than cold-dryness and more occurs often in the early period of autumn, which still inherits the heat from summer. Because the weather is still warm and the air lacks moisture. It is easy for people to get warm-dryness. Warm-dryness injures the lung and consumes body fluids, which results in the failure of lung qi to purify, along with symptoms such as headache, fever, dry cough with little phlegm or panting caused by counterflowing of qi, thirst, nasal dryness, red at the tip and side of the tongue, thin and white tongue coating. What is good at clearing the lung and moistening dryness are acrid, cool, sweet and moisten medicines, such as *sāng yè*, *xìng rén*, *shā shēn*, *mài dōng*, *shí gāo*, *ē jiāo*. The representative formulas are *Sāng Xìng Tāng* (Mulberry Leaf and Apricot Kernel Decoction, 桑杏汤), *Qīng Zào Jiù Fèi Tāng* (Clearing Dryness to Save the Lung Decoction, 清燥救肺汤).

Xìng Sū Sǎn (Apricot Kernel and Perilla Leaf Powder, 杏苏散)
Systematic Differentiation of Warm Diseases (*Wēn Bìng Tiáo Biàn*, 温病条辨)

[Ingredient]

Sū Yè (Folium Perillae)　(9 g)

Xìng Rén (Semen Armeniacae Amarum)　(9 g)

Bàn Xià (Rhizoma Pinelliae)　(9 g)

Fú Líng (Poria)　(9 g)

Jú Pí (Pericarpium Citri Reticulatae)　(4.5 g)

Qián Hú (Radix Peucedani)　(9 g)

Kǔ Jié Gěng (Bitter Radix Platycodonis)　(3 g)

Zhǐ Qiào (Fructus Aurantii)　(4.5 g)

Gān Cǎo (Radix Et Rhizoma Glycyrrhizae)　(3 g)

Shēng Jiāng (Rhizoma Zingiberis Recens)　3 slices

Dà Zǎo (Fructus Jujubae)　removes core, 3 pcs [no amount given in the original formula]

[Usage]   There is no instruction given in the original formula.

Modern instruction: prepared as a decoction.

[Action]   Relieve cold-dryness by dispersing, diffusing the lung and resolving phlegm.

[Indication]   This formula is used to treat externally-contracted cold-dryness, along with symptoms like slight headache, aversion to cold without sweating, cough with thin phlegm, nasal congestion, and throat discomfort, which leads to blockage when swallowing or breathing, a wiry pulse, white tongue coating.

[Formula Analysis]   This syndrome is caused by externally-contracted cold-dryness, failure of lung qi to diffuse and internal obstruction of phlegm-damp. *xìng rén* in the formula is bitter, warm and moist, which can disperse the lung, relieve cough and dissolve phlegm. In *Shen Nong's Classic of the Materia Medica* (*Shén Nóng Běn Căo Jīng*, 神农本草经), *xìng rén* is good at treating cough with counterflow qi ascent, *sū yè* is acrid and warm which can release the flesh and exterior, open and diffuse the lung qi, promoting cold-dryness relief from the exterior. These two are both the chief medicine. *Qián hú* is bitter, acrid and slightly cold, which can soothes wind, directs qi downward and dissolves phlegm which helps *xìng rén* and *sū yè* to produce their functions of dispersing, reaching the exterior and dissolving phlegm. *jié gěng* is bitter, acrid and neutral which can cause ascend while *zhǐ qiào* is bitter and slightly cold which can cause a descent. These two together can help *xìng rén* to diffuse the lung qi. These three are all deputy medicines.

As for assistant medicines, *bàn xià*, *jú pí* and *fú líng*, they can rectify qi and dissolve phlegm. *gān căo* and *jié gěng* can diffuse the lung and dispel phlegm. *Shēng jiāng* and *dà zăo*, as envoy medicines, can together harmonize *ying* and *wei* levels. All medicines used together can produce the functions of releasing the exterior, diffusing and dissolving so that the exterior can be released, phlegm can be dissolved, the lung qi can be regulated. This formula uses the method of treating diseases by bitter-warm and sweet-acrid medicines following the theory of "If dryness has encroached upon the interior, this is treated with bitter [flavor] and warm [qi]. To assist with sweet and acrid[flavor]" in the *Basic Questions-Comprehensive Discourse on the Essentials of*

the Most Reliable (*Sù Wèn-Zhì Zhēn Dà Yào Lùn*, 素问·至真要大论). Thus, it can be seen that disease caused by cold-dryness is the result of "a slight cold" in the early autumn. It is lesser when compared to the cold pathogen and it is easier to damage liquid and transform into heat.

[Clinical Application] This is the representative formula for treating cold-dryness, which suits the wind damage and cough caused by dryness qi in autumn the most.

Sāng Xìng Tāng (Mulberry Leaf and Apricot Kernel Decoction, 桑杏汤)
Systematic Differentiation of Warm Diseases (*Wēn Bìng Tiáo Biàn*, 温病条辨)

[Ingredient]

Sāng Yè (Folium Mori)　1 *qian* (3 g)

Xìng Rén (Semen Armeniacae Amarum)　1.5 *qian* (4.5 g)

Shā Shēn (Radix Adenophorae seu Glehniae)　2 *qian* (6 g)

Xiàng Bèi (Bulbus Fritillaria)　1 *qian* (3 g)

Xiāng Chǐ (Semen Sojae Praeparatum)　1 *qian* (3 g)

Zhī Pí (Fructus Gardeniae)　1 *qian* (3 g)

Lí Pí (Pyrus Bretschneideri Rehd)　1 *qian* (3 g)

[Usage] In the original formula, use two cups of water to decoct the medicines into one cup. If the patient's condition is severe, he should take one more dose.

Modern usage: Prepared as a decoction.

[Action] Relieve warm-dryness by dispersing qi, cooling and moistening the lung [metal].

[Indication] This formula is used to treat externally-contracted warm-dryness, along with symptoms like headache and fever, thirst, dry throat and nasal dryness, dry cough without phlegm or with little sticky phlegm, red at the tip and side of the tongue, thin white and dry coating, the right pulse is rapid and large.

[Formula Analysis] This syndrome is caused by externally-contracted warm-dryness and lung *yin* being scorched. *Sāng yè* in the formula can relieve dryness-heat by dispersing qi. *Xìng rén* can moisten dryness and relieve cough. They

are both chief medicines. *Xiāng chǐ* helps *sāng yè* to vent heat by dispersing. *Xiàng bèi* helps *xìng rén* to relieve cough and dissolve phlegm. *shā shēn* has the functions of moistening the lung to relieve cough and engender fluids. These three all belong to the deputy medicines. *Zhī pí* is light that belongs to upper *jiao*, and it can clear lung heat, *lí pí* can clear heat, moisten dryness, relieve cough and dissolve phlegm. They are both assistant medicines. All medicines used together can relieve dryness-heat by dispersing on the exterior, cool and moisten the lung metal on the interior, which reflects the method of treating diseases by acrid-cool medicine. Once the dryness-heat is relieved, fluids of the lung can be engendered again. Then the syndrome can be cured. In this formula, the dosage of all the medicines is light. Wú Jú-Tōng believes that "the dosage of light formula [*qīng jì*] should be controlled at a proper degree, if it is used too much, other symptoms will occur", because "threatening the diseases are in the upper *jiao*, light medicine like feathers [nature] are the best".

[Clinical Application]　This formula which has the function of cooling and moistening dryness by dispersing qi, is the representative formula for treating externally-contracted warm-dryness and cough caused by lung dryness. According to editors' clinical experience, if warm dryness damages the lung and exterior heat is not severe, we could remove *xiāng chǐ*, *zhī pí* in this formula and add *yù zhú*, *tiān huā fěn* to nourish yin and promote fluid production. If heat damages yang collateral causing the coughing of blood, we should remove *xiāng chǐ* and add *bái máo gēn*, *qiàn cǎo tàn* to cool the blood and staunch bleeding.

Qīng Zào Jiù Fèi Tāng (Relieve Dryness of the Lung Decoction, 清燥救肺汤) *Precepts for Physicians* (*Yī Mén Fǎ Lǜ*, 医门法律)[83]

[Ingredient]

Sāng Yè (Folium Mori)　which has been through frost, nourished by metal qi so it's soft, moist and not easy to wither. Remove branches and stems, 3 *qian* (9 g)

Shí Gāo (Gypsum Fibrosum)　calcined, which has the function of purifying and is extremely good at clearing lung heat, 2.5 *qian* (8 g)

Gān Cǎo (Radix et Rhizoma Glycyrrhizae)　which is good at harmonizing

the stomach and generating metal, 1 *qian* (3 g)

Rén Shēn (Radix et Rhizoma Ginseng)　which can generate stomach fluid and benefit lung qi, 0.7 *qian* (2 g)

Hú Má Rén (Fructus Cannabis)　dry-fried and grinded, 1 *qian* (3 g)

Zhēn Ē Jiāo (Colla Corii Asini)　0.8 *qian* (3 g)

Mài Mén Dōng (Radix Ophiopogonis)　remove the plumule from lotus seed 1.2 *qian* (4 g)

Xìng Rén (Semen Armeniacae Amarum)　soaking, remove the seed coat and radicle, fry them till the medicines become yellow, 0.7 *qian* (2 g)

Pí Pá Yè (Folium Eriobotryae)　one leaf, remove fuzz by brushing, soak it in honey, fry it with liquid adjuvant till the medicine become yellow (3 g)

[Usage]　In the original book, it uses a bowl of water to decoct the medicine until six-tenths of the decoction remains. Boil them two to three times and take it while the decoction is hot.

Modern usage: Prepared as a decoction.

[Action]　Clear dryness and moisten the lung.

[Indication]　This formula is used to treat warm dryness attacking the lung, along with symptoms like headache, fever, hacking cough without phlegm, panting caused by qi counterflow, dry throat, thirst and nasal dryness, chest oppression and rib-side pain, thin white and dry coating, red at the tip and side of the tongue, a deficient, large and rapid pulse.

[Formula Analysis]　The climate in autumn is dry, and the dryness-heat hurts the lung. In this formula, *Sāng yè,* as the chief medicine, is light and cold which can diffuse and vent the dryness-heat pathogen in the lung. The calcined *shí gāo* is the deputy medicine, which is acrid-sweet and cold, and extremely good at clearing lung heat and can help the chief medicine to cure the causes of disease as well. *Difficult Issues-the Fourteenth Issue* (*Nàn Jīng-Dì Shí Sì Nàn,* 难经·第十四难) says, "If the lung is injured, [we] should boost qi". Stomach-earth is the mother of lung-metal, so this formula uses *gān cǎo* to bank up earth to generate metal. *Rén shēn* can

promote fluid production of the stomach and nourish the qi of the lung. There are *má rén, ē jiāo, mài mén dōng* together to moisten the lung and enrich fluids, so the lung gets nourished and moistened then can it perform its function. There's a theory in the book *Basic Questions-Discourse on How the Qi in the Depots Follow the Pattern of the Seasons* (*Sù Wèn-Zàng Qì Fǎ Shí Lùn*, 素问·脏气法时论) says, "The lung [tends to] suffer from adverse flow qi which can be stopped by bitter[flavor]". So in this formula, it uses the bitterness of *xìng rén* and *pí pá yè* to direct the lung qi downward and discharge it. Once the lung qi is directed downward, the fire will be subdued. Then the counterflow will disappear, coughing will also be stopped. These medicines above are all assistants. Also, *gān cǎo* harmonizes the action of all the medicines in this formula, so we use it as the envoy medicine. In this way, the dryness-heat of lung-metal can be cleared and moistened, the lung qi which counterflows can be purified and descended, so the various symptoms caused by lung dryness can be treated. That's why this formula is called "*Qīng Zào Jiù Fèi Tāng* (Relieve Dryness of the Lung Decoction)".

[Clinical Application]　　This formula is the representative formula for treating lung damage caused by warm dryness. Based on the original formula, we can add *bèi mǔ, guā lóu* if the patient has lots of phlegm. We can add *shēng dì huáng* if the patient has blood exhaustion. If the patient has intense heat, we can use *xī jiǎo, líng yáng jiǎo* or *niú huáng*.

Section 2　Formulas that enriches the yin and moistens internal dryness

Formulas of nourishing and moistening internal dryness are suitable for internal dryness syndrome of fluid consumption of *zang-fu* organs caused by various reasons. This syndrome can be caused by severe damage to fluids because of sweat promotion, vomiting induction, or purgative method. Or it is caused by lack of essence and blood aeipathia. Or it is caused by yin damage because of warm pathogens turning into dryness. Internal dryness can influence different parts of the body, due to the different

parts being influenced. There are also different symptoms and treatment methods. For instance, when there is an upper attack of dryness, the lung is to be blamed, along with symptoms like dry cough with less phlegm, dry throat and expectoration of blood. When there is a middle attack of dryness, the stomach is to be blamed, along with symptoms like marasmus, thirst, belching and poor appetite. When there is a lower attack of dryness, the kidney is to be blamed, along with symptoms like flaccid and weak legs, *xiāo kě* [wasting-thirst] or constipation caused by fluid exhaustion.

The treatment principles of internal dryness can be generalized as saving lung fluid to treat upper dryness, increasing stomach fluid to treat middle dryness, and enriching yin blood to treat lower dryness. The main point of treating internal dryness is to nourish and moisten with sweet-cold medicine, preferring soft and moist medicines while bitter-dry medicines are strictly forbidden. *xuán shēn*, *shēng dì huáng*, *mài dōng* and *bǎi hé* are commonly used as main medicines. The representative formulas are *Yǎng Yīn Qīng Fèi Tāng* (Yin-Nourishing and Lung-Clearing Decoction, 养阴清肺汤), *Bǎi Hé Gù Jīn Tāng* (Lily Bulb Metal-Securing Decoction, 百合固金汤), *Mài Mén Dōng Tāng* (Ophiopogon Decoction, 麦门冬汤) and *Zēng Yè Tāng* (Humor-Increasing Decoction, 增液汤).

Yǎng Yīn Qīng Fèi Tāng (Yin-Nourishing and Lung-Clearing Decoction, 养阴清肺汤)

Jade Key to the Secluded Chamber (*Chòng Lóu Yù Yào*, 重楼玉钥)[84]

[Ingredient]

Dà Shēng Dì (Radix Rehmanniae) 2 *qian* (12 g)

Mài Dōng (Radix Ophiopogonis) 1.2 *qian* (7 g)

Shēng Gān Cǎo (Radix et Rhizoma Glycyrrhizae) 0.5 *qian* (3 g)

Xuán Shēn (Radix Scrophulariae) 1.5 *qian* (9 g)

Bèi Mǔ (Bulbus Fritillaria) 0.8 *qian*, remove the plumule from lotus seed (4.5 g)

Dān Pí (Cortex Moutan) 0.8 *qian* (4.5 g)

Bò He (Herba Menthae) 0.5 *qian* (3 g)

Chǎo Bái Sháo (Radix Paeoniae Alba)   0.8 *qian* (4.5 g)

[Usage]   There is no instruction given in the original formula.

Modern usage: Prepared as a decoction.

[Action]   Nourish yin, clears lung, resolve toxicity and dissipate pathogens.

[Indication]   This formula is used to treat diphtheria, along with symptoms like white, curd-like phlegm[①] (白如腐) in the throat, difficult to be wiped off, swelling and painful throat, may have a fever at first or not, dry nose and lips, coughing or not, breathing along with noise, sounds like wheezing but not asthma, a rapid weak pulse or a thready and rapid pulse.

[Formula Analysis]   The syndrome of diphtheria mainly occurs because the patient has yin deficiently. There is heat accumulation inside the body, contracted dryness and epidemic toxin, internal and external dryness. This formula uses a heavy dosage of *dà shēng dì* for nourishing yin and clearing heat. It is the chief medicine. *Xuán shēn* can nourish yin and promote fluid, drain fire and resolve toxins. *mài dōng* can nourish yin and clear lung [heat]. The book *Pouch of Pearls* (*Zhēn Zhū Náng*, 珍珠囊) describes it as "good at treating lurking fire in the lung". They are both deputy medicines. *Dān pí* can clear heat and cool the blood. *Chǎo bái sháo* can boost yin and nourish the blood. *Bèi mǔ* can moisten the lung and resolve phlegm, clear heat and dissipate masses. A small quantity of *bò he* is acrid-cool and dissipating and it can dredge the exterior and benefit the throat, those are all assistant medicines. *Shēng gān cǎo* can drain fire and resolve toxins and harmonizes the function of all medicines in this formula, as the envoy medicine. This formula has the function of nourishing yin, clearing lungs, resolving toxins and dissipating pathogens.

[Clinical Application]   This formula is commonly used to treat diphtheria. Usually, we advise the patient to take one dose daily. But if the syndrome is severe, it can be taken twice daily. If the heat toxin of the patient is severe, *tǔ niú xī* can be added to drain fire and resolve toxins which has a very significant effect.

---

① 白如腐 curd-like substance, in western medicine, it is white pseudo membrane.

Bǎi Hé Gù Jīn Tāng (Lily Bulb Metal-Securing Decoction, 百合固金汤)
Medical Formulas Collected and Analyzed (*Yī Fāng Jí Jiě*, 医方集解)
(*This formula is quoted from Zhao Ji-an's formulas*)

[Ingredient]

Shēng Dì Huáng (Radix Rehmanniae) 2 *qian* (6 g)

Shú Dì Huáng (Radix Rehmanniae Praeparata) 3 *qian* (9 g)

Mài Dōng (Radix Ophiopogonis) 1.5 *qian* (4.5 g)

Bǎi Hé (Bulbus Lilii) 1 *qian* (3 g)

Sháo Yào (Radix Paeoniae) dry-fried, 1 *qian* (3 g)

Dāng Guī (Radix Angelicae Sinensis) 1 *qian* (3 g)

Bèi Mǔ (Bulbus Fritillaria) 1 *qian* (3 g)

Shēng Gān Cǎo (Radix et Rhizoma Glycyrrhizae) 1 *qian* (3 g)

Xuán Shēn (Radix Scrophulariae) 0.8 *qian* (2.4 g)

Jié Gěng (Radix Platycodonis) 0.8 *qian* (2.4 g)

[Usage] There is no instruction given in the original formula.

Modern usage: Prepared as a decoction.

[Action] Nourish yin, clears heat, moisten the lung and dissolve phlegm.

[Indication] This formula is used to treat yin deficiency of the lung and kidneys, along with symptoms like deficiency-fire flaming upward, dryness and pain of the throat, cough and panting, blood in the phlegm, vexing heat in the five centers (chest, palms and soles), red tongue with little coating, a thready and rapid pulse.

[Formula Analysis] The syndrome of this formula is caused by yin deficiency in the lung and kidney. In this formula, *bǎi hé* and s*hēng dì huáng* are sweet-bitter and slightly cold, which can nourish yin and clear heat, moisten the lung and relieve cough. *Shú dì huáng* is sweet and slightly warm, which can enrich yin and supplement the blood. These three are all chief medicines. The two deputy medicines: *mài dōng* is sweet and cold, which can assist *bǎi hé* in nourishing yin and clearing heat, moistening the lung and relieving cough, *xuán shēn* is salt and cold, which helps *shēng dì huáng* and *shú dì huáng* to enrich yin and supplement liquid so the

deficiency-fire can be restricted. When metal is deficient, which cannot restrict wood, then the wood fire will rebel against metal. So this formula uses *dāng guī* and *bái sháo* to nourish and harmonize the blood to calm the liver. *Bèi mǔ* can moisten the lung, relieve cough and dissolve phlegm. These three are all assistant medicines. *Shēng gān cǎo* can clear heat and drain fire and harmonize the actions of all medicine in this formula. A small quantity of *jié gěng* together with *shēng gān cǎo* can clearing the throat and carrying all the medicines upward, they are the channel envoy medicines of the lung channel. This formula can enrich yin and moisten the lung, regulate metal and water. Thus the yin and fluids can be gradually enriched and deficiency-fire can disappear. Therefore the lung (metal), is protected, that is why this formula is called *Bǎi Hé Gù Jīn Tāng* (Lily Bulb Metal-Securing Decoction).

[Clinical Application]   This formula is commonly used to treat cough caused by yin deficiency of the lung and kidney. If there is lot of phlegm, base on the original formula, we can add *guā lóu pí* to clear metal [lung] and dissolve phlegm. If the patient has severe panting, we can remove *jié gěng* which has a rising function. If the patient has hemoptysis, we should also remove *jié gěng*, add *bái jí*, *bái máo gēn* and *xiān hè cǎo*.

Mài Mén Dōng Tāng (Ophiopogon Decoction, 麦门冬汤)
Essentials from the Golden Cabinet (*Jīn Guì Yào Lüè*, 金匮要略)

[Ingredient]
Mài Mén Dōng (Radix Ophiopogonis)   7 *sheng* (15 g)

Bàn Xià (Rhizoma Pinelliae)   1 *sheng* (4.5 g)

Rén Shēn (Radix et Rhizoma Ginseng)   3 *liang* (9 g)

Gān Cǎo (Radix et Rhizoma Glycyrrhizae)   2 *liang* (6 g)

Jīng Mǐ (Oryza Sativa L)   3 *he* (15 g)

Dà Zǎo (Fructus Jujubae)   12 pcs (4 pcs)

[Usage]   Mix the six with 1 *dou* 2 *sheng* (2200ml) water, boil them into 6 *sheng*, drink warmly, three times daily.

Modern usage: Prepared as a decoction.

[Action]　Nourish and moisten the lung, direct counterflow downward and lower qi.

[Indication]　This formula is used to treat lung *wěi* (萎), along with symptoms like dysphoria, cough, drool foaming at the mouth, shortness of breath, panting, dryness and pain of the throat, red tongue with little coating, a deficient and rapid pulse.

[Formula Analysis]　This formula is used to treat lung *wěi*, in which the disease's location is in the lung while the origin [cause] is in the stomach. Because the earth is the mother of metal and the stomach governs fluids. When stomach fluid is insufficient, deficiency-fire will flame upward, lung yin will get scorched. The lung is considered as a delicate viscus, the son of stomach-earth. When the fluids in the stomach cannot be transported to the lung, the lung cannot be moistened or nourished, and then there will be fluid exhaustion and dryness. That is how the lung get withered gradually. This formula uses a heavy dosage of *mài mén dōng*. It is sweet-cold, clear and moist, it belongs to the lung and stomach channels which can enrich yin and promote fluid production, enrich fluid and moisten dryness to clear deficiency-fire, as the chief medicine. *Rén shēn*, *gān cǎo*, *jīng mǐ*, *dà zǎo* are all deputy medicines, which can boost stomach qi, nourish stomach yin and make center qi sufficient, so fluids can return to the lung spontaneously, then the lung can be nourished. That is what is called "bank up earth to generates metal". A small dosage of *bàn xià* which is an assistant medicine can direct counterflow downward and lower qi, dissolve phlegm-drool, Though its nature is acrid-warm, when combined with a heavy dosage of *mài mén dōng*, it will not be too drying. Moreover, when *mài mén dōng* is with *bàn xià*, it can produce its function of nourishing without being too cloying. If used together, they can be in a status of antagonism and complementation. *Gān cǎo* can moisten the lung and promote the throat, harmoniz the actions of all medicines in a formula, as the envoy medicine. Although there are only six medicines in this formula, they rank in order and produce moistening and descending functions. They can promote stomach fluid, moisten lung dryness, descend counterflow qi and stop turbid spit. This formula reflects the method of "supplementing the mother when the son is deficient".

[Clinical Application]

1. This formula is used to treat "qi counterflow that makes the throat uncomfortable", physicians of later generations all believe it is the main formula to treat lung *wěi* caused by deficiency-fire. In *Emergency Formulas to Keep up One's Sleeve* (*Zhǒu Hòu Bèi Jí Fāng*, 肘后备急方), there is a record of using this formula to treat "keeping spitting drool because of lung *wěi*". According to the editor's clinical experience, we can add *běi shā shēn* and *yù zhú* to the original formula if the patient has severe fluid consumption caused by lung *wěi*. If the patient has severe qi deficiency, we can add *sheng huáng qí* and *shān yào*. If the patient spits lot of drool, we can add *fú líng*.

2. This formula has a good effect on treating vomiting and hiccup caused by stomach yin deficiency and the loss of the harmonizing and descending function of stomach.

Zēng Yè Tāng (Fluids-Increasing Decoction, 增液汤)
Systematic Differentiation of Warm Diseases (*Wēn Bìng Tiáo Biàn*, 温病条辨)

[Ingredient]

Xuán Shēn (Radix Scrophulariae)　1 *liang* (30 g)

Mài Dōng (Radix Ophiopogonis)　keep the plumule, 8 *qian* (24 g)

Xì Shēng Dì (Radix Rehmanniae)　8 *qian* (24 g)

[Usage]　In the original formula, it uses 8 cups of water and decocts them until there are only 3 cups of water remaining. Ask the patient to drink all the decoction if he/she is very thirsty. If the patient does not urinate, take more decoction.

Modern usage: Prepared as a decoction.

[Action]　Generate fluids and moisten dryness.

[Indication]　This formula is used to treat *yangming* warm disease, along with symptoms like insufficiency of body fluids, constipation for multiple days, thirst, dry and red tongue, thin, faint and a rapid pulse or a deep weak pulse.

[Formula Analysis]　*Yangming* includes the stomach and intestines. Constipation caused by *yangming* warm disease mainly has these two reasons: heat

accumulation or fluid dry up, [we] must differentiate the mechanisms of the disease whether it is due to deficiency or due to excess. If the syndrome is mainly caused by an intense yang pathogen that belongs to the excess pattern of heat bind, we should use *Chéng Qì Tāng* (Purgative Decoction) to purge the heat out and preserve yin. While if the syndrome is caused by febrile disease, which consumes fluids, fluids dry up and the intestines become dry. There will be a failure to conduct and transmit. *Systematic Differentiation of Warm Diseases* (*Wēn Bìng Tiáo Biàn*, 温病条辨) believes that "if there are many dry fluids and only a little heat bind" or "there are insufficient fluids to moisten the intestines which cause the occurrence of constipation", we cannot use *Chéng Qì Tāng* to consume the patient's fluids. In this formula, The large dosage of the chief medicine, *xuán shēn* which is bitter and cold, can nourish yin and clear heat, increase body fluids and moisten dryness. *Mài dōng* is sweet and cold, which can increase body fluids and moisten dryness. *Xì shēng dì* is sweet, bitter and cold, which can nourish yin and moisten dryness, supplement without being too cloying. They are both assistant medicines. These three medicines together can enrich yin and moisten dryness, especially for the intestines, in which constipation can be solved spontaneously. That is why this formula is called "*Zēng Yè Tāng* (Fluids-Increasing Decoction)". This formula reflects the method of using cold, bitter and sweet medicines. It can promote fluid production to treat constipation. However, when we use it, many medicines is necessary to produce the desired effect.

[Clinical Application] This formula has the function of increasing body fluids and moistening dryness. It cannot only treat liquid damage caused by febrile disease or constipation caused by intestinal dryness, but also can be used to treat internal damage and yin deficiency. The critial points of pattern differentiation includ constipation, thirst, dry and red tongue, thready, faint and rapid pulse or deep weak pulse.

Chapter 13

Digestive and Evacuative Formulas

Any formula which has the function of promoting digestion and reducing (food) stagnation (*shí jī* 食积), resolving concretions and (food) stagnation to treat food accumulation stomach cavity *pǐ*, concretions and conglomerations (lower abdominal masses; *zhēng jiǎ*, 癥瘕) and accumulations and gatherings (abdominal masses, *jī jù*, 积聚) is called Digestive and Evacuative Formulas. It belongs to the dispersion method among the eight methods. Commonly use *shān zhā, shén qǔ, mài yá, zhǐ shí, bīng láng, biē jiǎ* as main medicines. The representative formulas include *Bǎo Hé Wán* (Harmony-Preserving Pill, 保和丸), *Zhǐ Zhú Wán* (Immature Bitter Orange and Atractylodes Macrocephala Pill, 枳术丸), *Mù Xiāng Bīng Láng Wán* (Costus Root and Areca Pill, 木香槟榔丸), *Shī Xiào Wán* (Sudden Smile Pill, 失笑丸), and *Biē Jiǎ Jiān Wán* (Turtle Shell Decocted Pill, 鳖甲煎丸).

Bǎo Hé Wán (Harmony-Preserving Pill, 保和丸)
Teachings of [Zhu] Dan-xi (Dān Xī Xīn Fǎ, 丹溪心法)

[Ingredient]

Shān Zhā (Fructus Crataegi)   6 *liang* (180 g)

Shén Qǔ (Massa Medicata Fermentata)   2 *liang* (30 g)

Bàn Xià (Rhizoma Pinelliae)   3 *liang* (90 g)

Fú Líng (Poria)   3 *liang* (90 g)

Chén Pí (Pericarpium Citri Reticulatae)   1 *liang* (30 g)

Lián Qiào (Fructus Forsythiae)   1 *liang* (30 g)

Lái Fú Zǐ (Semen Raphani)   1 *liang* (30 g)

[Usage]   In the original formula, grind the ingredients into a powder and forms them into pills which are as big as *wú tong zǐ* (Semen Firmianae). The patient should take 70–80 pills with plain boiled water each time.

Modern usage: Grind the ingredients into a powder and form them into pills, the standard dosage is 6–9 g with warm water or prepared them as a decoction made with *chǎo mài yá* each time. Also, we could decoct the medicine with water and with a proportionate adjustment in dosage.

[Action]   Promote digestion and harmonize the stomach.

[Indication]   This formula is used to treat food accumulation, along with symptoms like stuffiness [*pǐ*] and fullness feeling in the chest and diaphragm, abdominal distention along with occasional pain, putrid-smelling belching and acid regurgitation, poor appetite and vomiting, diarrhea, thick, greasy and yellow tongue coating and a slippery pulse.

[Formula Analysis]   The book *Basic Questions-Further Discourse on the Five Depots* (*Sù Wèn-Wǔ Zàng Bié Lùn*, 素问·五脏别论) says, "the six *fu* organs can convey and transform but cannot store things". Overeating and excessive consumption of alcohol and meat or fatty food may lead to food accumulation in the middle[stomach], which causes indigestion syndrome.

In this formula, a large dosage of *shān zhā* which is sweet and slightly warm, is good at removing accumulation caused by the meat-type food. *The Grand Compendium of Materia Medica* (*Běn Cǎo Gāng Mù*, 本草纲目) says, "it can assists digestion and eliminate the accumulation of meat". That's why it is the chief medicine. There are two deputies. *Shén qǔ*, sweet-acrid and warm. It is instrumental in reducing the stagnant accumulation of alcohol and food; *lái fú zǐ* is sweet-acrid, which can facilitate the qi and reduce the accumulation caused by wheaten (gluten) foods and smooth the chest and diaphragm. The three medicines above are used together to resolve all sorts of food accumulation. Meanwhile, food accumulation in the middle *jiao* will lead to the production of dampness and phlegm. *bàn xià* which is acrid-warm dries dampness and dispels phlegm, facilitating the qi and dissipating the masses. *chén pí*, acrid-bitter and warm, dries dampness and dissolves phlegm,

which is good at promoting the movement of the qi and harmonizing the center. Bland and neutral *fú líng* can fortify the spleen, harmonize the center, dissolve phlegm and eliminate dampness. When there is food accumulation, it readily gives rise to heat from constraints. *Lián qiào* is bitter-cold and aromatic, which can dissipate masses and clear heat. These four are all assistant medicines. The compatibility of various medicines can resolve food accumulation, and then the stomach qi and is harmonized. Though the primany function of this formula is to digest and resolve, the properties of the medicines are all neutral. Which is why it is named "*Bǎo Hé*".

[Clinical Application]   This formula is a neutral one among all the digestion-promoting and stagnation-resolving formulas, which is suitable for those who have food accumulation in the middle portion of the stomach cavity with sufficient healthy qi. If the patient has severe food accumulation, we can add *hòu pò*, *zhǐ shí* to resolve the accumulation. If the patient has severe food accumulation transforming into heat, *huáng qín* and *huáng lián* can be added to clear the heat. If the patient has constipation, *dà huáng* can promote defecation and remove stagnation.

Zhǐ Zhú Wán (Immature Bitter Orange and Atractylodes Macrocephala Pill, 枳术丸)

Clarifying Doubts about Damage from Internal and External Causes (*Nèi Wài Shāng Biàn Huò Lùn*, 内外伤辨惑论)

(*This formula is quoted from* Zhang Yuan-su's[85] *formulas*)

[Ingredient]

Bái Zhú (Rhizoma Atractylodis Macrocephalae)   2 *liang* (60 g)

Zhǐ Shí (Fructus Aurantii Immaturus)   fry them with bran until it become yellow, remove the flesh or pulp, 1 *liang* (30 g)

[Usage]   In the original formula, grind the ingredients into a powder, wrap the rice with *hé yè* and boil them, then mix the powder with the rice and makes them into pills that are as big as *wú tong zǐ* (Semen Firmianae). Take 50 pills each time, mainly with rice-soup.

Modern usage: Pills, the patient should take 6–9 g with warm water each time.

Decoct the medicines with water, and with a proportionate adjustment in dosage.

[Action]   Fortify spleen and disperse *pǐ*.

[Indication]   This formula is used to treat spleen-stomach weakness, along with symptoms like indigestion, *pǐ* and fullness.

[Formula Analysis]   The spleen governs transportation and transformation and the stomach governs the intake of food and drinks. In this formula, *bái zhú* is bitter-sweet and warm, which can fortify the spleen and dry dampness to help the transformation. It is the chief medicine. *Zhǐ shí* as the deputy medicine is bitter and slightly cold which can promote qi and resolve food stagnation, disperse accumulation and *pǐ*. The dosage of *bái zhú* is twice as much as the dosage of *zhǐ shí*, so this formula mainly aims at supplementing, reflecting dispersing from supplementing. The book *Clarifying Doubts about Damage from Internal and External Causes* (*Nèi Wài Shāng Biàn Huò Lùn*, 内外伤辨惑论) says, "The meaning of using *bái zhú* is not to digest food quickly, but to strengthen and protect stomach qi as primacy". *Hé yè* is used to promote the ascension and nourishment of the clear qi of the spleen and stomach which helps *bái zhú* to fortify the spleen and supplement the stomach at the same time. Also together with *zhǐ shí*, one can raise the clear [yang], one can direct the turbid downward. The clear [yang] can be raised, and the turbid [yin] can be directed downward. Then qi movement is regulated, and the fullness can disperse. This treatment method is in accordance with the theory that "the spleen qi should be raised to be healthy, and the stomach qi should be descended to be harmony", so it is the assistant medicine. This formula can disperse and supplement at the same time, but mainly aims at supplementing. Also, it can ascend and descend at the same time, but mainly aims at ascending. Though this formula is simple, it has a good method of using medicines. We shouldn't look down on it just because it's neutral and easy.

[Clinical Application]   This formula varied by Zhang Yuan-su from *Zhǐ Zhú Tāng* (Immature Bitter Orange and Atractylodes Macrocephala Decoction, *zhǐ shí* seven pcs, *bái zhú* two *liang*), which is in the book *Essentials from the Golden Cabinet* (*Jīn Guì Yào Lüè*, 金匮要略). *Zhǐ Zhú Tāng* originally was used to treat cases where "the patient feels like there's rigidity below the heart which is as big as a plate. And

the edge is smooth, caused by water [retention]". Because there's water amassment below the heart (stomach area), it should be eliminated urgently. And *zhǐ shí* in large dosage is used to expel water by purging, dissipating masses and dispersing *pǐ* [fulless]. And *bái zhú* is used to bank up earth to control water which regards its function of supplementing as an adjuvant. But the syndrome of this formula is the failure of spleen to transport and indigestion which should be treated slowly. That is why the physician has changed the decoction into pills. Also, the dosage of *bái zhú* is twice before and it can fortify the spleen and help with transportation and transformation which mainly aims at supplementing combined with *zhǐ shí*. Decoction and pills have different significance of application. We should differentiate them properly in the clinic and avoid misuse.

Mù Xiāng Bīng Láng Wán (Costus Root and Areca Pill, 木香槟榔丸)
Confucians' Duties to Their Parents (*Rú Mén Shì Qīn*, 儒门事亲[86])

[Ingredient]

Mù Xiāng (Radix Aucklandiae)   1 *liang* (30 g)

Bīng Láng (Semen Arecae)   1 *liang* (30 g)

Qīng Pí (Pericarpium Citri Reticulatae Viride)   1 *liang* (30 g)

Chén Pí (Pericarpium Citri Reticulatae)   1 *liang* (30 g)

É Zhú (Rhizoma Curcumae)   scorching, 1 *liang* (30 g)

Huáng Lián (Rhizoma Coptidis)   dry-fried with bran, 1 *liang* (30 g)

Huáng Bò (Cortex Phellodendri Chinensis)   3 *liang* (90 g)

Dà Huáng (Radix et Rhizoma Rhei)   3 *liang* (90 g)

Xiāng Fù Zǐ (Rhizoma Cyperi)   dry-fried, 4 *liang* (120 g)

Qiān Niú (Semen Pharbitidis)   4 *liang* (120 g)

[Usage]   In the original formula, grind the ingredients into a powder and form into pills with water, as bean size, and take 30 pills each time with the fresh ginger decoction.

Modern usage: Grind the ingredients into a powder and form into pills with water; take 6 g each time, 2–3 times daily, with a decoction of *shēng jiāng* or warm water.

[Action] Promote the movement of qi and guide out stagnation.

[Indication] This formula is used to treat the internal retention of food stagnation, along with symptoms like abdominal *pǐ* [fullness] and distending pain, constipation, red-white dysenteric diarrhea, abdominal urgency with rectal heaviness, yellow greasy tongue coating, an excess pulse.

[Formula Analysis] Intemperate diet leads to food accumulation and stagnation, which in turn aggravates the congestion and stagnation of the qi mechanism, abnormal transmission and transformation. In this formula, *mù xiāng* belongs to the *sanjiao* qi level, commanding the ascending and descending of all kinds of qi, is especially good at moving stagnant qi of the stomach and intestines. *Bīng láng*, which enters the spleen, stomach and large intestine channels, is particularly good at promoting the movement of qi. These two chief medicines are both bitter-acrid and warm, which promote the movement of qi, transform stagnation and abdominal distention, and can also treat abdominal urgency with rectal heaviness. *Qiān niú, dà huáng* both can discharge heat. They have a strong function of purging food accumulation and removing stagnation through the bowels. Both are deputy medicines. *Qīng pí* breaks stagnant qi and resolves food stagnation, *chén pí* can rectify qi and dry dampness. Among the assistants, *xiāng fù* can rectify qi, together with *mù xiāng*, it can produce the effect of soothing the stagnation and harmonizing the center, *é zhú* can move qi and disperse stagnation in [qi aspect of] the blood, disperse accumulation to relieve the pain, which is good at treating food indigestion and abdominal pain, *huáng lián* and *huáng bǎi* can clear heat, dry dampness and relieve dysentery. Making a comprehensive view of this formula, we are aware that it uses *mù xiāng* and *bīng láng* as the name of this formula, but with plenty of herbs that have the function of promoting qi that aims at removing stagnation, purging accumulation, and discharging heat downward. It makes qi move again freely, reduces the accumulation and stagnation, clears the dampness and heat, and then all the symptoms can be relieved.

[Clinical Application] This formula contains harshly-acting herbs and has a strong power to purge accumulation. It is good at treating symptoms like internal

retention of food accumulation and stagnation, which constrain into damp-heat, qi movement obstruction and excess of both pathogenic qi or healthy qi.

Shī Xiào Wán (Sudden Smile Pill, 失笑丸) A.k.a. *Zhǐ Shí Xiāo Pǐ Wán* (Immature Bitter Orange and Glomus-Dispersing Pill, 枳实消痞丸) *Secrets from the Orchid Chamber* (*Lán Shì Mì Cáng*, 兰室秘藏)

[Ingredient]

Gān Jiāng (Rhizoma Zingiberis) 1 *qian* (3 g)

Zhì Gān Cǎo (Radix Et Rhizoma Glycyrrhizae Praeparata Cum Melle) 2 *qian* (6 g)

Mài Yá Miàn (Fructus Hordei Germinatus) 2 *qian* (6 g)

Bái Fú Líng (Poria) 2 *qian* (6 g)

Bái Zhú (Rhizoma Atractylodis Macrocephalae) 2 *qian* (6 g)

Bàn Xià Qǔ (Rhizoma Pinelliae Fermentata) 3 *qian* (9 g)

Rén Shēn (Radix Et Rhizoma Ginseng) 3 *qian* (9 g)

Hòu Pò (Cortex Magnoliae Officinalis) fry them with liquid adjuvant, 4 *qian* (12 g)

Zhǐ Shí (Fructus Aurantii Immaturus) 5 *qian* (15 g)

Huáng Lián (Rhizoma Coptidis) 5 *qian* (15 g)

[Usage] Grind the ingredients into a powder, soak in water, and mix with flour formed into pills as big as *wú tóng zǐ* (Semen Firmianae) and steamed. The patient should take 50–70 pills each time with water and take them after meals [at least 2 hours before or after meals].

Modern usage: Mix the ground powder with water and flour [like the usage mentioned above] and rounds into pills, 6–9 g each time, take them twice a day with warm water. Nowadays, you can also decoct the medicines in the water, and with a proportionate adjustment in dosage.

[Action] Disperse *pǐ* and eliminate fullness, fortify the spleen and harmonize the stomach.

[Indication] This formula is used to treat spleen-stomach deficiency along

with mutual clumping of chills and fever, *pǐ* and fullness feeling below the heart, poor digestion, sleepiness and fatigue, greasy and yellow tongue coating.

[Formula Analysis] A weak and deficient spleen-stomach will lose control of ascending and descending, mutual of chills and fever, qi congestion and dampness accumulation until phlegm and food inter-obstruction. In this formula, *zhǐ shí* is heavily used. It is bitter and slightly cold that can dissipate accumulation and disperse *pǐ*, enter into the spleen-stomach channel, as the chief medicine. *Hòu pò* is bitter-acrid and warm, which can lower qi and eliminate fullness, acting as the deputy medicine. These two medicines aim at treating the main syndrome *pǐ* and fullness below the heart. If used together they can strengthen the effect of dispersing *pǐ* and eliminating fullness. *Huáng lián* is bitter-cold, which can clear heat and dry dampness, drain the heart and disperse *pǐ*. *Bàn xià qū* is acrid-warm which can dry dampness and dispel phlegm, disperse *pǐ* and dissipate accumulation. A small usage of *gān jiāng* which is very acrid-hot, can warm the center and dissipate cold. These three combined medicines correspond with the method of acrid medicines opening and bitter medicines promoting descent, and they can help *zhǐ shí and hòu pò* to produce the effect of dissipating masses and dispersing *pǐ*. *Mài yá miàn* is salty and neutral and it can promote digestion and harmonize the center. But for pathogens to invade, qi must first be deficient. So *rén shēn, bái zhú, fú líng* and *zhì gān cǎo* are added to supplement qi and fortify the spleen, reinforce healthy qi to dispel pathogens. Those medicines are all assistants. *Zhì gān cǎo* can harmonize the actions of all medicines and act as the envoy medicine. The flour used here is not only for forming the pills, but also can nourish the spleen and stomach and promote digestion.

Making a comprehensive view of this formula, we can discover that the *zhǐ shí*, *hòu pò* and *huáng lián* are used in large dosages, which shows this formula mainly has a bitter and cooling nature; good at dispersing *pǐ*, draining heat and drying dampness. As for *rén shēn, bái zhú, fú líng,* and *zhì gān cǎo*, they are used to reinforce healthy qi and dispel pathogens, protecting healthy qi from being hurt by too many dispersing medicines and making sure that supplementing won't interfere with a dispelling pathogen.

[Clinical Application]   This formula is based on *Bàn Xià Xiè Xīn Tāng* and *Zhǐ Zhú Tāng*. The dialectical point for this formula is that the *pǐ* syndrome below the heart, which is a deficiency-excess complex, along with a cold-heat complex with heat predominating over cold, excess predominates over deficiency syndrome. If the cold pathogen is in predominance and the tongue coating is white-greasy, the dosage of *huáng lián* should be reduced, and the dosage of *gān jiāng*, should be increased or we can add medicines such as *chén pí*, *mù xiāng* and *shā rén* to rectify qi and warm the center.

Biē Jiǎ Jiān Wán (Turtle Shell Decocted Pill, 鳖甲煎丸)
Essentials from the Golden Cabinet (*Jīn Guì Yào Lüè*, 金匮要略)

[Ingredient]

Biē Jiǎ (Carapax Trionycis)   fry them with liquid adjuvant, 12 *fen* (90 g)

Shè Gān (Rhizoma Belamcandae)   scorching, 3 *fen* (22.5 g)

Huáng Qín (Radix Scutellariae)   3 *fen* (22.5 g)

Chái Hú (Radix Bupleuri)   6 *fen* (45 g)

Shǔ Fù (Porcellio Sp.)   fry, 3 *fen* (22.5 g)

Gān Jiāng (Rhizoma Zingiberis)   3 *fen* (22.5 g)

Dà Huáng (Radix Et Rhizoma Rhei)   3 *fen* (22.5 g)

Sháo Yào (Radix Paeoniae)   5 *fen* (37.5 g)

Guì Zhī (Ramulus Cinnamomi)   3 *fen* (22.5 g)

Tíng Lì (Semen Lepidii)   fry, 1 *fen* (7.5 g)

Shí Wéi (Folium Pyrrosiae)   fry, 1 *fen* (7.5 g)

Hòu Pò (Cortex Magnoliae Officinalis)   3 *fen* (22.5 g)

Mǔ Dān (Cortex Moutan)   5 *fen* (37.5 g)

Qú Mài (Herba Dianthi)   2 *fen* (15 g)

Líng Xiāo Huā (Flos Campsis)   3 *fen* (22.5 g)

Bàn Xià (Rhizoma Pinelliae)   1 *fen* (7.5 g)

Rén Shēn (Radix Et Rhizoma Ginseng)   1 *fen* (7.5 g)

Zhé Chóng (Eupolyphaga Seu Steleophaga)   fry 5 *fen* (37.5 g)

Ē Jiāo (Colla Corii Asini)   fry them with liquid adjuvant, 3 *fen* (22.5 g)

Fēng Cháo (Nidus Vespae)   fry them with liquid adjuvant, 4 *fen* (30 g)

Chì Xiāo (Mirabilitum Rubra)   12 *fen* (90 g)

Qiāng Láng (Geotrupidae)   6 *fen* (45 g)

Táo Rén (Semen Persicae)   2 *fen* (15 g)

[Usage]   In the original formula, grind those 23 medicines into a powder. Take 1 *dou* of ashes of wood and soak in 5 *dou* of *qing jiu* (glutinous rice wine) until half of the liquid is absorbed by the ashes. Then add *biē jiǎ* into them, boil them until it looks like glue. After filtrating the herbs out, add all the other medicines, and roll them into pills as big as *wú tóng zǐ*. Take 7 pills before meals, three times a day.

Modern usage: Make the rest of the medicines (all of them except *biē jiǎ*) into powder and decoct them with the juice made by boiling *biē jiǎ* with Shaoxing rice wine. Roll them into pills. The patient is advised to take 3–6 g before meals with warm water, three times a day.

[Action]   Disperse concretions and remove accumulation.

[Indication]   This formula is used to treat malaria which has not been cured for a long time but generates the accumulated below the left ribside and form aggregation-accumulation[or concretions and conglomerations], which is called malaria with splenomegaly (a.k.a. mother-of-malaria). This formula is also used to treat abdominal mass below the rib-side, which is hard when pressed, and immovable when pushed, along with symptoms like irregular pain or alternating chills and fever.

[Formula Analysis]   The reason for forming malaria with splenomegaly is that the pathogen of malaria has stayed in *shaoyang* for a long time. The healthy qi gradually becomes insufficient and the pathogen stays inside. The longer the pathogen lingers, the more there will be contention between the pathogen of cold-heat, phlegm-dampness and qi-blood. It will accumulate below the left rib-side to finally forms aggregation-accumulation. In *Basic Questions-Comprehensive Discourse on the Essentials of the Most Reliable (Sù Wèn-Zhì Zhēn Dà Yào Lùn*, 素问·至真要大论) says, "what is firm cut it, what has settled remove it, what is knotted disperse it, what stays in place attack it". This formula uses a large dosage of *biē jiǎ*, which is

neutral and can soften hardness, dissipate masses and disperse concretions. The book *Shen Nong's Classic of the Materia Medica* (*Shén Nóng Běn Cǎo Jīng*, 神农本草经) records it "governs hard-accumulated, cold-heat concretions and conglomerations of heart and abdomen", so it's the chief medicine. *Dà huáng, sháo yào, zhé chóng, táo rén, chì xiāo, mǔ dān, shǔ fù, fēng cháo, qiāng láng* and *líng xiāo huā* are deputy medicines. They're used to promote blood [circulation] and purge the stasis in blood levels. *Hòu pò, bàn xià, tíng lì* and *shè gān* are used to drive qi downward and dispel phlegm, working at the qi level. *Shí wéi* and *qú mài* can promote urination to get rid of dampness through the urine. *Chái hú* and *guì zhī* can dredge and free *ying-wei*, dissipate masses and dispel stasis. *Gān jiāng* and *huáng qín* can harmonize yin and yang, regulate cold and warm medicines. *Rén shēn* and *ē jiāo* can boost qi and nourish the blood, reinforce the healthy qi and consolidate root. The medicines above are all assistant medicines. As for the ashes of wood, it is warm and related to qi while rice wine is hot and relates to the blood. They used together can accompany other ingredients to produce the effect of dispersing concretions and removing accumulation, as the envoy medicines. In this formula, cold and warm medicines are both used to treat the disease with both attack and supplementation. This formula can rectify qi and blood, dispel phlegm and dampness, with many methods of treating. Indeed it is the main formula for acute situations. In the original formula, it advises the patient to "take seven pills before meals, three times a day", which reflects the formula's function of slowly dispersing concretions, and then gradually eliminating the concretions and conglomerations without hurting the middle.

[Clinical Application]

1. In *Important Formulas Worth a Valuable Prescriptions of Emergency* (*Bèi Jí Qiān Jīn Yào Fāng*, 备急千金要方), *Biē Jiǎ Jiān Wán* uses 12 slices of *biē jiǎ*, and is added 3 *fen* of *hǎi zǎo*, 1 *fen* of *dà jǐ* but without *shǔ fù, chì xiāo. biē jiǎ* is decocted with all the other medicines and they are made into pills. The pills are especially good at softening hard masses and expelling water.

2. This formula isn't merely used to treat malaria with splenomegaly. The patient has shaped concretions and conglomerations that are not moving when being pushed,

along with symptoms like qi-blood stagnation and coagulation which have not been cured for a long time.

3. Though there are medicines for reinforcing healthy qi in this formula, it still mainly aims at dispelling pathogens. As for those who have been ill for a long time, we could use supplementing formulas at the same time.

Chapter 14

Qi-Regulating Formulas

Formulas that can regulate the qi, promote qi, or direct qi downward are frequently used to treat syndromes like qi stagnation, qi counterflow, etc, They are called qi-regulating formulas.

Section 1　Formulas that promotes the movement of qi

Those formulas have the effect of promoting qi flowing and resolving constraints. They are suitable for the syndromes like constraint and stagnation of the qi mechanism. Due to the stagnation of qi and the abnormal ascend and descend, there are symptoms such as chest oppression, abdominal pain, vomiting, rib-side pain and plum-stone qi. Commonly used acrid-aromatic and can rectify qi medicines such as *xiāng fù*, *sū gěng*, *mù xiāng*, *wū yào* along with medicines that are bitter-warm and can break stagnant such as *qīng pí*, *bīng láng*, *hòu pò*, which are often used together to constitute a formula. The constraint and stagnation of qi usually influence different parts of the body and lead to many different symptoms, so the compatibility formula should be flexible. For instance, if phlegm combines with qi stagnation, the phlegm-dissolving medicines should be used, the medicine which can unblock yang, dissipate masses and dispell phlegm can be added. If qi stagnation combiness with coldness, rectify qi and dispel coldness at the same time. If there is heat along with qi stagnation, medicines for rectifying qi and dispelling heat should be applied. If there is blood stasis, we should rectify qi while dissolving blood stasis. The representative formulas include *Yuè Jú Wán* (Constraint-Resolving Pill, 越鞠丸),

Jīn Líng Zǐ Săn (Toosendan Powder, 金铃子散), *Bàn Xià Hòu Pò Tāng* (Pinellia and Officinal Magnolia Bark Decoction, 半夏厚朴汤) and *Guā Lóu Xìe Bái Bái Jiǔ Tāng* (Trichosanthes and White Wine Decoction, 瓜蒌薤白白酒汤).

Yuè Jū Wán (Escape Restraint Pill, 越鞠丸) A.k.a *Xiōng Zhú Wán* (Chuanxiong-Cangzhu Pill, 芎术丸)
Teachings of [Zhu] Dan-xi (*Dān Xī Xīn Fǎ*, 丹溪心法)

[Ingredient]

Cāng Zhú (Rhizoma Atractylodis)　　(9 g)

Xiāng Fù (Rhizoma Cyperi)　　(9 g)

Chuān Xiōng (Rhizoma Chuanxiong)　　(9 g)

Shén Qǔ (Massa Medicata Fermentata)　　(9 g)

Zhī Zǐ (Fructus Gardeniae)　　(9 g)

[Usage]　In the original formula, the ingredients are ground into a powder and formed into pills with water, which is as big as a mung bean size.

Modern usage: Make ingredients into pills, take 6 g of pills each time, twice a day with warm water. It may also be prepared as a decoction, and the dosage should depend on the original formula and the patient's situation.

[Action]　Promote the movement of qi and release stagnation.

[Indication]　This formula is used to treat six stagnation, including qi stagnation, blood stagnation, phlegm stagnation, fire stagnation, dampness phlegm and food stagnation, along with symptoms like *pǐ* and fullness of chest and diaphragm, abdominal distending pain, acid swallowing and vomiting, food indigestion, a greasy, slightly yellow tongue coating.

[Formula Analysis]　Zhu Dan-xi once said, "If one's qi and blood are in harmony, he'll be healthy. If one has stagnation, all sorts of diseases will occur". The meaning of this formula is to move qi and resolve stagnation. When qi flows, it can promote blood transportation, and once qi is moving smoothly, the phlegm, fire, dampness and food stagnation can be resolved. In this formula, *xiāng fù* can promote the movement of qi and resolve stagnation, acting as the chief medicine. *Chuān xiōng*

can invigorate blood and move qi to treat blood stagnation; *cāng zhú* dries dampness and activates the spleen to treat dampness stagnation. *Shén qǔ* can promote digestion and harmonize the stomach, which is used for food stagnation. *Zhī zǐ* can clear heat and drain fire, which is used to treat fire stagnation, which also can constrain the properties of warm-dryness of other medicine and make all the stagnation resolved without causing fire and heat. These four medicines are all assistant-envoy medicines. Once qi is normalized and blood is harmonized, dampness-fire can be cleared and food stagnation can be dissolved, then the phlegm stagnation will be resolved too. So there's no need to add phlegm-dissolving medicines. It reflects the method of treating the root of the disease. There are five medicines in this formula [but] used to treat six stagnation, disperse binding stagnation of qi. That is why this formula is called "*Yuè Jú* (Constraint-Resolving)".

[Clinical Application]　This is the most common formula used to treat six stagnation. However, one still needs to adapt the formula [dosage] according to clinical presentations. For example, *xiāng fù* should be used as the chief medicine when one is qi constraint. For blood constraint, *chuān xiōng* is used as the chief medicine, *cāng zhú* is the most used when one has dampness constraint, *zhī zǐ* is used as the chief medicine when one has fire constraint, *shén qǔ* is used as the chief medicine when one has food constraint. For qi constraint, we could add *mù xiāng*, *bīng láng*; add *táo rén*, *hóng huā* for blood constraint, add *fú líng*, *bái zhǐ* for dampness constraint, add *huáng qín*, *qīng dài* for fire constraint, add *hǎi shí*, *nán xīng*, *guā lóu* for phlegm and add *shān zhā*, *mài yá* for food constraint.

Jīn Líng Zǐ Sǎn (Melia Toosendan Powder, 金铃子散)
Collection of Writings on the Mechanism of Disease, Suitability of Qi, and the Safeguarding of Life as Discussed in the 'Basic Questions'
(*Sù Wèn Bìng Jī Qì Yí Bǎo Mìng Jí*, 素问病机气宜保命集)

[Ingredient]

Jīn Líng Zǐ (Fructus Toosendan)　1 *liang* (30 g)

Yán Hú Suǒ (Rhizoma Corydalis)　1 *liang* (30 g)

232

[Usage] In the original formula, grind the ingredients into a powder, take 3 *qian* of the powder with rice wine each time.

Modern usage: Ground the medicines into power, take 9 g each time with (rice) wine or warm water. Or make it into a decoction, with a proportionate reduction in the dosage of the ingredients.

[Action] Soothe liver, drain heat, promote qi and alleviate pain.

[Indication] This formula is used to treat liver qi stagnation which transforms into fire. The symptoms like intermittent epigastric and hypochondriac pain, hernial pain (*shàn qì*, 疝气), or menstrual pain is aggravated by the ingestion of hot food or beverage, vexation and agitation, accompanied by irritability, a bitter taste in the mouth, a red tongue with yellow coating, a rapid pulse.

[Formula Analysis] Liver governs the free flow of qi and stores the blood. Its channel passes through the genital area, reaches the lower abdomen. It is next to the stomach, connecting with the gallbladder, crossing the diaphragm upwards, covering the rib-sides. *Jīn líng zǐ*, also called *chuān liàn zǐ*, bitter and cold, which can soothe the liver and discharge heat, rectify qi to relieve pain, as the chief medicine. *Yán hú suǒ* is acrid and warm, invigorating blood, promoting qi and relieving pain, as the assistant-envoy medicine. The combination of the two medicines can treat all kinds of pain caused by liver qi stagnation, qi constraint transforming into fire and blood stagnation.

[Clinical Application]

1. According to the editor's clinical experience, for the treatment of dysmenorrhea in women, which is caused by constraint and stagnation of liver qi, this formula is very effective with *Xiāo Yáo Sǎn* (Free Wanderer Powder). The medicines like *xiāng fù*, *yù jīn* and *dān shēn* can be added.

2. This formula added with *wū yào*, *lì zhī hé*, *jú hé*, *xiǎo huí xiāng* and *qīng pí* can treat hernial pain. If the pain was caused by a pathogenic cold, *wú zhū yú* and *ròu guì* could be added to warm the liver and dissipate the cold.

Bàn Xià Hòu Pò Tāng (Pinellia and Officinal Magnolia Bark Decoction, 半夏厚朴汤)

Essentials from the Golden Cabinet (*Jīn Guì Yào Lüè*, 金匮要略)

[Ingredient]

Bàn Xià (Rhizoma Pinelliae)   1 *sheng* (12 g)

Hòu Pò (Cortex Magnoliae Officinalis)   3 *liang* (9 g)

Fú Líng (Poria)   4 *liang* (12 g)

Shēng Jiāng (Rhizoma Zingiberis Recens)   5 *liang* (15 g)

Gān Sū Yè (Folium Perillae)   2 *liang* (6 g)

[Usage]   In the original formula, use 7 *sheng* of water and decoct them until 4 *sheng* remaining. Take four times a day, that is three times during the day and one time at night.

Modern usage: Usually prepared as a decoction.

[Action]   Promote the flow of qi and open stagnation, direct counterflow downward and resolve phlegm.

[Indication]   This formula is used to treat the binding constraint of seven emotions, accumulation of phlegm-drool, along with symptoms like something obstructed in the throat, which is unable to be expectorated out or swallowed it, or chest oppression and shortness of breath, a white-moist or white greasy tongue coating.

[Formula Analysis]   If one has qi stagnation that leads to inhibition of the body fluids, which accumulate and turns into phlegm-drool, it will lodge in the throat. That is why the patient feels like there's something obstructed in the throat. This is so-call plum-pit qi (*méi hé qì* 梅核气). In this formula, the two bitter, acrid, warming and downward-directing medicines: *bàn xià* can direct counterflow downward and dissolve phlegm, lower qi and dissipate masses; *hòu pò* can lower qi and dry dampness. Both are chief medicines; *fú líng* can dissolve phlegm and drain dampness. *sū yè* can move qi and dissipate constraints, *shēng jiāng* can dissolve phlegm, direct counterflow downward and can resolve toxins of *bàn xià*. They are all assistant-envoy medicines. The combination of medicines can promote qi and open constraints,

directing counterflow downward and dissolving phlegm. Then the syndrome of the binding constraint of phlegm and qi can be resolved spontaneously.

[Clinical Application] This formula is commonly used to treat plum-stone qi. It has a good effects on symptoms of mutual-obstruct of phlegm and qi. If we add *dà zǎo* into this formula, this formula would turn into *Sì Qì Tāng* (Four-Seven Decoction), Formulary of the Pharmacy Service for Benefiting the People in the Taiping Era (*Tài Píng Huì Mín Hé Jì Jú Fāng*, 太平惠民和剂局方) quoted from *Simple Book of Formulas* (*Yì Jiǎn Fāng*, 易简方[87]). This last formula is used for almost the same indications as *Bàn Xià Hòu Pò Tāng* and has a better effect when treating patients who have phlegm-dampness of a lesser degree.

Guā Lóu Xiè Bái Bái Jiǔ Tāng (Trichosanthes and White Wine Decoction, 瓜蒌薤白白酒汤)

Essentials from the Golden Cabinet (Jīn Guì Yào Lüè, 金匮要略)

[Ingredient]

Guā Lóu Shí (Fructus Trichosanthis)   1 pc, pounding, (15 g)

Xiè Bái (Bulbus Allii Macrostemi)   half *sheng* (9 g)

Bái Jiǔ (White Wine)   7 *sheng*

[Usage] In the original formula, decoct the three medicines together until 2 *sheng* of liquid remains. The patient is advised to take the decoction after warming it up.

Modern usage: It is usually prepared as a decoction.

[Action] Unblock yang and dissipates clumps. Promote the flow of qi and resolve phlegm.

[Indication] This formula is used to treat chest *bì* along with symptoms like panting, coughing and pitting, pain in chest and back, shortness of breath, a white, greasy coating, a deep-slow or deep-tight pulse.

[Formula Analysis] *Bì* is caused by the blockage. The chest *bì* is the blocking and obstructing of qi movement in the chest. The reason is that the yang qi coagulates in the chest, which leads to the body's fluid failure to distribute, so it

coagulates into phlegm. In this formula, *guā lóu* is sweet-cold, which can open the chest coagulation and dissipate masses, move qi and dispel phlegm. *Miscellaneous Records of Materia Medica* (*Běn Cǎo Bié Lù*, 本草别录) says it can "treat chest *bì*". That's why it's the chief medicine. *Xiè bái* is acrid-bitter and warm, which can soothe qi and unblock yang, lower qi and dissipate masses, *The Grand Compendium of Materia Medica* (*Běn Cǎo Gāng Mù*, 本草纲目) says it can "treat stabbing pain caused by chest *bì*", and it is the deputy medicine. *Bái jiǔ* (white wine) is acrid-warm, which can help medicine go upwards to strengthen *guā lóu* and *xiè bái*'s effect of unblocking yang and dissipating masses. All these medicines together can diffuse and unblock the yang qi in the chest and dispel turbid phlegm. Then chest *bì* can be resolved.

[Clinical Application]　This formula is the main formula used to treat chest *bì*. In this formula, *guā lóu* is the whole fruit parts of *guā lóu*. Nowadays *bái jiǔ* (white wine) is rice wine. Yellow rice wine can also be used. The usual dosage is 30–60 ml. According to Professor Wang Mian-zhi's experience, we can also use *shēng jiāng* to replace *bái jiǔ*. Professor Wang believes it's better to use fresh *xiè bái* than dried one because fresh one has mucous on it, which can have a better effect of unblocking qi with this acrid medicine.

Section 2　Formulas that directs rebellious qi downward

Formulas of directing rebellious qi downward are mainly used to treat the syndrome of lung and stomach loss of descent and ascending-counterflow of qi. The lung governs purification and descent, which is similar to the stomach qi. So ascending-counterflow of qi movement manifests in two aspects: the upward reversal of lung qi and the upward reversal of stomach qi. For upward reversal of lung qi, there are symptoms like panting and cough. To direct qi downward and relieve panting, *sū zǐ*, *xìng rén*, *bàn xià*, *kuǎn dōng huā* as the main medicines are usually used to treat this syndrome. And for upward reversal of stomach qi, there are symptoms like belching, vomiting, and hiccups. To harmonize the stomach and direct the counterflow

downward, *xuán fù huā*, *dài zhě shí*, *bàn xià*, *jú pí*, *dīng xiāng* and *shì dì* as the main medicines are usually used to treat this syndrome.

This disease of ascending-counterflow of qi has different syndromes like cold-heat and deficiency-excess, so there are different combinations of descending qi methods. For instance, if the healthy qi deficiency along with ascending counterflow of qi movement, medicines for descending qi and supplementing should be used together. If the patient has ascending counterflow of qi movement without deficiency of healthy qi, medicines for lowering qi and directing counterflow downward should be mainly used. But we should be careful not to hurt the healthy qi while directing it downward. If there is deficiency-heat, deficiency-cold along with ascending counterflow of qi movement, medicines for clearing and supplementing or warming and supplementing should be used together with medicines for descending qi. If there's phlegm-heat or cold-fluid along with ascending counterflow of qi movement, medicines for clearing and removing or warming and removing should be used together with medicines for descending qi. In clinical, we should apply medicines according to the patient's condition. The representative formulas are *Sì Mò Tāng* (Four Milled Ingredients Decoction, 四磨汤), *Sū Zǐ Jiàng Qì Tāng* (Perilla Fruit Qi-Descending Decoction, 苏子降气汤), *Dìng Chuǎn Tāng* (Arrest Wheezing Decoction, 定喘汤), *Sān Zǐ Yǎng Qīn Tāng* (Three-Seed Filial Devotion Decoction, 三子养亲汤), *Xuán Fù Dài Zhě Tāng* (Inula and Hematite Decoction, 旋覆代赭汤), *Jú Pí Zhú Rú Tāng* (Tangerine Peel and Bamboo Shavings Decoction, 橘皮竹茹汤), *Dīng Xiāng Shì Dì Tāng* (Clove and Persimmon Decoction, 丁香柿蒂散).

Sì Mò Tāng (Four Milled-Herb Decoction, 四磨汤)
Formulas to Aid the Living (*Jì Shēng Fāng*, 济生方)

[Ingredient]

Rén Shēn (Radix Et Rhizoma Ginseng)　(9 g)

Bīng Láng (Semen Arecae)　(9 g)

Chén Xiāng (Lignum Aquilariae Resinatum)　(3 g)

Tiān Tāi Wū Yào (Radix Linderae)　(9 g)

[Usage]   In the original formula, the four medicines are milled with water, until 7 *zhan* remain. Decoct them by boiling 3–5 times, the patient should take the decoction while it's warm.

Modern usage: Usually prepared as a decoction and with a proportionate reduction in the dosage of the ingredients.

[Action]   Break stagnation and direct rebellious qi downward, reinforce healthy qi in the meantime.

[Indication]   This formula is used to treat internal damage caused by the seven emotions, along with symptoms like the abnormal rising of qi and panting, oppression and result in no desire to eat.

[Formula Analysis]   When there's internal damage caused by the seven emotions, liver qi will be transverse and counterflow. When the lung is invaded, there will be panting; if the spleen and stomach are influenced, there will also be oppression and no desire to eat. For this syndrome, its branch lies in the lung and spleen-stomach and its root lies in the liver. In this formula, *chén xiāng* is the chief medicine, which is warm but not dry, moving but not discharging. It can not only direct counterflow downward but also can receive kidney qi, so that the qi will counterflow. *Bīng láng* can break stagnant qi and direct counterflow downward, *wū yào* can normalize qi and direct counterflow downward. They used together assist *chén xiāng* to direct counterflow downward and these two are deputy medicines. But with the medicines of descending and breaking qi are easy to consume the healthy qi to so *rén shēn* is added in this formula to boost qi and reinforce healthy qi, making sure that counterflow qi can be descended without hurting healthy qi. In the original formula, these four medicines are all milled and decocted with water, so this formula has strong power and can produce an effect rapidly. That's why it's called "*Sì Mò Tāng* (Four Milled Ingredients Decoction)".

[Clinical Application]   This formula is used to treat syndromes like panting and poor appetite caused by qi counterflow failing to descend. The root cause is due to the seven emotions. If the patient is strong, *zhǐ ké* can be used to replace *rén shēn* to strengthen the function of directing counterflow downward.

Sū Zǐ Jiàng Qì Tāng (Perilla Fruit Decoction for Directing Qi Downward, 苏子降气汤)

Formulary of the Pharmacy Service for Benefiting the People in the Taiping Era (*Tài Píng Huì Mín Hé Jì Jú Fāng*, 太平惠民和剂局方)

[Ingredient]

Zǐ Sū Zǐ (Fructus Perillae)   2.5 *liang* (9 g)

Bàn Xià (Rhizoma Pinelliae)   washed with soup seven times, 2.5 *liang* (9 g)

Chuān Dāng Guī (Radix Angelicae Sinensis)   removes the residue of rhizome from the root, 1.5 *liang* (6 g)

Gān Cǎo (Radix et Rhizoma Glycyrrhizae)   fry with liquid adjuvant 2 *liang* (6 g)

Qián Hú (Radix Peucedani)   removes the residue of rhizome from the root, 1*liang* (4.5 g)

Hòu Pò (Cortex Magnoliae Officinalis)   scrap off the coarse layer of bark, fry it with ginger Juice, 1 *liang* (4.5 g)

Ròu Guì (Cortex Cinnamomi)   removes the skin 1.5 *liang* (3 g)

According to another record, there's also *chén pí* in this formula. It removes the white inner surface of the exocarp, 1.5 *liang*.

[Usage]   In the original formula, the medicines are ground into a powder, decoct 2 *qian* each time with 1.5 *zhan* water and add three pieces of *shēng jiāng*, five leaves of *sū yè*. Decoct them together until eight-tenths remains. Before drinking the decoction, remove the sediment and warm it. The patient can take the decoction at any time.

Modern usage: Add three pieces of *shēng jiāng*, one piece of *dà zǎo*, 3 g of *sū yè* into the medicines and decoct them with water.

[Action]   Direct rebellious qi downward, calm panting and dissolve phlegm, warm the kidney to improve qi reception and return qi to its source.

[Indication]   This formula is used to treat upper excess and lower deficiency, along with symptoms like phlegm-drool, panting, cough and shortness of breath,

oppression of chest and diaphragm, constipation, lumbago and feet weakness, fatigue and bad appetite and a white-greasy coating.

[Formula Analysis] The syndrome of this formula is upper excess with lower deficiency caused by phlegm obstructing, and failure of the kidney to receive qi. In this formula, *sū zǐ* is warm, moist and descending, which is good at directing qi downward and has the function of benefiting the diaphragm and loosening intestines, so it's the chief medicine. *Bàn xià* can lower qi and dissolve phlegm. *hòu pò* can lower qi and calm panting. *qián hú* can direct qi downward and dispel phlegm. These three are deputy medicines that can help the chief medicine to strengthen the function of directing qi downward, calming panting and dispelling phlegm to treat upper excess. Because this syndrome has a lower deficiency, *ròu guì* is used to warm the kidney to improve qi reception and help to return qi to its source; then yang qi is sufficient, there can be qi transformation and phlegm can be dispelled. *Dāng guī* has two functions, and one is to treat cough and qi counterflow, *Shen Nong's Classic of the Materia Medica* (*Shén Nóng Běn Cǎo Jīng*, 神农本草经) believes it governs "cough and qi counterflow"; the other is to nourish the blood and moisten dryness to counter the effect of the other dry [nature] medicines in this formula that may damage the yin and consume blood, *dāng guī* can moisten the intestines to promote defecation. If there's yang deficiency, the patient is easy to catch a wind-cold, so *shēng jiāng* and *dà zǎo* are used to harmonize *ying* and *wei* levels. *Sū yè* is used to dissipate external coldness. The above are assistant medicines. *Gān cǎo* is used to harmonize the actions of all the medicines as the envoy. The combination of these medicines can promote and supplement, dry and moisten, and mainly direct qi downward, calm panting and dissolve phlegm, and warm kidney to improve qi reception and return qi to its original house as a supplement. The root and branch are treated simultaneously while treating upper and the branch is the main purpose. In this formula, *sū zǐ* is the chief medicine and the main purpose is to descend qi. That's why this is called *Sū Zǐ Jiàng Qì Tāng* (Perilla Fruit Qi-Descending Decoction).

[Clinical Application] This formula is used to treat cough and panting caused by upper excess and lower deficiency. Some believe there's no *ròu guì* but

chén xiāng in this formula which makes it less powerful in warming the kidney but more powerful in improving qi reception and relieving panting according to the records of *Medical Formulas Collected and Analyzed* (*Yī Fāng Jí Jiě*). And according to the editor's clinical experience, this formula can produce a better effect when *ròu guì* and *chén xiāng* are used together.

Dìng Chuǎn Tāng (Arrest Wheezing Decoction, 定喘汤)
Multitude of Marvelous Formulas for Sustaining Life
(*Shè Shēng Zhòng Miào Fāng*, 摄生众妙方[88])

[Ingredient]

Bái Guǒ (Semen Ginkgo)   21 pcs, remove the skin, break it into a piece, make it light-brown by stir heating (12 g)

Má Huáng (Herba Ephedrae)   3 *qian* (9 g)

Sū Zǐ (Fructus Perillae)   2 *qian* (6 g)

Gān Cǎo (Radix et Rhizoma Glycyrrhizae)   1 *qian* (3 g)

Kuǎn Dōng Huā (Flos Farfarae)   3 *qian* (9 g)

Xìng Rén (Semen Armeniacae Amarum)   remove the seed coat and radicle 1.5 *qian* (6 g)

Sāng Bái Pí (Cortex Mori)   fry them with water-diluted vitality, 3 *qian* (9 g)

Huáng Qín (Radix Scutellariae)   fry slightly, half *qian* (4.5g)

Fǎ Bàn Xià (Rhizoma Pinelliae Praeparatum)   3 *qian* (9 g)

[Usage]   In the original formula, decoct the medicines with 3 *zhong*[①]of water until 2 remain, take the decoction 2 times, each time one *zhong*. The ginger is not needed. The patient can take it slowly, without time limits.

Modern usage: Usually prepared as a decoction.

[Action]   Diffuse the lung and direct qi downward, relieve panting and dissolve phlegm.

[Indication]   This formula is used to treat the wind-cold fettering the exterior, symptoms like a large amount of yellow and sticky sputum, coughing accompanied

---

① zhong 盅 , handleless cup; wine cup, the capacity is 30ml.

by panting, or aversion to cold, fever, yellowish and greasy coating, slippery and rapid pulse.

[Formula Analysis]　If the patient has phlegm-heat and retained phlegm with an external wind-cold pathogen invading, it can be constrained and transformed into heat. In this formula, *má huáng* can diffuse the lung, relieve panting and disperse wind-cold, *bái guǒ* can astringe the lung, relieve panting and eliminate turbid phlegm. These two combined together, can not only reinforce the effect of relieving panting, but *bái guǒ* also can counterbalance the disadvantages of *má huáng's* dispersing effect from dissipating the lung qi. They are both the chief medicines. *Xìng rén, sū zǐ, bàn xià* and *kuǎn dōng huā* can direct qi downward and dissolve phlegm, relieve cough and panting, as the deputy medicines. *Sāng bái pí* combined with *huáng qín* are used as assistant medicines to clear lung heat and relieve panting. The combination of those medicines has the effect of dispersing lung and lowering qi, resolving phlegm and calming panting. As Wang Xu-gao said, "The method of treatment is to disperse the exterior cold, clear the diaphragm heat, to descend qi and eliminate phlegm, and moisten the lung. This formula is the most suitable.".

[Clinical Application]　This formula is formed based on the *Sān Ào Tāng* (Rough and Ready Three Decoction) but add *sāng bái pí, huáng qín, bàn xià, sū zǐ, kuǎn dōng huā* and *bái guǒ*, which are used to treat wheezing and panting caused by externally contracted wind-cold and internal phlegm-heat accumulation.

Sān Zǐ Yǎng Qīn Tāng (Three-Seed Filial Devotion Decoction, 三子养亲汤)
Comprehensive Medicine According to Master Han (*Hán Shì Yī Tōng,* 韩氏医通)[89]

[Ingredient]

Zǐ Sū Zǐ (Fructus Perillae)　(9 g)

Bái Jiè Zǐ (Semen Sinapis)　(6 g)

Lái Fú Zǐ (Semen Raphani)　(9 g) (In the original formula, the dosage was not given.)

[Usage]　In the original formula, these three medicines are washed clean. Then fry them lightly, and break them into pieces. Adjust their dosage according to the main

symptom. The one with the higher dosage is the chief medicine. [but] Each formula's dosage should not be over three *qian*. Warp them with a raw silk bag and then boil them in water. The patient can drink the decoction instead of water. The medicines should not be decocted too much. If the patient has constipation, a small amount of honey can be added before drinking. If the patient has a wintercold, three slices of *shēng jiāng* can be boiled together.

Modern usage: It is usually prepared as a decoction.

[Action] Lower qi and direct rebellious qi downward, resolve phlegm and promote digestion.

[Indication] This formula is used to treat cough and qi counterflow, along with symptoms like profuse phlegm and chest *pǐ* [depression], poor appetite, a white-greasy coating, a slippery pulse.

[Formula Analysis] This formula is originally designed for the elderly with cough, qi counterflow and profuse phlegm, chest depression. In this formula, *zǐ sū zǐ* is used to lower qi and disperse phlegm, relieve cough and calm panting. *Bái jiè zǐ* can disinhibit qi and eliminate phlegm. *Lái fú zǐ* can lower qi and dispel phlegm, relieve stagnation and promote digestion. These three medicines can normalize qi, dissolve phlegm and digest food, calm cough and qi counterflow. They all can dissolve phlegm, and each of them can show their specialty in the meantime. In clinical practice, depend on the severity of the three aspects, qi, phlegm or food stagnation, then use the target medicine as the chief medicine and the rest as the assistant-envoy medicines. In the original book, these three "*zǐ* (子)" (which has the same pronunciation as the son in Chinese) are used to serve a parent. Hence, it's called "*Sān Zǐ Yǎng Qīn Tāng* (Three-Seed Filial Devotion Decoction)".

[Clinical Application]

1. This formula is commonly used for treating phlegm accumulation and chest *pǐ* [depression], cough and qi counterflow. It can be used for men and women, old and young, and especially good for the elderly. However, this formula is ultimately a remedy for treating the branch, not the root, so it's not suitable for those with qi deficiency. The elderly usually have an inner deficiency, which is the source of

phlegm. Once the symptoms are relieved, we should immediately change to use formulas that can supplement qi and fortify the spleen. Otherwise, the overuse of this formula will lower qi and promote digestion too much and hurt the middle qi.

2. According to the editor's clinical experience, for those with yang deficiency, phlegm-fluid accumulation inside the body, cough, qi counterflow, this formula combined with *Líng Guì Zhú Gān Tāng*, *Èr Chén Tāng* (Two Matured Substances Decoction) to treat the root and the branch can have a great effect.

Xuán Fù Dài Zhě Tāng (Inula and Hematite Decoction, 旋覆代赭汤)
Treatise on Cold Damage (*Shāng Hán Lùn*, 伤寒论)

[Ingredient]

Xuán Fù Huā (Flos Inulae)   3 *liang* (9 g)

Rén Shēn (Radix et Rhizoma Ginseng)   2 *liang* (6 g)

Shēng Jiāng (Rhizoma Zingiberis Recens)   5 *liang* (15 g)

Bàn Xià (Rhizoma Pinelliae)   half *sheng* washed (9 g)

Dài Zhě Shí (Haematitum)   1 *liang* (6 g)

Dà Zǎo (Fructus Jujubae)   12 pcs, break them off with hands (4 pcs)

Gān Cǎo (Radix et Rhizoma Glycyrrhizae)   fry them with liquid adjuvant, 3 *liang* (9 g)

[Usage]   In the original formula, decoct the medicines with one *dou* of water until 6 *sheng* remains; after removing the sediment, decoct the medicines again until 3 *sheng* remains. The patient should take 1 *sheng* of the decoction while it's still warm, three times a day.

Modern usage: It is usually prepared as a decoction.

[Action]   Direct rebellious qi downward and transform phlegm, augment the qi and harmonize the stomach.

[Indication]   This formula is used to treat phlegm obstruction caused by stomach deficiency and stomach qi counterflow, causing symptoms like *pǐ* and hardness below the heart, consistent belching, or hiccup, nausea and vomiting, a white-glossy coating and a wiry, deficient pulse.

[Formula Analysis]   The stomach governs the intake of food and drinks, preferring to descend. When stomach qi is weak, there's internal turbid phlegm obstruction, which is manifests with *pǐ* and hardness below the heart. If one has stomach deficiency and qi counterflow, there will be consistent belching. It is better to direct the counterflow qi downward, dissolve turbid phlegm and supplement stomach deficiency. In this formula, *xuán fù huā* can lower qi and disperse phlegm, direct counterflow downward and relieve belching. *Dài zhě shí* is used to direct counterflow downward with heavy sedatives which can treat belching and vomiting. These two combined can have a good effect of directing counterflow downward and they are both chief medicines. *Bàn xià* can direct counterflow downward and dispel phlegm, disperse *pǐ* and dissipate masses, *shēng jiāng* can lower qi, dispel phlegm and resolve toxins of *bàn xià*. These two can increase the formula's effect of directing counterflow downward and dispelling phlegm and they are deputy medicines. For deficiency of stomach qi *rén shēn* is used to supplement and boost stomach qi. *Dà zǎo* boosts qi and supplements the center; they are both assistant medicines. *Zhì gān cǎo* can boost qi and supplement the center, harmonize the actions of all the medicines in this formula, as the envoy medicine. And when *rén shēn*, *dà zǎo* and *gān cǎo* are used together, the power of boosting qi and harmonizing the stomach can be strengthened. This formula treats the root and the branches at the same time, [but] it mainly aims at treating the branches more than treating the root. After taking this formula, qi counterflow can be directed downward, turbid phlegm can be dissolved and stomach qi can be harmonized. Thus, all the symptoms can be relieved.

[Clinical Application]   Syndromes such as stomach cavity *pǐ*, belching, hiccup, regurgitation, vomiting caused by stomach deficiency, phlegm obstruction, and qi counterflow can all be treated by using this formula. If stomach deficiency is not severe, we can reduce the dosage of *rén shēn*, *dà zǎo* and *gān cǎo* because they are sweet and easily create congestion. If the patient has a lot of phlegm, we can add *fú líng* and *chén pí* to dissolve it. If one has severe *pǐ* and hardness below the heart, we can add *shā rén* to lower qi and harmonize the stomach. As for those who have a severe hiccup, we can add *dīng xiāng* and *shì dì* to warm the stomach and direct counterflow downward.

Jú Pí Zhú Rú Tāng (Tangerine Peel and Bamboo Shavings Decoction, 橘皮竹茹汤)

Essentials from the Golden Cabinet (*Jīn Guì Yào Lüè*, 金匮要略)

[Ingredient]

Jú Pí (Pericarpium Citri Reticulate)   2 *sheng* (9 g)

Zhú Rú (Caulis Bambusae in Taenia)   2 *sheng* (9 g)

Dà Zǎo (Fructus Jujubae)   30 pcs (5 pcs)

Shēng Jiāng (Rhizoma Zingiberis Recens)   half *jin* (9 g)

Gān Cǎo (Radix et Rhizoma Glycyrrhizae)   5 *liang* (6 g)

Rén Shēn (Radix Et Rhizoma Ginseng)   1 *liang* (3 g)

[Usage]   In the original formula, decoct the medicines with 1 *dou* of water until 3 *sheng* remains. The patient should take 1 *sheng* of the decoction while it's warm, three times a day.

Modern usage: It is usually prepared as a decoction.

[Action]   Harmonize the stomach and direct rebellious qi downward, clear heat and augment the qi.

[Indication]   This formula is used to treat stomach deficiency with heat, along with qi counterflow without descending, hiccuping or belching, a white-thin coating but a little bit yellow, a deficient while slightly rapid pulse.

[Formula Analysis]   For those who have a long-term illness with stomach deficiency, along with stomach heat, which causes disharmony of the stomach and failure of the descending function, qi counterflow, so there will be a hiccup and belching. In this formula, *jú pí* can rectify qi, harmonize the stomach and direct counterflow downward, *Shen Nong's Classic of the Materia Medica* (*Shén Nóng Běn Cǎo Jīng*, 神农本草经) says it's good at "lowering qi". *Zhú rú* is good at clearing stomach heat without attacking and leading to the cold lingering. It is the main medicine to treat vomiting and qi counterflow caused by stomach deficiency. These two are both chief medicines. *Rén shēn* can supplement and boost stomach qi together with *jú pí*; there is supplementation within moving. *Shēng jiāng* can harmonize the stomach and direct qi counterflow downward, together with *zhú rú*;

there is warmth within clearance; they are both deputy medicines. *Dà zǎo* and *gān cǎo* can boost qi, supplement the center and slow the stomach qi counterflow, as assistant-envoy medicines. This formula combines the clear [method], supplement [method] accompanied with direct counterflow downward [method], but mainly aims at directing counterflow downward, clearing without generating too much cold and supplementing without creating stagnation. This formula can normalize qi and clear heat, harmonize the stomach, so it's the most suitable one for hiccups and belching caused by stomach deficiency.

[Clinical Application] This formula is commonly used to treat hiccups and belching caused by stomach deficiency along with heat and qi counterflow without descending. If the stomach qi is not deficient, we can remove *rén shēn*, *dà zǎo* and *gān cǎo*. If there is too much phlegm, we can add *bàn xià* and *fú líng*. If the patient can't stop vomiting, we can add *pí pá yè*. If the stomach yin is insufficient with red tongue, little coating, we can add *mài dōng* and *shí hú*.

Dīng Xiāng Shì Dì Tāng (Clove and Persimmon Calyx Decoction, 丁香柿蒂汤) *Symptoms, Causes, Pulses, and Treatment* (*Zhèng Yīn Mài Zhì*, 症因脉治)[90]

[Ingredient]

Dīng Xiāng (Flos Caryophylli)　(3 g)

Shì Dì (Calyx Kaki)　(6 g)

Rén Shēn (Radix et Rhizoma Ginseng)　(3 g)

Shēng Jiāng (Rhizoma Zingiberis Recens)　(6 g) (In the original formula, the dosage was not given)

[Usage] Decoction. (In the original formula, the instruction was not given)

Modern usage: It is usually prepared as a decoction.

[Action] Warm the middle burner and augment qi, dissipate cold and direct rebellious qi downward.

[Indication] This formula is used to treat stomach qi deficiency and cold, failure of harmony and descending, along with symptoms like a hiccup, stomach *pǐ*, a pale tongue, a white coating, a deep, slow pulse.

[Formula Analys] When stomach qi is deficient and obstructed by a cold pathogen, it fail to transport, and there will be a cold obstruction and qi counterflow, inducing a hiccup. In this formula, *dīng xiāng* warms the middle and dissipates cold, which is good at directing the counterflow downward, *shì dì* can direct qi downward and relieve hiccups, they are both main medicines. *Rén shēn* is the deputy medicine to supplement the center and boost qi. *Shēng jiāng* is the assistant medicine to warm the middle and dissipate cold. These four medicines used together can make the center yang qi healthy and sufficient, so hiccup will be relieved.

[Clinical Application] This formula is commonly used to treat hiccups caused by stomach qi deficiency-cold and qi counterflow without descending. If one has severe hiccups, *dāo dòu zǐ* can be added to prevent it. If the patient has qi stagnation and phlegm obstruction at the same time, *chén pí*, *bàn xià* and *chén xiāng* can be added to rectify qi and dissolve phlegm, direct counterflow downward and relieve hiccup. This formula can also be used to treat vomiting caused by stomach cold and qi counterflow.

Chapter 15

Blood-Regulating Formulas

The blood-regulating formula is composed of blood-regulating medicines with functions of invigorating the blood or stanching the bleeding to treat blood stasis or hemorrhage.

Section 1   Formulas that invigorates the blood and dissolves stasis

The blood-regulating formula is suitable for a series of syndromes caused by stagnation of blood stasis. Since the locations of the stasis are different, the pathogens are varied, and the syndromes are also different. Like blood amassment in the lower *jiao*, manifested with distended pain or stiffness in the lesser abdomen, urinary incontinence, agitation and delirium, mania; or amenorrhea, painful menstruation, stasis, flooding and spotting, pain in the lower lateral abdomen that the patient refuses pressure, deep and choppy pulse with strength; or lochiorrhea after delivery, pain in the lower abdomen; or blood stasis leading to headache, chest pain, abdominal pain; or distended pain because of blood stasis from trauma; or qi deficiency and blood stasis after apoplexy, leading to hemiplegia, facial paralysis.

All the patients with the conditions above should be treated with formulas that invigorate the blood and dissolve stasis to remove and expel the blood stasis according to the states of the specific diseases. The common medicines that invigorate the blood and dissolve the blood stasis are *dà huáng, táo rén, hóng huā, chì sháo, chuān xiōng, wǔ líng zhī, dān pí, dān shēn, etc.* To form the formula, combining the medicines that regulate qi to strengthen the function of invigorating the blood and dissolving

the blood stasis because that qi is the commander of blood, qi flow promotes blood transportation.

In addition, according to the cold or heat, excess or deficiency of the disease, the corresponding medicines should be allocated together. For example, for patients with cold sydrome, medicines that warm the channels and dissipate cold should be combined, since the blood moves with warmth and congeals with cold; blood stasis and heat intertwined should be treated with clearing stasis heat medicines to conduct stasis heat to go downward, and there will be a way out for the pathogen; for patients who have deficiency of healthy qi with stasis, boosting qi and nourishing blood medicines should be combined so that the pathogen can be dispelled without harming the healthy qi. As for the pregnant woman with blood stasis, doctors should apply medicines to dissolve the stasis but with a light dosage so that the stasis can be removed without affecting the fetus; when most of the stasis has been removed, the patient should stop taking the formula. The typical formulas are *Táo Hé Chéng Qì Tāng* (Peach Kernel Qi-Guiding Decoction, 桃核承气汤), *Guì Zhī Fú Líng Wán* (Cinnamon Twig and Poria Pill, 桂枝茯苓丸), *Xuè Fǔ Zhú Yū Tāng* (Blood Mansion Stasis-Expelling Decoction, 血府逐瘀汤), *Bǔ Yáng Huán Wǔ Tāng* (Yang-Supplementing and Five-Returning Decoction, 补阳还五汤), *Fù Yuán Huó Xuè Tāng* (Original Qi-Restoring and Blood-Moving Decoction, 复元活血汤), *Wēn Jīng Tāng* (Channel-Warming Decoction, 温经汤), *Shēng Huà Tāng* (Engendering and Transforming Decoction, 生化汤).

Táo Hé Chéng Qì Tāng (Peach Kernel Qi-Guiding Decoction, 桃核承气汤)
Treatise on Cold Damage (*Shāng Hán Lùn*, 伤寒论)

[Ingredient]

Táo Rén (Semen Persicae)   50 pics without the peel and tip (12 g)

Guì Zhī (Ramulus Cinnamomi)   without peel, 2 *liang* (6 g)

Dà Huáng (Radix et Rhizoma Rhei)   4 *liang* (12 g)

Máng Xiāo (Natrii Sulfas)   2 *liang* (6 g)

Gān Cǎo (Radix et Rhizoma Glycyrrhizae)   liquid-fried, 2 *liang* (6 g)

[Usage] Decoction. The original text advises using seven liters of water, two and a half liters before boiling, removing the sediment, and then adding *máng xiāo*, and then heating it up slightly. The text also specifies that it should be drunk warm in three doses per day before meals. If the formula is effective, the stools should become slightly loose.

Modern usage: Decocted by water, filter, melting the *máng xiāo*, take it warm.

[Action] Break up blood, expel stasis and discharge heat.

[Indication] Blood amassment in the lower *jiao*, spasmodic pain in the lesser abdomen, uninhibited urination, vexation and delirium, quasi-mania. And for women: blood stasis and painful menstruation, amenorrhea, deep and excess pulse.

[Formula Analysis] The pathogenic heat of cold damage hasn't been released, and transmitted to the lower *jiao*, contending with blood with binding of stasis and heat, leading to the syndrome of blood amassment in the lower *jiao*. This formula is *Guì Zhī Tāng* with *táo rén* and *guì zhī*. use the bitter, sweet and neutral *táo rén* to treat the binding of stasis and heat, breaking up blood, expelling stasis. In *Shennong's Classic of Materia Medica* (*Shén Nóng Běn Cǎo Jīng*, 神农本草经) says it "treats stasis and blood block". *Pouch of Pearls* (*Zhēn Zhū Náng*, 珍珠囊) says it "breaks up blood amassment"; *dà huáng* is bitter and cold, purging the stasis and discharging the heat. The *Shennong's Classic of Materia Medica* (*Shén Nóng Běn Cǎo Jīng*, 神农本草经) says it is "good at dispelling stasis, blood block, cold and heat [manifestations]". *Pouch of Pearls* (*Zhēn Zhū Náng*, 珍珠囊) says it "discharges all the excessive heat and blockage", to use the two medicines together to treat the stasis and heat at the same time as chief medicine. *Guì zhī* is acrid, sweet and warm, warming the blood and meridians and dispersing the blood stasis in the lower *jiao*, helping *táo rén* to break up blood and dispel stasis. *máng xiāo* is bitter and extreme cold, entering the blood level, softening hardness, dissipate masses and moisten the dryness, helping *dà huáng* to purge stasis and discharge heat as deputy medicines. *Zhī gān cǎo* harmonizes the stomach and alleviates the strong flavors of other medicines to dispel the pathogen without harming the healthy qi as an assistant and envoy medicine. combine all the medicines, cold and hot, to break up blood, dispell stasis

and discharge heat, which is a good formula for treating blood stasis in the lower *jiao*. For the original formula, take it warm before meals leading the potency downward with a swift effect. Patients usually have diarrhea after taking medicines, which is just for promoting defecation, probably without blood stool. The diarrhea is to make outlets for the pathogen and relieve all the symptoms.

[Clinical Application]   This formula is commonly used to treat the combination of blood stasis and heat. For women with static heat, amenorrhea and dysmenorrhea, we can combine *Sì Wù Tāng* (Four Substances Decoction). If also with qi stagnation, *xiāng fù, zhǐ shí, qīng pí* can be added to regulate qi and break stagnation. This formula can also be used for postpartum lochia, lesser abdominal pain, serious dyspnea and pant. We often combine it with *Shī Xiào Sǎn* (Sudden Smile Powder) to invigorate the blood and remove the blood stasis.

Guì Zhī Fú Líng Wán (Cinnamon Twig and Poria Pill, 桂枝茯苓丸)
Essentials from the Golden Cabinet (*Jīn Guì Yào Lüè*, 金匮要略)

[Ingredient]

Guì Zhī (Ramulus Cinnamomi)

Fú Líng (Poria)

Mǔ Dān (Cortex Moutan)   without the core

Táo Rén (Semen Persicae)   without the peel and tip

Sháo Yào (Radix Paeoniae)   stewed

same dosage for each one (9 g)

[Usage]   The original text advises grinding the ingredients into a powder, forming them into pills the size of rabbit droppings with honey, and take three times daily before meals.

Modern usage: All the ingredients are ground into a powder, made into pills with honey, 1.5–6 g per serving, twice a day. Take it with warm water before eating. Or as a decoction, 9 g each, decocted in water, one dose per day.

[Action]   Dissolve the stasis and concretions.

[Indication]   For the women who have concretions (*zhēng*, 癥) for a long time,

less than 3 months of conception and spotting with purple, black and dark blood. Or a woman who has lesser abdominal masses, painful under pressure with a choppy pulse. Or a woman who has blood stasis and amenorrhea, abdominal pain during menstruation, dystocia, stillbirth, postpartum lochia retention and abdominal pain which refuses pressure.

[Formula Analysis] Concretions are visible and symptomatic, formed by coagulated blood stasis in the abdomen. The causes are cold and dampness, in the formula, *guì zhī* is acrid, sweet and warm, which warms the blood and meridians. *fú líng* is sweet and bland, percolating dampness and supplementing healthy qi; these two are chief medicines. Blood stasis generates heat if it stagnates for a long time, therefore *dān pí*, *sháo yào* are used to cool the blood and dissipate blood stasis and dissolve stasis and concretions, *táo rén* is good at breaking blood, dispelling stasis to promote regeneration as the assistant medicine together with former two. this formula. The combination of cold and warm herbs, considering both pathogen and healthy qi, is a moderate formula to remove blood stasis and concretions. The original formula used honey to alleviate the potency, remove the concretions without harming the fetus. And the administration is limited to taking one pill a day as big as rabbit excrement. If it have no effect, add to three pills, preserving the primordial fetal qi. This formula is characterized by relieving the concretions, due to the falt that the chronic diseases are not easy to cure immediately and should be treated gradually, slowly relieving the concretions can not only make the stasis be dispelled to promote regeneration, but also nourish and keep the patient safe and sound. To eliminate blood stasis and concretions without disregarding the injury of the fetus, we should treat the disease first. Just as the theory of *Basic Questions-Comprehensive Discourse on the Policies and Arrangements of the Six Principal [Qi]* (*Sù Wèn-Liù Yuán Zhèng Jì Dà Lùn*, 素问·六元正纪大论) says, "If there is a hardening, there will be no harm [to the woman] and [the fetus] will not be harmed either"; "Massive accumulations; massive agglomerations. They can be offended. Weaken them to a degree of just over one-half and then stop (the treatment). If this (limit) is exceeded, (mother and child) will die".

[Clinical Application] This formula is for activating blood circulation

and removing blood stasis. In addition to the treatment of concretions and spotting, it can also be used to treat abdominal pain caused by concretions, blood stasis, dysmenorrhea, dystocia, retention of placenta, stillbirth, postpartum lochia retention, abdominal pain that refuses pressure and so on, also, for surging vanquished blood, it leads to shortness of breath and panting. All the symptoms caused by blood stasis are suitable for this formula.

Xuè Fǔ Zhú Yū Tāng (Blood Mansion Stasis-Expelling Decoction, 血府逐瘀汤) *Correction on the Errors of Medical Works* (*Yī Lín Gǎi Cuò*, 医林改错) [91]

[Ingredient]

Dāng Guī (Radix Angelicae Sinensis)   3 *qian* (9 g)

Shēng Dì (Radix Rehmanniae)   3*qian* (9 g)

Táo Rén (Semen Persicae)   4 *qian* (12 g)

Hóng Huā (Stigma Croci)   3 *qian* (9 g)

Zhǐ Ké (Fructus Aurantii)   2 *qian* (6 g)

Chì Sháo (Radix Paeoniae Rubra)   2 *qian* (6 g)

Chái Hú (Radix Bupleuri)   1 *qian* (3 g)

Gān Cǎo (Radix et Rhizoma Glycyrrhizae)   2 *qian* (6 g)

Jié Gěng (Radix Platycodonis)   1.5 *qian* (4.5 g)

Chuān Xiōng (Rhizoma Chuanxiong)   1.5 *qian* (4.5 g)

Niú Xī (Radix Achyranthis Bidentatae)   3 *qian* (9 g)

[Usage]   Decocted by water.

Modern usage: Same as original usage.

[Action]   Invigorate blood and dissolve blood stasis, move qi and relieve pain.

[Indication]   Blood stasis in the chest leads to headache, prolonged chest pain, stabbing pain in a certain location, or hiccups, retching, irritability, dreaminess, insomnia, palpitation, fever at night, dark red tongue with stasis macule and spots on the sides, choppy pulse.

[Formula Analysis]   Wang Qing-ren[92] said, "Above the diaphragm, the cavity is filled with blood, thus called the house of blood" and "The house of blood

is the area below the chest and the diaphragm". It can be seen that the house of blood that Wang refered to is in the chest. In the formula, *dāng guī*, *táo rén* and *hóng huā* invigorate the blood and dissolve stasis, used as the chief medicines; *chì sháo* and *chuān xiōng* help the chief medicines to invigorate the blood and dissolve stasis, *shēng dì* coordinates the *dāng guī* to nourish and invigorate blood, so as to dissolve stasis without harming the yin blood. They are all deputy medicines; *zhǐ ké* is descending and *jié gěng* is ascending, widening the chest and regulating the qi so that the activated qi drives blood, *jié gěng* can ship the medicines upwards so that the medicine can acts on the chest, *chái hú* soothes qi and resolves constraint, raises the lucid yang, works with *zhǐ ké*, which is good at regulating qi and dissipating masses, *niú xī* breaks up blood and dispells stasis, which is good at inducing the stasis flow downward. The medicines above are all assistant medicines; *gān cǎo* alleviates the urgent conditions, promotes blood qi and harmonizes the actions of all medicines, and is used as envoy medicine. Combining all the medicines, it can promote blood circulation without the consideration of blood consumption, move qi without the harm of yin, treat the house of blood stasis by dissolving it and dispelling downward. All the symptoms can be healed, hence it is named "Blood Mansion Stasis-Expelling Decoction".

[Clinical Application]   This formula is a commonly used prescription for the treatment of blood stasis in the chest. According to the clinical experience of Wang Qing-ren, this formula can be used to treat headache, chest pain, chest oppression, morning sweating, food passing [feeling] behind the chest, heart inner heat called lantern disease, visual distortion, impatience, dreaminess, hiccups (common name *kǎ tè* 咯忒), water choke, insomnia, baby night crying, palpitation, which are commonly called liver qi disease, retching, night fever.

Fù Yuán Huó Xuè Tāng (Original Qi-Restoring and Blood-Moving Decoction, 复元活血汤)

Illumination of Medicine (*Yī Xué Fā Míng*, 医学发明[93])

[Ingredient]

Chái Hú (Radix Bupleuri)   half *liang* (15 g)

Guā Lóu Gēn (Trichosanthis Radix)   3 *qian* (9 g)

Dāng Guī (Radix Angelicae Sinensis)   3 *qian* (9 g)

Hóng Huā (Flos Carthami)   2 *qian* (6 g)

Gān Cǎo (Radix et Rhizoma Glycyrrhizae)   2 *qian* (6 g)

Chuān Shān Jiǎ (Squama Manitis)   blast-fried 2 *qian* (6 g)

Dà Huáng (Radix et Rhizoma Rhei)   wine maceration 1 *liang* (30 g)

Táo Rén (Semen Persicae)   50 pics wine macerated, without peel and tip, ground, (15 g)

[Usage]   The original text advises to coarsely grind the herbs, except *táo rén*, as big as hemp beans, and take 1 *liang* as a draft in a mixture of 1 *zhan* water and half *zhan* wine. Cook together to seven-tenths, remove the sediment, and warmly drink it before a meal. Take diarrhea lightly as the sign to stop drinking the rest of the decoction.

Modern usage: Boil the formula with three-quarters of the water and a quarter of yellow rice wine, take it warm on an empty stomach.

[Action]   Invigorate blood and dispel stasis, unblock collaterals and dissipate masses.

[Indication]   Trauma caused by falls, blood stasis accumulated under the rib-side, causing insufferable pain.

[Formula Analysis]   The liver stores blood, and the foot *jueyin* liver channel passes through the rib-side. When the patients fall from a height or get trauma by fall or fights, the blood stasis lingers under the rib-side, the blood and qi are blocked, causing unbearable pain. In the formula, *chái hú* leads all the medicines into the liver meridian as chief medicine; *dāng guī* invigorates the blood; *gān cǎo* relaxes tension and pain, supplements qi and engenders blood, used as deputy medicines;

chuān shān jiǎ breaks up stasis and unblocks the collaterals; *guā lóu gēn* moistens the dryness and dispels stasis, *Shennong's Classic of Materia Medica* (*Shén Nóng Běn Cǎo Jīng*, 神农本草经) says *guā lóu gēn* can "heal the fracture", *Ri Hua Zi Master Medica* (*Rì Huá Zǐ Běn Cǎo*, 日华子本草[94]) says it can "Dispell the blood stasis caused by dispersion"; *táo rén* and *hóng huā* dispel stasis and generate [new]. The envoy medicine *dà huáng* is processed by wine, flushing the stasis coagulation and vanquished blood, leading the stasis to move downward, removing the stagnant pathogen to promote regeneration. Processed with wine which nature is moving, it can help the formula to invigorate the blood and unblock the collaterals. All medicines combined, the blood stasis can be dispelled, and the new blood can be generated and the pain can be alleviated. Just like Zhang Bing-cheng said, "Dispel the pathogen, generate the new, the pain can be relieved and the spirit can be recovered". So the formula was named "Original Qi-Restoring and Blood-Moving Decoction".

[Clinical Application]   This formula is commonly used in oral administration in traumatology, whose indication is trauma and injury, a syndrome of pain caused by stagnated blood stasis. If the pain is severe, 3 to 6 g powder of *sān qī* can be added, or add *rǔ xiāng*, *yù jīn*, *yán hú suǒ* to enhance the effect of promoting blood circulation and relieving pain. However, for injuries caused by falls with blood stasis and stagnation of qi, *xiāng fù*, *yù jīn*, *jú luò* can be added to invigorate the qi and motivate the blood with a good effect.

Bǔ Yáng Huán Wǔ Tāng (Yang-Supplementing and Five-Returning Decoction, 补阳还五汤)
Correction on the Errors of Medical Works (*Yī Lín Gǎi Cuò*, 医林改错)

[Ingredient]

Huáng Qí (Radix Astragali Praeparata cum Melle)   raw, 4 *liang* (60 g)

Guī Wěi (Radix Angelicae Sinensis)   2 *qian* (6 g)

Chì Sháo (Radix Paeoniae Rubra)   1.5 *qian* (4.5 g)

Dì Lóng (Pheretima)   remove dirt, 1 *qian* (3 g)

Chuān Xiōng (Rhizoma Chuanxiong)   1 *qian* (3 g)

Táo Rén (Semen Persicae)   1 *qian* (3 g)

Hóng Huā (Flos Carthami)   1 *qian* (3 g)

[Usage] Decoction.

Modern usage: The same as the original.

[Action] Replenish the vital energy, promote blood circulation for removing obstruction in collaterals.

[Indication] Hemiplegia after stroke, oblique mouth and eyes, sluggish speech, angular salivation, dry stool, frequent urination, enuresis, pale tongue with white coating, slow and weak pulse.

[Formula Analysis] In *Spiritual Pivot-Needling the True and the Pathological* (*Líng Shū-Cì Jié Zhēn Xié*, 灵枢·刺节真邪) says, "The deficient pathogen tends to invade half of the body when it moves forwards, lingers in the *ying-wei* level, when the *ying-wei* level fades then the true qi weakens, left with the pathogenic qi, leading to hemilateral withering". Hemilateral withering is hemiplegia. In the formula, a large dosage of *huáng qí* is used to supplement the original qi, to boost the qi and invigorate the blood as chief medicine; *guī wěi* motivates the blood as deputy medicine; a small amount of *chì sháo, chuān xiōng, táo rén, hóng huā* help *guī wěi* to activate blood and harmonize *ying*; *dì lóng* can dredge channels and activate collaterals. The combination of these medicines has the effect of nourishing vitality, promoting blood circulation and dredging collaterals. Qi belongs to yang, and this formula is good at replenishing qi and returning fifty percent of its lost vitality to treat hemiplegia, hence it's named "Yang-Supplementing and Five-Returning Decoction".

[Clinical Application] This formula is mainly used for the treatment of hemiplegia after stroke. Deficiency of qi and blood stasis are the pathogenesis. Pale tongue and weak pulse, are the key points of syndrome differentiation. The dosage of *huáng qí* should be heavy, while the dosage of medicines that invigorates the blood and unblocks the collaterals should be light. A heavy dosage of medicines to supplement qi will help promote blood circulation and dredge collaterals, while less use of medicine that invigorates the blood and unblocks the collaterals will dispel the pathogen without harming healthy qi, which is satifactory to both sides.

Shī Xiào Sǎn (Sudden Smile Powder, 失笑散)
Formularies of the Bureau of Formulary of the Pharmacy Service for Benefiting the People in the Taiping Era (*Tài Píng Huì Mín Hé Jì Jú Fāng*, 太平惠民和剂局方)

[Ingredient]

Pú Huáng (Pollen Typhae)　deep fried

Wǔ Líng Zhī (Faeces Trogopterori)　ground with wine, clean out the dirt

the same dosage of the two above

[Usage]　Grind the ingredients and mix with vinegar 2 *qian,* boil the mixture into a paste. Then stew the paste with a cup (*zhan*) of water until moderately boiled. Take it warm before meals.

Modern usage: Grind all the medicines into a powder, and 6 g each time, take it after mixing with yellow rice wine or vinegar; or 6–12 g every day, wrap-boiling.

[Action]　Motivate the blood, dispel the blood stasis and relieve the pain.

[Indication]　Blood stasis stagnation, dysmenorrhea, amenorrhea, uterine bleeding with purple blood and clots, lower abdomen pain which refuses pressure, or postpartum lochiorrhea, postpartum blood sickness. And this formula is for all the syndromes of blood stasis blockage, painful heart and abdomen, a choppy pulse.

[Formula Analysis]　All the diseases that can be treated by this formula are caused by blood stasis and unsmooth blood circulation. In the formula, *pú huáng* is sweet and neutral, which can motivate blood and dispel blood stasis, *Shennong's Classic of Materia Medica* (*Shén Nóng Běn Cǎo Jīng*, 神农本草经) says it can "dispel the blood stasis", *The Compendium of Materia of Medica* (*Běn Cǎo Gāng Mù*, 本草纲目) says it can "cool and motivate the blood, relieve all the pain in the heart and abdomen". Also, it can be used to stanch the blood, treating the bleeding symptoms, so that it attacks without curtailing the body; *wǔ líng zhī* is sweet and warm, which enters the liver meridian and blood level, unblocks the blood vessels, dispels the stasis and relieves the pain, the two reinforce each other and both are chief medicines. Mixed it with rice vinegar, it tastes sour and enters the liver, which not only helps *pú huáng* and *wǔ líng zhī* remove the stasis and motivate the blood but also suppresses the fishy and

animal smells of *wǔ líng zhī*, Chen Cang-qi's *Supplement to "The Materia Medica"* (*Běn Cǎo Shí Yí*, 本草拾遗[95]) says, "it treats the postpartum dizziness...eliminates the malignant toxin". Thus, *wǔ líng zhī* is assistant and envoy medicine. Combining the two to form the formula, they play the role of dispelling the stasis and relieving the pain, and promoting regeneration. The predecessors used this formula each time the patients felt that their symptoms are eliminated without realizing it, and they couldn't help but laugh dumbly, which led to the name 'Sudden Smile Powder'.

[Clinical Application] This formula is commonly used to treat the pain caused by blood stasis, especially the blood stasis in the liver meridian. If added with *dāng guī*, *chì sháo*, *shēng dì*, *táo rén*, *hóng huā*, *dān shēn* and so on, the effect of motivating the blood and dispelling the stasis will be even better; if added with *rǔ xiāng* and *mò yào*, the effect of relieving the pain will be obvious. For patients with qi stagnation, the formula can be added with *xiāng fù* and *yù jīn*, or combined with *Jīn Líng Zǐ Sǎn* (Toosendan Powder).

Wēn Jīng Tāng (Channel-Warming Decoction, 温经汤)
Essentials from the Golden Cabinet (*Jīn Guì Yào Lüè*, 金匮要略)

[Ingredient]

Wú Zhū Yú (Fructus Evodiae)   3 *liang* (9 g)

Dāng Guī (Radix Angelicae Sinensis)   2 *liang* (6 g)

Chuān Xiōng (Rhizoma Chuanxiong)   2 *liang* (6 g)

Sháo Yào (Radix Paeoniae)   2 *liang* (6 g)

Rén Shēn (Radix et Rhizoma Ginseng)   2 *liang* (6 g)

Guì Zhī (Ramulus Cinnamomi)   2 *liang* (6 g)

Ē Jiāo (Colla Corii Asini)   2 *liang* (6 g)

Dān Pí (Cortex Moutan) remove the core   2 *liang* (6 g)

Shēng Jiāng (Rhizoma Zingiberis Recens)   2 *liang* (6 g)

Gān Cǎo (Radix et Rhizoma Glycyrrhizae)   2 *liang* (6 g)

Bàn Xià (Rhizoma Pinelliae)   half *sheng* (9 g)

Mài Dōng (Radix Ophiopogonis)   remove the core, 1 *sheng* (12 g)

[Usage]　Decoct the 12 medicines with 1 *dou* of water, boil them until 3 *sheng* left, take it warm in three times.

Modern usage: Decocted by water.

[Action]　Warm the meridians and dissipate the coldness, nourish the blood and dispel the blood stasis.

[Indication]　Deficient cold in the *Chong* and *Ren Meridian*, blood stasis stagnation, irregular menstruation or profuse menstruation, late menstruation, flooding and spotting, bleeding, fever at dusk, cold pain in the lesser abdomen, abdomen fullness, vexing heat in the palms, dry lips and mouth. Also cold in the lesser abdomen, infertility for females.

[Formula Analysis]　*Chong* Meridian is the sea of blood, and *Ren* Meridian governs the fetus; the two both originate from the uterus. And the channel's running course is in the lesser abdomen. *Basic Questions-Discourse on Regulating the Conduits* (*Sù Wèn-Tiáo Jīng Lùn*, 素问·调经论) says, "The blood and qi prefer warmth and are averse to cold. When meeting cold, the two stop flowing. When meeting warmth, the two dissipate". In the formula, *wú zhū yú* and *guì zhī* warm the meridians and dissipate the cold. As chief medicines, *wú zhū yú* is good at warming the liver and relieving the pain and *guì zhī* is good at warming and unblocking the blood vessels. *Dāng guī*, *chuān xiōng*, *sháo yào* and *ē jiāo* nourish the blood and regulate menstruation, remove blood stasis and generate the new, used assistant medicines. *Dān pí* not only helps *guì zhī*, *dāng guī*, *chuān xiōng* motivate the blood, dispel the blood stasis, but also clears the constraint heat in blood level, *The Compendium of Materia of Medica* (*Běn Cǎo Gāng Mù*, 本草纲目) says, it can "treat the hidden fire in blood and relieve the vexing heat"; *Chong* Meridian is attached to *yangming*, thus *rén shēn*, *gān cǎo* and *mài dōng* boost stomach qi and nourish stomach yin to replenish the middle qi, which can transfer to blood; *bàn xià* directs the counterflow of the stomach downward, calming the surging; *shēng jiāng* warms the liver and harmonizes the stomach, and resolves the toxin. The medicines above serve as assistant medicines. *Gān cǎo* can also harmonize all the other medicines as envoy

medicine. All the medicines combined, warm and cold, tonifying and motivating, mainly warm tonifying to make the blood and qi move with warmness. When the blood circulation is smooth, the blood stasis will dispell and the new will generate, all the syndromes will be healed, which is the reason for the name "Channel-Warming Decoction".

[Clinical Application]   This formula is an ancestral formula to regulate menstruation, mainly used in the deficient cold in *Chong* and *Ren* Meridian, irregular menstruation caused by blood stasis, cold pain in the lesser abdomen and irregular uterine bleeding.

Shēng Huà Tāng (Engendering and Transforming Decoction, 生化汤) *Complete Works of Jingyue* (*Jǐng Yuè Quán Shū*, 景岳全书) quoted the Kuai Ji shi clan ancestral formula

[Ingredient]
Dāng Guī (Radix Angelicae Sinensis)   5 *qian* (15 g)

Chuān Xiōng (Rhizoma Chuanxiong)   2 *qian* (6 g)

Táo Rén (Semen Persicae)   10 without peel, tip and kernels (4.5 g)

Jiāo Jiāng (Rhizoma Zingiberis Recens)   3 *fen* (1 g)

Gān Cǎo (Radix et Rhizoma Glycyrrhizae)   liquid-fried, 5 *fen* (1.5 g)

[Usage]   Bite the medicines, add two cups of water and two *dà zǎo*, decoct the formula until eight-tenths boiled and take it warm.

Modern usage: Decocted by water.

[Action]   Warm the meridians and motivate the blood, dissolve the stasis and generate the new.

[Indication]   Postpartum lochiorrhea, blood stasis blockage, pain in the lower abdomen.

[Formula Analysis]   The lochia is the blood and turbid fluids left in the uterus after delivery, which should be expelled outside the body. In the formula, *dāng guī* supplements and motivates blood, dissolves the blood stasis and generates

the new, used as chief medicine; *chuān xiōng* is acrid and warm, which can dissipate and unblock, motivate blood and qi, used as deputy medicine; a little of *táo rén* to dissolves the stasis and generates the new; *páo jiāng* warms the meridian and dissipates cold, helps *dāng guī* to promote the new, *chuān xiōng*, *táo rén* to dissolve blood stasis; thus the blood can move with warmness. *Basic Questions-The discourse on Regulating the Conduits* (*Sù Wèn-Tiáo Jīng Lùn*, 素问·调经论) says, "Cold makes it difficult [for blood and qi] to flow and warmth removes [stagnation of blood and qi]"; using sweet liquid-fried *gān cǎo* and *dà zǎo* mildly invigorating blood and dissolving stasis, supplementing the deficiency and tonifying the spleen, harmonizing all the medicines. Combining all the medicines conducts the effect of warming the meridians and motivating the blood, dissolving the blood stasis and promoting the new. Just as *Treatise on Blood Syndromes* (*Xuè Zhèng Lùn*, 血证论[96]) says, it can "dissolve the blood stasis and generate the new, commonly used after delivery", so this formula is named "Engendering and Transforming Decoction".

[Clinical Application]　　This formula is commonly used after delivery. However, the nature of the medicines is relatively warm, so they should be used for patients with postpartum cold congealing and blood stasis. It's not suitable for the patients with blood heat and stasis.

Section 2　Formulas that stanches bleeding

The bleeding-stanch formula is suitable for blood syndromes like hematemesis, nosebleed, hemoptysis, bloody stool, hematuria, uterine bleeding caused by blood outflow from the vessels and meridians. The typical medicines to stanch the blood are *dà jì*, *xiǎo jì*, *cè bǎi yè*, *máo gēn*, *huái huā*, *zào zhōng huáng tǔ*, *ē jiāo* or *ài yè*. However, blood syndrome is complicated with different causes of cold and heat, deficiency and excess, different locations and different conditions like mild, severe, chronic and acute. Therefore, the use of the bleeding-stanch formula is according to the specific situation. Generally speaking, if it is caused by blood heat, it is appropriate

to cool the blood and stanch the bleeding; if the patients with yang deficiency that is unable to retain blood, it is appropriate to warm the yang and stanch the bleeding; for the deficiency in *Chong* Meridian and *Ren* Meridian, the tonifying and stanch bleeding treatment should be used; for massive hemorrhage, symptomatic treatment should be taken in acute conditions and the key is to stanch the bleeding; for qi desertion following blood loss, the original qi should be supplemented so that the yin growing while yang generating, qi and blood can be supplemented for chronic bleeding and the key is to treat the root, or treat the root and branch simultaneously. The typical formulas are *Shí Huī Săn* (Ten Charred Substances Powder, 十灰散), *Huái Huā Săn* (Sophora Flower Powder, 滑石散), *Huáng Tǔ Tāng* (Yellow Earth Decoction, 黄土汤), *Xiǎo Jì Yǐn Zǐ* (*Field Thistle Drink*, 小蓟饮子), *Jiāo Ài Tāng* (Donkey-Hide Gelatin and Mugwort Decoction, 胶艾汤).

Shí Huī Săn (Ten Charred Substances Powder, 十灰散)
Divine Book of Ten Medicine Formulas (*Shí Yào Shén Shū*, 十药神书[97])

[Ingredient]

Dà Jì (Herba Cirsii Japonici)

Xiǎo Jì (Herba Cirsii)

Hé Yè (Folium Nelumbinis)

Cè Bǎi Yè (Cacumen Platycladi)

Bái Máo Gēn (Rhizoma Imperatae)

Qiàn Cǎo (Radix Et Rhizoma Rubiae)

Shān Zhī (Fructus Gardeniae)

Dà Huáng (Radix Et Rhizoma Rhei)

Dān Pí (Cortex Moutan)

Zōng Lǚ Pí (Petiolus Trachycarpi)

all in the same dosage

[Usage] Burn all the medicines into ashes, ground them into a fine powder, wrap them with paper, cover them with a bowl for one night, aim to remove the fire

toxin. Use the white lotus root juice or radish juice to grind the Beijing ink stick, and get about half a bowl of ink, mix it with the powder, and take the mixture 5 *qian* after meals.

Modern usage: Burn all the medicines into a powder and mix with lotus root or radish juice and Beijing ink, each time 9–15 g; or the formula can be taken as a decoction, boil with water, the dosage proportion refers to the original formula.

[Action]   Cool the blood and stanch bleeding.

[Indication]   Frenetic movement of hot blood, hematemesis, hemoptysis.

[Formula Analysis]   Hematemesis and hemoptysis are caused mainly by intense heat, damaging the blood network vessels and straying blood out of the meridians. The heat leads to chaotic blood movement. In the formula, *dà jì, xiǎo jì, cè bǎi yè, máo gēn, qiàn cǎo, shān zhī* are all the medicines to cool blood and stanch bleeding, and *zōng lǚ pí* stanches bleeding with astringency, *hé yè* disperses stasis and stanches bleeding, *dà huáng* is descending, which can discharge excessive heat in blood level and dispel blood stasis. This formula is mainly to cool the blood and stanch bleeding, added with medicines to dissolve the stasis, making the bleeding stanched without leaving the stasis. In the formula, all the medicines are burnt to preserve nature to strengthen the action to stanch bleeding with astringency, just like Ge Ke-jiu says, "Generally blood moves with heat, congeals with coldness, stanches with the black, which is a theorem." Mix it with the juice of lotus root or radish and Beijing ink reinforces the effect of clearing heat, directing the qi downward and stanching the blood. The ten medicines are all burnt to ashes for preserving nature, and ground into a powder, thus it is named "Ten Charred Substances Powder", and this formula is the top one in the *Divine Book of Ten Medicine Formulas* (*Shí Yào Shén Shū*, 十要神书), so it is also named "A Ten Charred Substances Powder".

[Clinical Application]   This formula mainly treats hematemesis, hemoptysis caused by frenetic movement of hot blood. It is also a formula for treating the symptoms in acute conditions. After stanching bleeding, we should regulate the patients' bodies according to syndromes so that the effect can be consolidated.

Huái Huā Sǎn (Sophora Flower Powder, 槐花散)
Formulas of Universal Benefit from My Practice (Pǔ Jì Běn Shì Fāng, 普济本事方[98])

[Ingredient]

Huái Huā (Flos Sophorae)　deep-fried

Bǎi Yè (Cacumen Platycladi)　pestled, baked

Jīng Jiè Suì (Spica Schizonepetae)

Zhǐ Qiào (Fructus Aurantii)　remove pulp, sliced, bran-fried

All in the same dosage

[Usage]　Grind the original formula into a powder and mix with clear rice soup, 2 *qian* together, take it before meals on an empty stomach.

Modern usage: Grind the medicines into a powder, take 6 g each time with hot water or rice soup; or used as a decoction, boil it with water, the dosage is determined according to the original formula.

[Action]　Clear the intestines and stanch bleeding, scatter wind and motivate qi.

[Indication]　Intestinal wind and visceral toxin, bloody stool with scarlet or dark purple color blood, red tongue with yellow coating and rapid pulse.

[Formula Analysis]　The predecessors reckoned that the scarlet blood in stool is caused by intestinal wind, and the visceral toxin causes the purple dark stool. For the mechanism, it is caused by wind-heat or damp-heat stagnated in the blood level of the large intestine, heat damaging the yin collaterals, just like *Golden Mirror of the Medical Tradition-Essential Teachings on Miscellaneous Diseases* (*Yī Zōng Jīn Jiàn-Zá Bìng Xīn Fǎ Yào Jué*, 医宗金鉴·杂病心法要诀) says, "the two syndromes of bloody stool, [includes] intestinal wind and visceral toxin, their [root] causes both are heat damaging the yin collaterals, the heat and wind combine to form intestinal wind, the blood in stool usually is clear; the heat and damp combine to form the visceral toxin, [then] the blood is usually turbid". In the formula, *huái huā* particularly clears the intestines, cools the blood and stanches bleeding, as the chief medicine; *bǎi yè* dries dampness and clears heat to help the chief medicine cool the blood and stanch bleeding as deputy medicine; *jīng jiè suì* scatters wind and regulates blood, *zhǐ ké*

eases the intestines as assistant medicines.

The combination of medicines can not only cool blood and stanch bleeding, but also clear the damp heat in the large intestine, scatter wind and move qi so that the blood can be stanched without the disadvantage of leaving blood stasis. Although there are many medicines in the formula, the compatibility is proper; thus it is used to treat intestinal wind, visceral and bloody stool with a specific effect. The original formula is mixed with rice soup, which the stomach-qi can be supplemented, the cold will not harm the middle qi.

[Clinical Application]   This formula is commonly used to treat intestinal wind, visceral toxin and hemorrhoidal bleeding. If there is intense heat in the large intestine, *huáng qín*, *huáng lián* and *dà huáng* can be added to clear the intestinal excessive heat; if there is profuse blood in the stool, *jīng jiè suì* can be dry-fried until charred, added with the charcoal of *dì yú* to strengthen the effect of clearing heat and stanching blood; if the blood in the stool persists for a long time, and the patient has deficiency, of blood we are supposed to add medicines to nourish the blood, such as *Jiā Jiǎn Sì Wù Tāng* (Four Substances Variant Decoction) in *Formulas to Save the Living* (*Jì Shēng Fāng*, 济生方), that is *Sì Wù Tāng* (Four Substances Decoction) without *sháo yào* and combine with this formula to treat the bloody stool caused by the intestinal wind with yin blood deficiency.

Huáng Tǔ Tāng (Yellow Earth Decoction, 黄土汤)
Essentials from the Golden Cabinet (*Jīn Guì Yào Lüè,* 金匮要略)

[Ingredient]
Gān Cǎo (Radix et Rhizoma Glycyrrhizae)   3 *liang* (9 g)

Gān Dì Huáng (Radix Rehmanniae Recens)   3 *liang* (9 g)

Bái Zhú (Rhizoma Atractylodis Macrocephalae)   3 *liang* (9 g)

Fù Zǐ (Radix Aconiti Lateralis Praeparata)   processed 3 *liang* (9 g)

Ē Jiāo (Colla Corii Asini)   3 *liang* (9 g)

Huáng Qín (Radix Scutellariae)   3 *liang* (9 g)

Zào Zhōng Huáng Tǔ (Terra Flava Usta)   half *jin* (30 g)

[Usage]　Boil the 7 medicines with water 8 *sheng* until the mixture is 3 *sheng* and take it warm twice a day.

Modern usage: Boil the *zào zhōng huáng tǔ* (*fú lóng gān* 伏龙肝) and mix it with water, and filter, use the solution to boil with the other herbs. Melted *ē jiāo* in the decoction, then take it warm.

[Action]　Warm yang and fortify the spleen, nourish the blood and stanch bleeding.

[Indication]　Deficient cold of the spleen qi, unable to contain the blood, manifested as bloody stool, or hematemesis, nose bleeding, dark purple blood, cold limbs, withered-yellow face, pale tongue and white coating with a deep, thready and weak pulse.

[Formula Analysis]　Spleen controls blood and deficient-cold spleen qi fails to control blood. In the formula, a large dosage of *zào zhōng huáng tǔ*, also named "oven earth", is acrid and slightly warm, good at warming the middle and stanching the blood, used as chief medicine. It is combined with *bái zhú, fù zǐ* to fortify the spleen and warm yang, to retrieve the blood-controlling action of spleen earth; *bái zhú* and *fù zǐ* are used as deputy medicines. With a large amount of bleeding, the yin blood is consumed, *shēng dì, ē jiāo* and *gān cǎo* are used to nourish the yin and blood and stanch bleeding. There is also bitter cold *huáng qín* stanching bleeding, *The Compendium of Materia of Medica* (*Běn Cǎo Gāng Mù*, 本草纲目) says it treats "all the bleeding syndrome", it can help *shēng dì, ē jiāo* to constrain the warm dryness of *zào zhōng huáng tǔ, bái zhú* and *fù zǐ* that might consume blood and cause bleeding. *Huáng qín* is considered as a paradoxical assistant; *gān cǎo* regulates the middle and harmonizes medicines, used as envoy medicine. The combination of hardness and softness, warm and cool, tonifies the spleen and warms yang without harming yin and causing bleeding, nourishs yin and blood without harming the spleen yang. Wu Ju-tong called this formula a "combination of sweet and bitter, softness and firmness [method]", which is a good match.

[Clinical Application]　This formula is mainly used for spleen qi deficiency-cold syndrome, which is unable to control the blood, leading to bloody stool,

hematemesis, nose bleeding. But now in the herbal pharmacy, there is no *zào zhōng huáng tǔ*, which can be replaced by *chì shí zhī*. For those with a poor appetite, *ē jiāo* can be replaced by *ē jiāo zhū* to reduce its greasy properties; for those with severe deficiency of qi, *rén shēn* or *dǎng shēn* can be added to supplement qi and contain blood; for the profuse bleeding, the blood-stopping medicines like *sān qī* can be added; for those with severe stomach and spleen deficient cold, *pào jiāng* can be added to warm the middle and stanch the blood.

Xiǎo Jì Yǐn Zǐ (Field Thistle Drink, 小蓟饮子)
Formulas to Save the Living (*Jì Shēng Fāng*, 济生方)

[Ingredient]

Shēng Dì (Radix Rehmanniae)　wash, 4 *liang* (24 g)

Xiǎo Jì (Herba Cirsii)　root (12 g)

Huá Shí (Talcum)　(12 g)

Mù Tōng (Caulis Akebiae)　(6 g)

Pú Huáng (Pollen Typhae)　deep-fried (6 g)

Dàn Zhú Yè (Herba Lophatheri)　(9 g)

Ǒu Jié (Nodus Nelumbinis Rhizomatis)　(12 g)

Dāng Guī (Radix Angelicae Sinensis)　removing stem, immersed by wine (6 g)

Shān Zhī (Fructus Gardeniae)　(9 g)

Gān Cǎo (Radix et Rhizoma Glycyrrhizae)　liquid-fried, all half *liang* (6 g)

[Usage]　Chew the original formula, 4 *qian* for each time, one and a half bowls of water, stew until eight-tenths boiled, filter the mixture and take it warm before meals with an empty stomach.

Modern usage: Decocted by water.

[Action]　Cool the blood and stanch the blood, promote water circulation and urination.

[Indication]　Intense heat in the lower *jiao*, blood strangury, frequent urination, inhibited reddish or bloody urine, red tongue, rapid pulse.

[Formula Analysis]　*Basic Questions-Discourse on Qi Recession (Sù Wèn-*

Qì Jué Lùn, 素问·气厥论) says, "when the uterus heat transmits to the bladder, [it causes] dysuria and hematuria". The intense heat in the lower *jiao* damages the yin collaterals, forcing the blood to flow into the bladder and urinating. There is pain for blood strangury, but no pain for hematuria. In the formula, *xiǎo jì* cools and stanches blood, dissolves stasis and generates the new; a large amount of *shēng dì* clears heat and cools blood, stanches blood and dissolves stasis; These two are the chief medicines. As the deputy medicines, the deep-fried *pú huáng* cools blood and stanches blood, and promotes water circulation; *ǒu jié* stanches blood with its astringency and it also dissolves stasis. The chief and the deputy medicines combined, the blood is stanched without leaving the stasis. *Basic Questions-Comprehensive Discourse on Phenomena Corresponding to Yin and Yang (Sù Wèn-īn Yáng Yīng Xiàng Dà Lùn* 素问·阴阳应象大论) says, "Pathogen in the lower requiring dredging therapy", the heat in the lower *jiao* should be dredged. Therefore *huá shí*, *mù tōng*, *dàn zhú yè* can be added to clear the heat and promote water circulation and urination. *shān zhī* (9 g) clears the intense heat in the lower *jiao*, getting out from the urine; *dāng guī* dissolves the stasis and generates the new, leading the blood back to the channels, to clear the heat and promote water circulation without harming the yin blood combined with *shēng dì*. *Zhì gān cǎo* can moderate pain or relax tension to harmonize all the medicines. By being combined in this way, this formula has the effect of cooling blood and stanching blood, promoting water circulation and urination.

[Clinical Application]　This formula stanches the blood and dissolves stasis, clearing and nourishing yin, which is a standard formula to treat the intense heat in the lower *jiao*, blood strangury, hematuria. Usually, the liquid-fried *gān cǎo* can be changed to the tip of *gān cǎo*, for it can straightly go to the penis, clear heat and relieve pain. For severe pain of blood strangury, 1.5 g of *hǔ pò* powder can be swallowed, which promotes water circulation and urination, stanches blood and dissolves the stasis. If the hematuria, blood strangury are unstoppable, add *bái máo gēn* (the fresher, the better), whose action is to cool blood and stanch blood, promote water circulation and urination.

Jiāo Ài Tāng (Donkey-Hide Gelatin and Mugwort Decoction, 胶艾汤)

Essentials from the Golden Cabinet (Jīn Guì Yào Lüè, 金匮要略)

[Ingredient]

Chuān Xiōng (Rhizoma Chuanxiong)　2 *liang* (6 g)

Ē Jiāo (Colla Corii Asini)　2 *liang* (6 g)

Gān Cǎo (Radix et Rhizoma Glycyrrhizae)　2 *liang* (6 g)

Ài Yè (Folium Artemisiae Argyi)　3 *liang* (9 g)

Dāng Guī (Radix Angelicae Sinensis)　3 *liang* (9 g)

Sháo Yào (Radix Paeoniae)　4 *liang* (12 g)

Gān Dì Huáng (Radix Rehmanniae Recens)　4 *liang* (12 g) [for *gān dì huáng*, there is no exact dosage in the book, completed according to the *Important Formulas Worth a Thousand Gold Pieces (Qīan Jīn Yào Fāng,* 千金要方)]

[Usage]　For the original book, the 7 medicines stewed with water 5 *sheng*, wine 3 *sheng* together until 3 *sheng* left, filter, add *ē jiāo* and melt it, take it warm with 1 *sheng*, three times a day. Keep taking it if the patient has not recovered.

Modern usage: Boil the medicines with two-thirds of water, one-third of yellow rice wine, filter the mixture and add *ē jiāo* to melt; take it warm.

[Action]　Nourish the blood and regulate menstruation, calm the fetus and stop the spotting.

[Indication]　*Chong* and *Ren Mai* deficiency, uterine bleeding, profuse dripping menstruation, bleeding after abortion, bleeding during pregnancy with abdominal pain.

[Formula Analysis]　*Chong* is the blood sea and *Ren* controls the uterus. Deficient *Chong* and *Ren* fail to contain the blood vessels. In the formula, *ē jiāo* is sweet and neutral, nourishing blood and stanching bleeding. *Shennong's Classic of Materia Medica (Shén Nóng Běn Cǎo Jīng,* 神农本草经) says it is responsible for "[when]Women uterus [is] bleeding, [should]calm the fetus"; *ài yè* is bitter, acrid and warm, warming the channels and stanching bleeding, *Miscellaneous Records of Famous Physicians (Míng Yī Bié Lù,* 名医别录) says it can treat "women blood spotting". The two are both important medicines for regulating menstruation and

calming fetus, stopping profuse uterine bleeding and stopping the spotting as chief medicines. *Gān dì huáng, sháo yào, dāng guī* and *chuān xiōng* nourish the blood and regulate menstruation, dissolve the stasis and regenerate to prevent leaving stasis while stanching bleeding, used as assistant medicines. Blood cannot be generated by itself, it is generated in the *yangming*, a sea of water and grain, *gān cǎo* supplements the earth, and nourishes blood and harmonizes all the medicines. The combination of *gān cǎo* and *ē jiāo* is good at stanching bleeding, combining with *sháo yào*, sour and sweet medicines boosting yin, moderating pain or relaxing tension and relieving pain; clear wine can lead the medicines to the blood vessels, stanch bleeding without leaving the stasis as envoy medicines. Combining all the medicines, take the manifestation and root cause into accout, block the source and clear the stream, nourish the blood and regulate menstruation, calm the fetus and stop the spotting.

[Clinical Application]　This formula is a crucial formula for stanching bleeding and calming the fetus, treating flooding and spotting, profuse menstruation, bleeding after abortion, abdominal pain during pregnancy. It also can be used in treating traumas during pregnancy, which leads to a restless fetus, bleeding and abdominal pain.

Chapter 16

Dampness-Expelling Formulas

The formula is composed of eliminate dampness medicines, which are good at promoting urination and percolating dampness, and relieving strangury and purging turbidity to expel dampness pathogens. Most formulas belong to the "dry [medicines] can eliminate dampness" of the "ten formula types".

Section 1　Formulas with aromatic medicines that remove dampness

Aromatic medicines decoction has the action of removing dampness as well as dispelling filth and purging turbidity. Dampness is heavy, turbid, sticky and qreasy. It is advisable to use aromatic medicines and bitter, warm and dry medicines to expel dampness and regulate for the syndromes of abdominal distension, belching, anorexia, weakness, and greasy coating caused by internal obstruction of damp-turbidity in the spleen and stomach. Commonly use *huò xiāng*, *cāng zhú*, *hòu pò*, *chén pí*, *bàn xià* to, like *Píng Wèi Sǎn* (Stomach-Calming Powder, 平胃散), *Huò Xiāng Zhèng Qì Sǎn* (Agastache Qi-Correcting Powder, 藿香正气散).

Píng Wèi Sǎn (Stomach-Calming Powder, 平胃散)
Analogous Medical Prescriptions Collection (*Yī Fāng Lèi Jù*, 医方类聚) quote from (*Jiǎn Yào Jì Zhòng Fāng*, 简要济众方)

[Ingredient]
Cāng Zhú (Rhizoma Atractylodis)　without rough peel, pounded into coarse powder, fried until brown, 4 *liang* (120 g)

Hòu Pò (Cortex Magnoliae Officinalis) without rough peel, ginger juice prepared, dry-fried

Chén Pí (Pericarpium Citri Reticulatae) wished and baked, 2 *liang* respectively (60 g)

Gān Cǎo (Radix et Rhizoma Glycyrrhizae) dry-fried, 2 *liang* (60 g)

[Usage] The original formula is pounded to powder, 2 *qian* every time, one cup of water, two slices of ginger, two pieces of *dà zǎo*, decoct it till water remains six-tenths, take out the residue, drink it before a meal.

Modern usage: Make into a powder, 6 g every time, decoct with water. The dosage should be increased or decreased according to the proportion of the original formula.

[Action] Dry dampness, fortify the spleen, smooth qi and harmonize the stomach.

[Indication] Internal obstruction of damp-turbidity in the spleen and stomach, abdominal distension, no appetite, blind and greasy taste, vomiting, belching and nausea, acid regurgitation laziness, somnolence, heavy body and pain joints, frequent diarrhea, white, thick and greasy coating, moderate pulse.

[Formula Analysis] The spleen governs transportation and transformation, which adores dryness and is averse to dampness. If attacked by dampness and turbid qi, or over-eating raw-cold and greasy food, it can lead to dampness obstruction in the spleen and stomach. This formula mainly uses bitter, warm and acrid *cāng zhú* to dry dampness and transport the spleen as the chief medicine. *Hòu pò* is bitter, warm and acrid, moving qi, removing dampness, and eliminating distension and fullness, used as deputy medicine. Acrid, bitter and warm *chén pí* can regulate qi, harmonize the stomach, dry dampness and tonify the spleen, used as assistant medicine. *Gān cǎo* supplements and boosts the spleen and stomach, harmonizes the actions of all medicines. *Shēng jiāng* and *dà zǎo* boost the stomach and harmonize the center. Those three medicines are envoy medicines. This formula can dry dampness and move qi, help the spleen govern transportation. The stomach qi will descend and all the symptoms will be healed themselves. It is named "stomach-calming, just as Zhang Jing-yue says "stomach-calming, treating uneven syndrome by even methods.

It is appropriate for those with stomach excessive [syndrome], to use acrid and bitter medicines to dry, eliminate and disperse dampness and stagnation."

[Clinical Application]

1. This formula is used to dry dampness and transport the spleen. The keys to differentiation include abdominal distension, poor appetite, white, thick and greasy coating, and moderate pulse. If the patient has poor appetite and digestion or diarrhea after eating, use dry-fried *shān zhā*, dry-fried *shén qū, jī nèi jīn* to promote digestion and resolve food stagnation. This is called *Zhā Qū Píng Wèi Sǎn* (Crataegi, Fermentata, Stomach-Calming Powder) recorded in *Treatise on Seasonal epidemic disease* (*Shí Bìng Lùn*, 时病论 [99]). If heat symptoms accompany it, manifested as yellow and greasy coating, bitter taste in the mouth, dryness feeling in the throat and no desire to drink, this is a damp-heat syndrome, It is preferable to use bitter and cold medicines, like *huáng qín, huáng lián* to clear heat and dry dampness.

2. This formula uses *gān cǎo, shēng jiāng, dà zǎo* to neutralize all the medicines, but it is better use less or not be cause such a combination in actual practice may aggravate the excessive dampness and be difficult to remove.

Huò Xiāng Zhèng Qì Sǎn (Agastache Qi-Correcting Powder, 藿香正气散) *Formulary of the Pharmacy Service for Benefiting the People in the Taiping Era* (*Tài Píng Huì Mín Hé Jì Jú Fāng,* 太平惠民和剂局方)

[Ingredient]

Huò Xiâng (Herba Agastachis)   without mud, 3 *liang* (90 g)

Dà Fù Pí (Pericarpium Arecae)   1 *liang* (30 g)

Bái Zhǐ (Radix Angelicae Dahuricae)   1 *liang* (30 g)

Zǐ Sū (Fructus Perillae)   1 *liang* (30 g)

Fú Ling (Poria)   without peel, 1 *liang* (30 g)

Bàn Xià Qū (Rhizoma Pinelliae Fermentata)   2 *liang* (60 g)

Bái Zhú (Rhizoma Atractylodis Macrocephalae)   2 *liang* (60 g)

Chén Pí (Pericarpium Citri Reticulatae)   without the white pith, 2 *liang* (60 g)

Hòu Pò (Cortex Magnoliae Officinalis)   without rough peel, ginger liquid-

fried, 2 *liang* (60 g)

    Jié Gěng (Radix Platycodonis)   2 *liang* (60 g)

    Gān Cǎo (Radix et Rhizoma Glycyrrhizae)   dry-fried, 2 *liang* (75 g)

[Usage] The original formula is fine powder, take 2 *qian* every time, one cup of water, 3 pieces of ginger, one *dà zǎo*, decoct it until water remains to seven-tenths, drink it when it is hot if needs to sweating, cover patient with a quilt, then decoct and drink again.

Modern usage: Make into powder, take 6–9 g every time, twice a day, add 3 slices of ginger, 1 piece of jujube, decocted with water. Or make into pill, take 6–9 g every time with warm water. Or make into decoction, decoct with water. The dosage should be reduced according to the proportion of the original formula.

[Action] Relieves the exterior, removes dampness, regulates qi and harmonizes center.

[Indication] Exogenous wind and cold, endogenous dampness and stagnation, aversion to cold, fever, distension and fullness in chest and diaphragm, abdominal pain, vomiting, borborygmus, diarrhea, white and greasy tough coating, soggy pulse.

[Formula Analysis] This formula applies to exogenous wind-cold and endogenous damp stagnation. Use the acrid, warm and aromatic *huò xiāng* to release the exterior, remove interior dampness, regulate qi and harmonize center, dispel filth and relieve vomiting. It is the chief medicine. *Zǐ sū* and *bái zhǐ* are aromatic medicines, having the action of removing dampness with aroma, can help chief medicine to release the exterior and dissolve cold. *Bàn xià qū* and *chén pí* can dry dampness, dispel phlegm, harmonize the stomach and direct counter-flow downward. *Hòu pò* and *dà fù pí* remove dampness, dissolve distension, lower qi, loosen the center to help expel turbidity and dampness. Those medicines are all deputy medicines. Failure of the spleen to transport leads to dampness stagnation, thus using *bái zhú* and *fú líng* to fortify the spleen and remove dampness. *Jié gěng* diffuse the lung and relieve the diaphragm to regulate the waterways and dispel dampness; those three medicines are assistant medicines. Dry-fried *gān cǎo* can boost qi, fortify the spleen and harmonize all the medicines, *shēng jiāng* and *dà zǎo* fortify the stomach and

harmonize the center as envoy medicines. Taking a panoramic view of this formula, it release the exterior, raise the clear and descend the turbid, reinforce the healthy qi, dispell the wind and cold outside, remove interior dampness, smooth the qi movement, harmonize the spleen and stomach. This formula uses *huò xiāng* as the chief medicine, which can boost healthy qi, so it is named *Huò Xiāng Zhèng Qì Sǎn* (Agastache Qi-Correcting Powder).

[Clinical Application]   This formula is a representative formula for aromatic medicines removing dampness; it also release the exterior. It is appropriate for the syndrome of exogenous wind-cold, endogenous dampness stagnation, dampness stagnation in the spleen and stomach, especially for those suffering from turbid dampness interior and wind-cold exterior, disharmony in the stomach and intestines, it is commonly used. It also has a specific curative effect on vomiting and diarrhea caused by mountain miasma and non-acclimatization.

Section 2   Formulas that clears heat and removes dampness

These formulas are good at clearing both dampness and heat. They are suitable for damp-heat, jaundice, heat strangury (*lin*), leg flaccidity and other syndromes caused by excess dampness and heat (including dampness generated from heat and damp-heat pouring downward). Heat is a yang pathogen and dampness is a yin pathogen. For clear away heat, bitter cold medicines are commonly used. For clear away dampness, bitter warm medicines or percolating-dampness bland ones are commonly used. There are common bitter cold medicines such as *zhī zǐ*, *dà huáng*, *huáng qín*, *huáng lián*, *huáng bǎi* and *lián qiào* and drying-dampness bitter warm medicines such as *hòu pò*, *bàn xià*, *huò xiāng*, *kòu rén* and *cāng zhú*, percolating-dampness bland medicines such as *huá shí*, *yì yǐ rén*, *tōng cǎo*. Typical formulas are like *Yīn Chén Hāo Tāng* (Virgate Wormwood Decoction, 茵陈蒿汤), *Sān Rén Tāng* (Three Kernels Decoction, 三仁汤), *Gān Lù Xiāo Dú Dān* (Sweet Dew Toxin-Removing Elixir, 甘露消毒丹), *Bā Zhèng Sǎn* (Eight Corrections Powder, 八正散), *Èr Miào Sǎn* (Two Mysterious Powder, 二妙散).

Yīn Chén Hāo Tāng (Virgate Wormwood Decoctio, 茵陈蒿汤)
Treatise on Cold Damage (*Shāng Hán Lùn*, 伤寒论)

[Ingredient]

Yīn Chén (Herba Artemisiae Scopariae)　6 *liang* (18 g)

Zhī Zǐ (Fructus Gardeniae)　14 pics, split (9 g)

Dà Huáng (Radix et Rhizoma Rhei)　2 *liang*, peeled (6 g)

[Usage]　Boil the *yīn chén* with 1 *dou* and 2 *sheng* water until 6 *sheng* water left, then add the other two medicines, boil until the mixture remains 3 *sheng*, filtered, take it when it is warm three times a day.

Modern usage: Decocted by water.

[Action]　Clear heat, drain dampness and abate jaundice.

[Indication]　Damp-heat jaundice, yellowish skin all over the body, bright yellow as orange, with sweat in the head without sweat in the body, difficult urination, slightly abdomen fullness, thirst, yellow greasy coating, deep excess or slippery rapid pulse.

[Formula Analysis]　The dampness entangles with the stasis heat inside; while the heat cannot externally overstep, damp heat cannot be discharged downward, and steaming damp-heat develops into yang jaundice. In the formula, a large amount of bitter *yīn chén* is used to discharge and descend, removing dampness, clearing heat and abating jaundice, *Shen Nong's Classic of the Materia Medica* (*Shén Nóng Běn Cǎo Jīng*, 神农本草经) says it can treat "jaundice caused by heat", *Miscellaneous Records of Famous Physicians* (*Míng Yī Bié Lù*, 名医别录) says it can "treat the overall yellowness in the body, difficult urination", it is good at clearing the liver gall bladder heat, and regulating the liver and gall bladder constraint, used as chief medicines; the deputy medicine, *zhī zǐ* is bitter cold, which drains fire and eliminates irritability, clears heat and drains dampness, expels damp heat from urine; a small amount of *dà huáng* can discharge the stasis heat, expel damp-heat from urine, act as assistant medicines, so *The Compendium of Materia of Medica* (*Běn Cǎo Gāng Mù*, 本草纲目) says it treats "dripping urine...jaundice"; *Compendium on Epidemic*

Febrile Diseases (*Wēn Rè Jīng Wěi*, 温热经纬) quotes Xu Ling-tai saying, "Boil the *yīn chén* first, then pathogen gets out from the urine, this is a secret method". Therefore, the original formula is followed by annotation: "disinhibit urine, the urine color like the gelditsia [fruit] juice, reddish color, the abdomen fullness will disappear overnight, [which indicate] the yellow [jaundice] dispelled through the urination." The compatibility of the three bitter medicines, discharge and descend, clear heat and drain dampness, opens a way out for the pathogen, so that jaundice can be cured spontaneously.

[Clinical Application] This formula is the main formula for treating yang jaundice with severe heat than dampness. The key to main differentiation is overall yellowness, bright yellow, inhibited urine, yellow and greasy coating. For the patients with short inhibited voiding of reddish urine, we can add *chē qián zǐ, zé xiè, Bì Yù Sǎn* (Jasper Jade Powder) to clear heat and drain dampness; for the patients with constipation, a large amount of *dà huáng* can be used to discharge heat and promote defecation; for the patients with loose stool, *dà huáng* should be removed and add *huáng lián. Medical Formulas Collected and Analyzed* (*Yī Fāng Jí Jiě*, 医方集解) named it "*Yin Chen Three Substances Soup*"; for the patients with serious abdominal fullness, the processed *xiāng fù, guǎng yù jīn*, coal of *shān zhā, jī nèi jīn* can be added to invigorate qi and motivate blood, disperse accumulation and remove stagnation.

Sān Rén Tāng (Three Kernels Decoction, 三仁汤)
Analysis of Warm Diseases (*Wēn Bìng Tiáo Biàn*, 温病条辨)

[Ingredient]

Xìng Rén (Semen Armeniacae Amarum)   5 *qian* (15 g)

Huá Shí (Talcum)   6 *qian* (18 g)

Tōng Cǎo (Medulla Tetrapanacis)   2 *qian* (6 g)

Kòu Rén (Fructus Amomi Rotundus)   2 *qian* (6 g)

Zhú Yè (Folium Phyllostachydis Henonis)   2 *qian* (6 g)

Yì Yǐ Rén (Semen Coicis)   raw 6 *qian* (18 g)

Bàn Xià (Rhizoma Pinelliae)   5 *qian* (15 g)

[Usage] Boil the formula with 8 bowls of *gan lan shui* (甘澜) [water with bubbles rolling on the surface] until 3 bowls left, take a bowl each time, three times a day.

Modern usage: Decocted by water.

[Action] Diffuse the qi movement, clear damp heat.

[Indication] The first stage of damp warmth, the pathogen in the qi level, headache and aversion to cold, body heaviness and pain, light yellow complexion, chest oppression without feeling hungry, fever in the afternoon, white tongue without feeling thirsty, wiry thready and soggy pulse.

[Formula Analysis] In the first stage of damp warmth [disease], the pathogen lingers at the qi level, and the dampness is heavier than the heat. In the formula, *xìng rén* is bitter and warm, good at opening the upper *jiao*, diffusing and governing lung qi to regulate the water passage. The lung governs all the qi in our body, the qi moves so the dampness can be removed; *kòu rén* is aromatic, acrid and warm, invigorating qi and dissolving dampness having, effects on the middle and upper *jiao*; raw *yì yǐ rén* is sweet, bland and slightly cold, which percolates dampness, enters the lung because of the white color, and enters the spleen with its sweet flavor, percolates dampness with its bland taste, discharges heat with its cold character. These two are serving as chief medicines. Bitter and warm *bàn xià*, *hòu pò* dry dampness, and help *xìng rén*, *kòu rén* diffuse the up and unblock the middle; *huá shí*, *tōng cǎo* are sweet, bland and cold, and help *yì yǐ rén* clear damp heat; *zhú yè* is acrid, bland, sweet and cold, which vents heat, percolates dampness as assistant medicines. Combining the medicines, the upper is diffused, the middle is uninhibited, and the lower is infiltrated. Then the pervasive dampness can be eliminated, among which the diffusing upper is the primany concern so that the qi mechanism is smooth, the dampness is dispelled and the heat is cleared, and all the symptoms are healed by themselves. *gan lan shui* is sweet, bland and light, which avoids generating dampness.

[Clinical Application] This formula commonly treats the early stage of damp warmth, the pathogen is in the qi level, and the dampness is heavier than the heat. If only just use bitter, acrid, warm and dry medicines to remove dampness, the heat will

aggravate; if just using the bitter cold to repulse the heat, the dampness will linger, it is most appropriate to use this formula to diffuse the triple *jiao*, disperse damp heat.

Gān Lù Xiāo Dú Dān (Sweet Dew Toxin-Removing Elixir, 甘露消毒丹)
(also named as *Pǔ Jì Xiāo Dú Dān*)
Supplement to 'Classified Case Records of Famous Physicians' (Xù Míng Yī Lèi Àn, 续名医类案) cited from Ye Tian-shi

[Ingredient]

Huá Shí (Talcum)   15 *liang* (450 g)

Huáng Qín (Radix Scutellariae)   10 *liang* (300 g)

Huò Xiâng (Herba Agastachis)   4 *liang* (120 g)

Yīn Chén (Herba Artemisiae Scopariae)   11 *liang* (330 g)

Shí Chāng Pú (Rhizoma Acori Tatarinowii)   6 *liang* (180 g)

Chuān Bèi Mǔ (Bulbus Fritillariae Cirrhosae)   5 *liang* (150 g)

Mù Tōng (Caulis Akebiae)   5 *liang* (150 g)

Huò Xiâng (Herba Agastachis)   4 *liang* (120 g)

Shè Gān (Rhizoma Belamcandae)   4 *liang* (120 g)

Lián Qiào (Fructus Forsythiae)   4 *liang* (120 g)

Bò He (Herba Menthae)   4 *liang* (120 g)

Bái Kòu Rén (Fructus Amomi Rotundus)   4 *liang* (120 g)

[Usage]   Grind the sun-cured medicines into powder. 3 *qian* each time, mix with hot water or *shén qū* and water, paste a pill as big as a marbles size, and melt it in hot water when taking it.

Modern usage: Suncured all the medicines, grind them into power, make into pills or power, 9 g each time, twice a day; or can be taken as a decoction, modify the dosage according to the original proportion.

[Action]   Clear heat and resolve toxins, dispel dampness and remove turbidity.

[Indication]   Damp warm pestilence, the pathogen in the qi level, [manifested as] fever and fatigue, chest oppression and abdominal distension, sore limbs and

swollen throat, allover yellowness, swollen lower cheek, thirst, short and reddish urine, vomiting and malaria, turbid urine, sores and ulcers, light white, or thick greasy or dry yellow coating.

[Formula Analysis]   This syndrome is caused by the attack of damp warm pestilence with the pathogen in the qi level, the heat is as intense as dampness, constraining qi movement. In the formula, a large amount of sweet, bland and cold *huá shí* is used as the chief medicine to dispel summer heat, promote urination and drain dampness. *Huáng qín* is bitter and cold, which clears heat and dries dampness. *Yīn chén* is bitter, neutral and slightly cold, which clears heat drains dampness. Both are deputy medicines. *Lián qiào*, *shè gān* are bitter and cold, which clear heat, resolve toxins, bitter and cold *mù tōng* clears heat and drains dampness; acrid warm and aromatic *shí chāng pú*, *huò xiāng*, *bái kòu rén* removes dampness and dispels filth, disseminates and facilitates the qi movement, to remove dampness. Damp-heat accumulates and steams, which is easy to generates phlegm; *chuān bèi mǔ* is bitter sweet, slightly cold, which clears phlegm heat; *bò he* is acrid and cool, diffusing and venting, making febrile pathogen come out from the inside. The above are all used as assistant medicines. With the compatibility of all the medicines, the cold and cool clears heat and resolves toxins, the bland percolates dampness and disperses damp-heat, the aromatic removes dampness and dispels filth; three methods are all completed. Among the three methods, heat-clearing is the main one, assisted with percolating dampness, and aromatization is supplemented; the primary and secondary methods are distinguished, which are used to treat the damp febrile turbid pathogen with a sound effect. This formula clears heat in dampness, percolates dampness below heat to eliminate the damp warm toxic pathogen, just like the descent of sweet dew clearing the summer heat, thus it is named "Sweet Dew Toxin-Removing Elixir".

[Clinical Application]   This formula is commonly used in the summertime. For damp warmth, summer-heat warmth, pestilence with the same heat and dampness, pathogen in the qi level, all can be treated with this formula; thus Wang Meng-ying recommends this formula as "the main formula to treat damp warmth and pestilence".

Bā Zhèng Săn (Eight Corrections Powder, 八正散)
Formulary of the Pharmacy Service for Benefiting the People in the Taiping Era
(*Tài Píng Huì Mín Hé Jì Jú Fāng,* 太平惠民和剂局方)

[Ingredient]

Chē Qián Zǐ (Semen Plantaginis)　1 *jin* (500 g)

Qú Mài (Herba Dianthi)　1 *jin* (500 g)

Biăn Xù (Herba Polygoni Avicularis)　1 *jin* (500 g)

Huá Shí (Talcum)　1 *jin* (500 g)

Gān Căo (Radix et Rhizoma Glycyrrhizae)　liquid-fried, 1 *jin* (500 g)

Mù Tōng (Caulis Akebiae)　1 *jin* (500 g)

Dà Huáng (Radix et Rhizoma Rhei)　roasted with flour, remove flour, slice and bake, 1 *jin* (500 g)

[Usage]　The original formula is powder; take 2 *qian* each time with a bowl of water, add *dēng xīn căo* and stew until seven tenth remain, filter and take it warm. The patient should lie down after taking it. Decrease the dosage for children.

Modern usage: Decoct by water and decrease the dosage according to the original proportion.

[Action]　Clear heat and discharge fire, promote urination and relieve strangury.

[Indication]　Damp-heat pouring downward, developing into heat strangury, blood strangury, stone strangury, frequent continuous dribbling urination with pain, yellow or reddish urine, or even dribbling urinary block, lower abdomen distension, with red tongue and yellow coating, rapid excess pulse.

[Formula Analysis]　Damp-heat pouring downward, storing in the bladder, leading to blockage in the water passage and developing into heat strangury. In the formula, bitter cold *qú mài* descends, clears heat and discharges fire, promotes urination and relieves strangury, *Shen Nong's Classic of the Materia Medica* (*Shén Nóng Běn Căo Jīng,* 神农本草经) says it can heal "mainly [treating] anuria and vomiting, dribbling and blockage, urinary stoppage", *Essentials of The Materia Medica* (*Běn Căo Bèi Yào,* 本草备要) says it can "eliminate the heat pathogen in bladder, it is the key medicine for treating strangury", used as the chief medicine;

Biǎn xù, bitter and neutral, clears heat and promotes urination, relieves strangury, in *The Compendium of Materia of Medica* (*Běn Cǎo Gāng Mù*, 本草纲目) calls it is "[good at] promoting urination", used as deputy medicines; *mù tōng* is bitter and cold, *chē qián zǐ* and *huá shí* are sweet and cold. All can clear heat, promote urination and relieve strangury. *shān zhī* is bitter and cold, discharging heat, clearing the triple *jiao*, guiding damp away from urination. Roasted *dà huáng* is bitter and cold, which descends, discharges fire and cools blood, removes damp-heat, promotes urination and relieves strangury, *Pouch of Pearls* (*zhēn zhū náng*, 珍珠囊) says *dà huáng* can "remove the damp heat in the lower *jiao*", *The Compendium of Materia of Medica* (*Běn Cǎo Gāng Mù*, 本草纲目) says it "treats continuous, dribbling urination". The above are all assistant medicines. Liquid-fried *gān cǎo* harmonizes all the medicines, prevents the too bitter and cold medicines from damaging the stomach qi, and moderates pain or relaxes tension, acting as envoy medicine. The above eight medicines clear heat and discharge fire, promote urination and relieve strangury, treat the damp-heat pouring downward strangury, "Heat should be treated with cold", as the straight treatment, it is made into powder and taken as a decoction, thus it is named "Eight Corrections Powder". Adding *dēng xīn cǎo* into the formula, which is light in flavor, has the effect of clearing heat and draining urination. Since it enters the heart and lung meridians, it clears the lung fire and subdues the heart fire. The lung is the source of qi transformation, and the heart is connected to the small intestine.

[Clinical Application] This bitter cold formula is commonly used to treat heat strangury by unblocking. The damp-heat pouring downward, continuous, dribbling urination, frequent urination with pain, or even dribbling urinary block, lower abdomen distension, all belong to excess heat syndrome, which can all be treated by this formula. For the blood strangury, *xiǎo jì*, *bái máo gēn* can be added to cool blood and stanch bleeding; for stone strangury, we can add *jīn qián cǎo*, *hǎi jīn shā*, *shí wéi, jī nèi jīn* to remove the stone and relieve strangury.

Èr Miào Sǎn (Two Mysterious Powder, 二妙散)
Essential Teachings of [Zhu] Dan Xi (Dān Xī Xīn Fǎ, 丹溪心法)

[Ingredient]

Huáng Bò (Cortex Phellodendri Chinensis)   deep-fried

Cāng Zhú (Rhizoma Atractylodis)   soaked by washing water of rice and deep-fry the same dosage each (there's no exact dosage of each in original book)

[Usage]   Boil the powder of the two medicines and take it with ginger juice. The two medicines both have a masculinity character, thus a little wine can be added to assist for the patients with excess exterior and qi.

Modern usage: Make into a powder or pills, 6 g each time with hot water or ginger juice, twice daily. It also can be used as a decoction and the dosage should be modified according to the disease situation.

[Action]   Clear heat and dry dampness.

[Indication]   Damp-heat pouring downward, flaccid lower limbs, or red swollen painful knees, leukorrhea and strangury turbidity, eczema in the genital, yellow greasy tongue coating.

[Formula Analysis]   Living in a damp environment for a long time, or getting soaked in the rain, or wading through water lead to steaming and stagnation of damp-heat, which would immerse the meridians and sinews, leading to slacken and extend of meridians and sinews, which is usually [mainifested as] the flaccidity of lower limbs and atrophy, [that is] *wěi*. In the formula, *huáng bǎi* is bitter and cold, which clears heat and dries dampness. *cāng zhú* is bitter and warm, which dries dampness. Together they clear heat and dry dampness, which is the best for the damp-heat pouring downward patients whose healthy qi is still sufficient. Just like Wang Jin-san said, "this is the pattern of *ǒu fāng* (偶方)[①] formula...treating the damp-heat in yin aspect with a good effect", thus it is named "Two Mysterious Powder".

[Clinical Application]   This formula is commonly used for treating damp-

---

[①]   *ou fang* (偶方): in ancient times, each medicine not only has its natures and tastes, but also has its direction, if there have two directions medicines in one formula, that is called *ou fang* (偶方), while if all the medicines are in the same directions, it is *ji fang* (奇方).

heat pouring downward. Generally speaking, the dosage of *huáng bǎi* and *cāng zhú* are equal. For patients with heavier heat than dampness, the dosage of *huáng bǎi* can be increased; for patients with stronger dampness than heat, the dosage of *cāng zhú* can be increased. According to the different clinical symptoms, it can be added with other medicines properly. For instance, add *chuān niú xī* and make them into pills, which is named *Sān Miào Wán* (Wonderfully Effective Three Pill) from *Correct Transmission of Medicine* (*Yī Xué Zhèng Zhuàn*, 医学正传)[100], treating damp-heat flowing downward, numbness of the feet, or as hot as fire; for damp-heat pouring downward, atrophy, numbness, swell and pain in the feet, difficult urination, *yì yǐ rén* can be added to percolate and drain dampness, remove the damp-heat from urination, named *Sì Miào Wán* (Wonderfully Effective Four Pill) from *Convenient Reader on Established Formulas* (*Chéng Fāng Biàn Dú*, 成方便读 [101]). Add *bīng láng* into this formula with the same dosage of each medicine, grind into powder and it is named *Sān Miào Wán* from *Golden Mirror of the Medical Tradition* (*Yī Zōng Jīn Jiàn*, 医宗金鉴), which is externally used for treating umbilical dampness (water) and eczema, and has the effect of clearing away heat, drying dampness and relieving itching.

Section 3　Formulas that promotes urination and percolates dampness

These formulas can promote urination and percolate dampness, which is suitable for syndromes like water and dampness retention, difficult urination, edema, dribbling urinary block, diarrhea. Using these formulas can dispel dampness from urination. The typical medicines for promoting urination and percolating dampness are *fú líng*, *zhū líng*, *zé xiè*, *huá shí* to form formula, such as *Wǔ Líng Sǎn* (Five Substances Powder with Pori, 五苓散), *Zhū Líng Tāng* (Polyporus Decoction, 猪苓汤), *Wǔ Pí Sǎn* (Five-Peel Powder, 五皮散).

Wŭ Líng Săn (Five Substances Powder with Poria, 五苓散)
Treatise on Cold Damage (*Shāng Hán Lùn*, 伤寒论)

[Ingredient]

Zhū Líng (Fructus Aurantii)   18 *zhu*, peel (9 g)

Zé Xiè (Rhizoma Alismatis)   1 *liang* 6 *zhu* (15 g)

Fú Líng (Poria)   18 *zhu* (9 g)

Guì Zhī (Ramulus Cinnamomi)   half *liang*, peeled (6 g)

Bái Zhú (Rhizoma Atractylodis Macrocephalae)   18 *zhu* (9 g)

[Usage]   Grind the five medicines into powder, mix with rice soup, and take it in small tablespoon [*fāng cùn bĭ*], three times a day. Patients must drink more warm water. The disease will recover after sweating.

Modern usage: Make it into a powder, take 6–9 g each time, twice a day, in an empty stomach with warm water or rice soup in an empty stomach. Or, boil with water and take the decoction.

[Action]   Transform qi and promote urination.

[Indication]

1. Exterior syndrome with water amassment inside, headache and slight fever, thirst and eagerness for water, or vomiting when drinking, epigastric *pĭ*, inhibited urination, tense abdomen with white greasy coating and floating pulse.

2. Edema, heavy body, diarrhea, inhibited urination, and cholera.

3. Phlegm rheum, throbbing below the navel, vomit phlegm-drool with dizziness of the head.

[Formula Analysis]   The exterior pathogen in the *taiyang* meridian is unsolved; it transmits to the *taiyang fu* organ–bladder, disturbing the bladder qi transformation and leading to water amassment in the lower *jiao*. In the formula, the main medicine *zé xiè*, sweet and cold, enters the bladder meridian, which can promote urination and percolate dampness; it is used as chief medicine; for deputy medicines, *fú líng* and *zhū líng* are sweet and bland, good at percolating dampness, unblocking water passage; the assistant medicine, *bái zhú* is bitter, sweet and warm, good at torifying spleen, drying dampness and promoting urination as banking up earth to

suppress the water; for envoy medicine, a small amount of *guì zhī,* which is acrid and sweet, can not only release the *taiyang* exterior, but also warm the bladder qi. The five medicines are combined to motivate qi and invigorate blood. The original formula is ground into powder and taken with rice soup. Require the patients to drink more warm water to induce sweating. Thus the sweat and urine are unblocked, and the exterior and interior are resolved.

[Clinical Application]

1. This formula is good at transforming qi and promoting urination, which can treat water stagnation, water amassment in the bladder, water counterflow, phlegm, edema, or diarrhea with its variant decoctions.

2. According to the experience of the predecessors, *guì zhī* is used to relieve the exterior. However, if there is no exterior syndrome, we can replace *guì zhī* with *ròu guì* for its effect of warming yang and transforming qi is better.

Zhū Líng Tāng (Polyporus Decoction, 猪苓汤)
Treatise on Cold Damage (*Shāng Hán Lùn,* 伤寒论)

[Ingredient]

Zhū Líng (Fructus Aurantii)   peel, 1 *liang* (9 g)

Fú Líng (Poria) 1 *liang* (9 g)

Zé Xiè (Rhizoma Alismatis) 1 *liang* (9 g)

Ē Jiāo (Colla Corii Asini) 1 *liang* (9 g)

Huá Shí (Talcum)   smashed, 1 *liang* (9 g)

[Usage]   Boil the five medicines with 4 *sheng* water. Firstly boil the four medicines until 2 *sheng* left, filter and add *ē jiāo* [melt]; take it warm for 7 *he*, three times a day.

Modern usage: Decocted by water.

[Action]   Promote urination, clear heat and nourish yin.

[Indication]   Deficiency of Yin binding with water heat, [leads to] inhibited urination, fever, thirst and desire for water, or vexation and insomnia, diarrhea, cough, vomiting.

[Formula Analysis] The *Shanghan* pathogen transmits to *yangming* or *shaoyang* and turns into heat, which hurts the yin and leads to water binding with heat. In the formula, *zhū líng* is sweet and neutral, percolating and draining dampness with its bland flavor, *Shen Nong's Classic of the Materia Medica* (*Shén Nóng Běn Cǎo Jīng*, 神农本草经) states that it "benefits the water pathway" and it is the chief medicine; *zé xiè* is sweet and bland, promoting urination, discharging heat with its cold character, used as deputy medicine; *huá shí* is sweet, cold and slippery, clearing heat with its coldness, smoothing the water passage, driving heat out from the urination; *ē jiāo* is sweet and neutral, nourishing yin and moistening dryness, preventing all the medicines from percolate and damage yin, as assistant medicines. The five medicines [works together can] are combined to promote urination without damaging yin, nourishing yin without constraining pathogen, removing water and relieving heat, recovering yin and eliminating irritability. So this formula was given the function of promoting urination, clearing heat, and nourishing yin; however, the promoting urination is still the primary purpose, clearing heat and nourishing yin is secondary.

[Clinical Application] The main indication of this formula is inhibited urination caused by deficiency of yin binding with water and heat, which is a half deficiency and half excess syndrome. For heat strangury, blood strangury, and bloody urine caused by deficiency of yin, water and heat binding, all can be treated by the variant decoctions of this formula, which is a way of treating branch and root simultaneously.

Wǔ Pí Sǎn (Five-Peel Powder, 五皮散)
(also named as Five-Peel Decoction) *Hua Shi Central Treasury Classic* (*Huá Shì Zhōng Zàng Jīng*, 华氏中藏经) [102]

[Ingredient]
Shēng Jiāng Pí (Cortex Zingiberis Rhizomatis, Exodermis Zingiberis Recens)

Sāng Bái Pí (Cortex Mori)

Chén Pí (Pericarpium Citri Reticulatae)

Dà Fù pí (Pericarpium Arecae)

Fú Líng Pí (Cutis Poriae)

Same dosage each

[Usage]   The formula is in coarse powder, take 3 *qian* each time with one and a half cup of water, stew until eight-tenths remain, filter and take it warm anytime. Avoid raw, cold, greasy food.

Modern usage: Decoct by water, and the dosage should be determined according to the original proportion.

[Action]   Promote urination and disperse swelling, regulate qi and fortify the spleen.

[Indication]   Edema, swollen head, face, four limbs, heavy limbs, heart and abdomen distension, rapid panting, inhibited urination with white greasy tongue coating.

[Formula Analysis]   The spleen belongs to earth and qi transports water. In the formula, *chén pí* is acrid, bitter and warm, which regulates qi, dissipates dampness, and harmonizes the middle and is a medicine of unblocking and dredging. *fú líng pí* is sweet and bland, which promotes urination, percolates dampness, disperses swelling, specializes in treating edema and anasarca, motivating qi and removing dampness. Since earth restricts water; these two medicines work as chief medicines. *Sāng bái pí* is sweet and cold, which drains the lung and directs qi downward, motivates water to disperse swelling, used as assistant medicines; *dà fù pí* is acrid and slightly warm, which can lower qi and disinhibit water; *shēng jiāng pí* is pungent and cool, which can induce diuresis to alleviate edema. The combination of the five medicines embodies the compatibility method of motivating qi and promoting urination so that when qi moves, water moves, aiming to in soothing the spleen qi, draining dampness and dispersing swelling. Those five medicines in this formula are all used the peel part, which means to promote skin [pí 皮] by peel and they are decocted in a powder, thus named "Five-Peel Decoction".

[Clinical Application]   This formula is a general formula for treating edema.

The critical points of pattern differentiation are swollen head, face, four limbs, heavy limbs, heart and abdomeninal distension, panting, inhibited urination. The pathogen is located in the spleen and lung. For patients with wind pathogen, *zǐ sū yè*, *qín jiāo*, *jīng jiè* and *fáng fēng* can be added; for the patients with swollen lumbar, water pouring downward, we can add *chì xiǎo dòu*, *yì yǐ rén*, *fáng jǐ*, *chē qián zǐ*, *zé xiè*, etc; for constipation and difficult urination, we can add *xìng rén*, *tíng lì zǐ*; for the patients with yin water, we can add *fù zǐ*, *guì zhī*; for the *yang* edema, we can add *mù tōng*, *huá shí*.

Fáng Jǐ Huáng Qí Tāng (Stephania Root and Astragalus Decoction, 防己黄芪汤)
Essentials from the Golden Cabinet (*Jīn Guì Yào Lüè*, 金匮要略)

[Ingredient]

Fáng Jǐ (Radix Stephaniae Tetrandrae)   1 *liang* (12 g)

Huáng Qí (Radix Astragali)   1 *liang* and 1 *fen*, remove stem (15 g)

Bái Zhú (Rhizoma Atractylodis Macrocephalae)   3 *fen* (9 g)

Gān Cǎo (Radix et Rhizoma Glycyrrhizae)   half *liang*, liquid-fried (6 g)

[Usage]   File the formula to get powder, take 5 *qian bi* each time with 4 slices of *shēng jiāng*, one piece of *dà zǎo*, half a cup of water, boil it until eight-tenths left, filter and take it warm.

Modern usage: Decocted by water, add *shēng jiāng* and *dà zǎo* (appropriate amount).

[Action]   Boost qi and dispel wind, strengthens spleen and promote urination.

[Indication]   Wind edema or wind-dampness, floating pulse and heavy body, sweat and aversion to wind, inhibited urination.

[Formula Analysis]   The wind edema and wind-dampness treated by this formula are caused by the insecurity of exterior qi, externally-contracted wind pathogen, and water stagnation in the striae and interstices. In the formula, a large amount of sweet and slightly warm *huáng qí* is used to boost qi and consolidate the exterior, promote urination. *Formula Collection* (*Yào Zhēng*, 药征) [103] says that it "treats the superior water in the skin". *Fáng jǐ* is acrid, cold and quite bitter, which

dispels wind and promotes urination, matching with *huáng qí*, exerts a strong effect to promote urination without harming the healthy qi. They are the chief medicines. For the deputy medicine, *bái zhú* is bitter, sweet and warm, strengthening spleen and drying dampness, helping *fáng jǐ* promote urination and assisting *huáng qí* consolidate the exterior and arrest sweating as the assistant medicine. *Gān cǎo* boosts qi and fortifies spleen, strengthens the spleen and stomach, removes the dampness, harmonizes all the medicines, alleviates the bitter acrid cold character of *fáng jǐ*, served as the envoy medicine; *shēng jiāng* and *dà zǎo* are acrid and sweet, with a dispersing effect, harmonizing *ying* and *wei* as envoy medicine. There are only six medicines in this formula, which can strengthen the healthy qi and remove pathogens, and complement each other. When the *wei* is strong and the exterior is consolidated, the wind pathogen will be prevented and will not re-enter; when the spleen qi is boosted, the dampness will be dredged out without accumulation. For deficiency in the exterior, wind edema and wind-dampness syndromes all can be cured. There is a postscript: "the patient feels like a worm moving under the skin after taking [the decoction]". This is the sign that *wei* yang is recovering, and wind-dampness is resolving. It is also: "the patient has ice-freezing sensation below the waist, then ask him to sit in the quilt, and wrap another quilt around the waist to warm and sweat slightly", which is the externally protect method to unblock the yang qi.

[Clinical Application]   This formula is commonly used to treat exterior deficiency combined with wind edema and wind-dampness. The main symptoms are edema, numbness in the four limbs and pain in the waist. The concurrent symptoms are floating pulse, aversion to wind and inhibited urination.

Section 4   Formulas that warmly resolves watery dampness

The formulas for warmly resolving watery dampness have the effect of warming yang and removing dampness, which is suitable for kidney affection by cold-dampness (*shèn zhuó*, 肾着), leg qi (*jiǎo qì*, 脚气) and phlegm, yin water caused by deficiency of yang and watery stagnation. The common yang-warming medicines are *gān jiāng*,

guì zhī and *fù zǐ*, combined with urination-promoting medicines like *bái zhú*, *fú líng* to form formulas. The typical formulas are *Shí Pí Sǎn* (Spleen-Strengthening Powder, 实脾散), *Líng Guì Zhú Gān Tāng* (Poria, Cinnamon Twig, Atractylodes Macrocephala and Licorice Decoction, 苓桂术甘汤), *Jī Míng Sǎn* (Rooster's Crow Powder, 鸡鸣散).

Shí Pí Sǎn (Spleen-Strengthening Powder, 实脾散)
Formulas to Aid the Living (*Jì Shēng Fāng*, 济生方)

[Ingredient]

Hòu Pò (Cortex Magnoliae Officinalis) peel, processed with ginger, deep-fried

Bái Zhú (Rhizoma Atractylodis Macrocephalae) remove pulp

Mù Xiāng (Radix Aucklandiae) without fire

Cǎo Guǒ (Fructus Tsaoko)

Dà Fù Zǐ (Arecae Semen) processed, remove peel and umbilicus

Fú Líng (Poria) peel

Gān Jiāng (Rhizoma Zingiberis) processed

1 *liang* above each (30 g)

Gān Cǎo (Radix et Rhizoma Glycyrrhizae) liquid-fried, half *liang* (15 g)

[Usage] Chew with the mouth, take 4 *qian* each time with 1 and a half cups of water, 5 slices of *shēng jiāng*, one *dà zǎo*, stew it until seven-tenths remained, filter and take it warm without time limitation.

Modern usage: Decocted by water with 5 slices of *shēng jiāng*, 1 *dà zǎo*. Other dosages are according to the original formula.

[Action] Warm yang and fortify the spleen, invigorate qi and promote urination.

[Indication] Yin edema, swelling of the limbs, especially in the lower part, chest and abdomen distension, heavy body with destructive appetite, cold hands and feet, not feeling thirsty, short and clear scanty urine, loose stool, pale tongue with greasy coating, deep slow or deep thready pulse.

[Formula Analysis] The spleen and kidney yang deficiency cause yin edema, qi does not transform to water, leading to water stagnation. In the formula, *fù*

293

zǐ and *gān jiāng* are very acrid and hot, warming the spleen and kidney, strengthening yang and suppressing yin, serving as chief medicines. *Bái zhú* and *fú líng* fortify the spleen and replenish qi, percolate and drain dampness with a bland flavour, used as deputy medicines. As assistant medicines, *hòu pò* relieves abdominal fullness, *mù xiāng* invigorates qi, *dà fù zǐ*, *bīng láng* invigorates qi and promotes urination, *cǎo guǒ* warms the middle and dries dampness, most subtly *mù guā*, restrains yin fluids with a sour flavor, removing dampness and harmonizing the middle with warmth, restraining the acrid and hot medicines in case that the yin is damaged, removing the water without harming fluids. The envoy medicines, *gān cǎo*, *shēng jiāng* and *dà zǎo* harmonize all the medicines and *ying* and *wei*. A large portion of *shēng jiāng* warms and disperses water qi. The combination of these medicines can warm the yang and strengthen the spleen, invigorate qi and promote urination, just like *Golden Mirror of the Medical Tradition* (*Yī Zōng Jīn Jiàn*, 医宗金鉴) says, "qi is the mother of water, earth is the defense of water, when qi moves then water moves, [when] the earth is firm then the water is restricted; thus the formula is named Spleen-Strengthening".

[Clinical Application]　This formula is essential for treating yin edema. In the formula, there are more medicines to warm the yang and invigorate qi, but the medicines to strengthen the healthy qi and boost qi are insufficient. For patients with weak breathing and low voice, deficient healthy qi, the formula should be modified. *Golden Mirror of the Medical Tradition* (*Yī Zōng Jīn Jiàn*, 医宗金鉴) claims that "add *fù zǐ* into *Lǐ Zhōng Tāng* (Center-Regulating Soup), and multiply the dosage of *fú líng* and use it as the chief medicine. The original qi is warmed to promote water, which is the best way".

Líng Guì Zhú Gān Tāng (Poria, Cinnamon Twig, Atractylodes Macrocephala and Licorice Decoction, 苓桂术甘汤)
Essentials from the Golden Cabinet (*Jīn Guì Yào Lüè*, 金匮要略)

[Ingredient]

Fú Líng (Poria)　4 *liang* (12 g)

Guì zhī (Ramulus Cinnamomi)　3 *liang* (9 g)

Bái Zhú (Rhizoma Atractylodis Macrocephalae)　3 *liang* (9 g)

Gān Cǎo (Radix et Rhizoma Glycyrrhizae)　2 *liang* (6 g)

[Usage]　Boil the four medicines with 6 *sheng* of water until 3 *sheng* left, filter and remove the sediment, and take it warm three times.

Modern usage: Decocted by water.

[Action]　Warm yang and dissolve rheum (fluid retention), fortify the spleen and dissolve the rheum.

[Indication]　Phlegm-fluid retention, propping fullness in the chest and rib-side, dizzy vision and palpitation, shortness of breath, cough, white slippery coating with wiry, slippery pulse or deep tight pulse.

[Formula Analysis]　Yang deficiency in the middle *jiao*, the spleen fails to transport and transform water, accumulating dampness and turning to phlegm-fluid retention. In the formula, a large amount of *fú líng* is used to fortify the spleen, percolate and drain dampness. *Shen Nong's Classic of the Materia Medica* (*Shén Nóng Běn Cǎo Jīng*, 神农本草经) says that "it treats the counterflow of qi in the chest...promotes urination", as the chief medicine. *Guì zhī* warms yang, transforms qi and promotes urination, used as deputy medicines. *Bái zhú* fortifies the spleen, dries dampness and promotes urination, as assistant medicine. *Zhì gān cǎo* harmonizes all the medicines, helping *fú líng*, *bái zhú* supplement the spleen and boost qi. Combined with *guì zhī*, it supports yang with the combination of acrid and sweet flavors, as envoy medicine. All the four medicines combined, the middle yang can recover and the qi can be activated, the function of the spleen is restored, then the fluid pathogen is eliminated, which is a method to treat the root. Also seen in *Essentials from the Golden Cabinet* (*Jīn Guì Yào Lüè*, 金匮要略), the formula is "for [the patients] with phlegm, should be treated with warm medicines to harmonize it", "for the ones with shortness of breath and slight edema, the pathogen should be removed from the urine". Thus, using warm medicines and promoting urination are important methods for treating phlegm-fluid retention.

[Clinical Application]　This formula essential for warming the yang and dissolving the rheum. For the patients with profuse phlegm, we can add prepared

bàn xià, *chén pí* to dry dampness and dissolves phlegm; for the patients with spleen deficiency, we can add *dǎng shēn* to boost qi and supplement the spleen.

Jī Míng Sǎn (Rooster's Crow Powder, 鸡鸣散)
Effective Medical Formulas Arranged by Category by Master Zhu
(*Lèi Biān Zhū Shì Jí Yàn Fāng*, 类编朱氏集验方)[104] *cited from Huai Tou Lao Bin*

[Ingredient]

Bīng Láng (Semen Arecae)   7 pic (12 g)

Chén Pí (Pericarpium Citri Reticulatae)

Mù Guā (Fructus Chaenomelis)   1 *liang* each, (9 g)

Wú Zhū Yú (Fructus Evodiae)   2 *qian* (3 g)

Jié Gěng (Radix Platycodonis)   half *liang* (4.5 g)

Zǐ Sū Yè (Folium Perillae) and Zǐ Sū Gěng (Caulis Perillae)   3 *qian* (6 g)

[Usage]   The original formula is coarse powder divided into eight parts. Boiled with three big bowls of water of the last night, simmered over a slight fire till half bowl left filter it, boil the sediment dregs with two boals of water, take one small bowl and mix the two decoctions, settle it beside the bed. In the next day around the five watches of the night (*wǔ gèng tiān*, 五更天), take the decoction to two or three times in cold, warm it a little bit in winter, and after drinking, ask the patient to eat a pancake. If he can't finish it immediately, suggest him to take it gradually in the next few days. After taking this medicine until dawn, the patient should defecate some black dung stool that indicates the cold damp qi which lingered in the kidney come out. The swollen feeling will disappear and the pain will be relieved around breakfast. Take food after the medicines works because this is not a diffusion formula, it doesn't have restraints.

Modern usage: Decocted by water, take it in the morning with an empty stomach 2–3 times in cold. The dosage can be changed according to the original proportion.

[Action]   Descend qi and direct turbidity downward, warm cold dampness.

[Indication]   Damp *jiǎo qì* (leg qi). The ankle is swollen and weak, inconvenience

of movement, numbness and cold pain, chest oppression and sickness; wind dampness invading the feet with unbearable pain, swollen sinews.

[Formula Analysis] *Spiritual Pivot-The Origin of All the Diseases* (*Líng Shū-Bǎi Bìng Shǐ Shēng*, 灵枢·百病始生) says, "the clear dampness invades the deficient [patient], the disease originates from the lower part". *Arcane Essentials from the Imperial Library* (*Wài Tái Mì Yào*, 外台秘要) says, "for *jiao qi* (leg qi), [it is]a disease caused by stagnation". Only diffusing [method] can treat stagnation. In the formula, a large amount of acrid, bitter and warm *bīng láng* is used to lower qi and remove dampness as chief medicine. As deputy medicine. *chén pí* is acrid, bitter and warm, which rectifies qi and dries dampness. *Mù guā* is sour and warm, which relaxes the sinews and quickens the collaterals, harmonizes the stomach and removes dampness. *Essential Readings in Medicine* (*Yī Zōng Bì Dú*, 医宗必读) says "it is the best for [treating] *jiao qi* (leg qi)". With assistant medicine *wú zhū yú*, which is acrid, bitter and very hot it lowers qi and disperses cold. *Shēng jiāng* is acrid and warm, which disperses cold and removes dampness. *zǐ sū yè* is acrid and aromatic and its aroma can vent the exterior and its warmth disperses the cold. It works with *chén pí* to motivate qi, with *mù guā* to disperse dampness. As the envoy medicine, *jié gěng* can go to upper *jiao* and diffuse the lung qi. Qi moves, then dampness removes. The clear ascending is good for lowering the turbidity. These medicines are going to open the upper, conduct the lower, dredge the middle. They work together to lower qi and descend turbidity, warm the cold dampness, driving the long-lingered cold dampness out of the body through stool, and exert an excellent effect on treating leg qi. The original formula is taken at five watches, which is the time for crow and sunrise, yang ascending and yin descending; the yin pathogen is dispersed along with the raise of yang. Take the formula with an empty stomach, thus the effect of medicines can be focused. Therefore, it is named "Rooster's Crow Powder"; take the medicines when it's cold; since cold dampness is a yin pathogen, taking it cold can follow the yin move, preventing the disadvantage of rejection, which is good for improving the effectiveness. Just like *Basic Questions-Comprehensive Discourse on the Five Regular Policies* (*Sù Wèn-Wǔ Cháng Zhèng Dà Lùn,* 素问·五常政大论) says, "treating the

cold with hot medicines, apply it cool", this is co-acting treatment.

[Clinical Application] This formula treats *jiao qi* (leg qi), swollen and weak feet, difficulty in moving, numbness and cold pain, and the curative effect is good. This formula can suppress the development of disease and avoid invading the heart.

Section 5 Formulas that dispels wind and overcomes dampness

The formulas are suitable for head and body heaviness, aversion to cold and slight fever caused by wind coldness in the exterior, or numbness, pain and *bì* syndrome in the lumbar region and knees. caused by wind-damp lingering in the sinews and bones, leading to the common medicines to dispel wind-damp are *qiāng huó*, *dú huó*, *fáng fēng* and *qín jiāo* to form the formula. For wind-damp impediment pain, we usually can combine medicines with nourishing the blood and activating the blood, such as *dāng guī*, *chuān xiōng*, *dì huáng*, *sháo yào*, with the method of "to treat wind first treat the blood; when the blood moves wind naturally disappears". Suppose the patient has a chronic disease with a deficiency in both the liver and kidney and insufficient healthy qi, in that case, we should add medicines to supplement if the healthy qi is harmed while dispelling pathogen, strengthening the healthy qi and dispelling the pathogen. The typical formulas are *Qiāng Huó Shèng Shī Tāng* (Notopterygium Dampness-Drying Decoction, 羌活胜湿汤), *Dú Huó Jì Shēng Tāng* (Pubescent Angelica and Mistletoe Decoction, 独活寄生汤).

Qiāng Huó Shèng Shī Tāng (**Notopterygium Dampness-Drying Decoction, 羌活胜湿汤**)
Treatise on Clarification of Perplexities About Internal and External Damage (***Nèi Wài Shāng Biàn Huò Lùn,*** 内外伤辨惑论)

[Ingredient]

Qiāng Huó (Rhizoma Et Radix Notopterygii)   1 *qian* (3 g)

Dú Huó (Radix Angelicae Pubescentis)   1 *qian* (3 g)

Găo Běn (Rhizoma Ligustici)   5 *fen* (1.5 g)

Fáng Fēng (Radix Saposhnikoviae) 5 *fen* (1.5 g)

Gān Cǎo (Radix et Rhizoma Glycyrrhizae) 5 *fen* (1.5 g)

Chuān Xiōng (Rhizoma Chuanxiong) 5 *fen* (1.5 g)

Màn Jīng Zǐ (Fructus Viticis) 3 *fen* (1 g)

[Usage] Chew, boil it with two cups of water until one cup is left, filter and take it warm with an empty stomach before meals.

Modern usage: Decocted by water.

[Action] Dispel wind and overcome dampness.

[Indication] Wind-damp in the exterior, heavy head and body, heavy pain in the spine, or pain all over the body, hard to turn around, with an aversion to cold, white greasy coating and floating moderate pulse.

[Formula Analysis] *Taiyang* governs the exterior of the body. *The Spiritual Pivot-Channel* (*Líng Shū-Jing Mai*, 灵枢·经脉) says "the foot *taiyang* bladder channel from the top of the head returns to the outside and branches out to descend along the nape, ...moves on both sides of the spine and reaches the center of the lower back." In the formula, *qiāng huó* is acrid, bitter and warm with light flavor and strong qi, good at ascending, *Encountering the Sources of the "Classic of Materia Medica"* (*Běn Jīng Féng Yuán*, 本经逢原) says, "it treats the contention between wind and dampness in *taiyang*, pain in the whole body". It has the effect to dispel wind and overcome dampness as the chief medicine. As deputy medicine, *dú huó* is acrid and bitter, slightly warm, helping *qiāng huó* unblock the body, dispelling wind and overcoming dampness. *Encountering the Sources of the "Encountering the Sources of the Classic of Materia Medica"* (*Běn Jīng Féng Yuán*, 本经逢原) says that "there are descending in the ascending, reaching and unblocking the whole body to disperse wind-damp". As assistant medicine, *gǎo běn* is acrid and warm, dispersing and ascending, particularly to the head, dispelling wind and overcoming dampness. *Pouch of Pearls* (*zhēn zhū náng*, 珍珠囊) says "it treats *taiyang* headache and parietal headache". *Fáng fēng* is acrid, sweet and slightly warm, good at dispelling wind pathogen, overcoming dampness and relieving pain. *Chuān xiōng* is acrid and warm, dispersing and ascending, raising the clear yang and dispelling wind-damp, as

important medicine to treat headache. Besides, it is good at treating *taiyang* headache with *qiāng huó*. *Màn jīng zǐ* is acrid, bitter and neutral, light and floating, ascending and dispersing, dispelling wind-damp to relieve headache. As envoy medicine, *zhì gān cǎo* harmonizes all the medicines and relaxes tensions with sweet flavor so that the wind medicine would not disperse too much and the damp pathogen getting out from slight sweating. The formula's original dosage are low, meaning "light [medicines] can eliminate repletion". Taking this formula is suitable for promoting sweating, better with slight sweating to dispel the wind-damp pathogen; if inducing sweating heavily, the wind qi is eliminated but the dampness left, the disease cannot be cured.

[Clinical Application]　This formula is not only used to treat wind-damp in the exterior, headache and head heaviness, pain in the lumbar and spine, but also exert a good effect on treating wind damage headaches. *Medical Formulas Collected and Analyzed* (*Yī Fāng Jí Jiě*, 医方集解) remarks, "though this decoction is named dampness-drying, it is actually a universal formula in wind damage headache".

Dú Huó Jì Shēng Tāng (Pubescent Angelica and Mistletoe Decoction, 独活寄生汤)
Valuable Prescriptions of Emergency (*Bèi Jí Qiān Jīn Fāng*, 备急千金方)

[Ingredient]

Dú Huó (Radix Angelicae Pubescentis)　3 *liang* (9 g)

Sāng Jì Shēng (Herba Taxilli)　2 *liang* (6 g)

Dù Zhòng (Cortex Eucommiae)　2 *liang* (6 g)

Niú Xī (Radix Cyathulae)　2 *liang* (6 g)

Xì Xīn (Radix Et Rhizoma Asari)　2 *liang* (6 g)

Qín Jiāo (Radix Gentianae Macrophyllae)　2 *liang* (6 g)

Fú Líng (Poria)　2 *liang* (6 g)

Guì Xīn (Cinnamomi Cortex Rasus)　2 *liang* (6 g)

Fáng Fēng (Radix Saposhnikoviae)　2 *liang* (6 g)

Chuān Xiōng (Rhizoma Chuanxiong)　2 *liang* (6 g)

Rén Shēn (Radix et Rhizoma Ginseng)　2 *liang* (6 g)

Gān Cǎo (Radix et Rhizoma Glycyrrhizae) 2 *liang* (6 g)

Dāng Guī (Radix Angelicae Sinensis) 2 *liang* (6 g)

Sháo Yào (Radix Paeoniae) 2 *liang* (6 g)

Gān Dì Huáng (Radix Rehmanniae Recens) 2 *liang* (6 g)

[Usage] Chew the fifteen medicines in the original formula and decoct with a *dou* of water until 3 *sheng* of water left, take it warm for three times.

Modern usage: Decocted by water.

[Action] Supplement the liver and kidney, tonify qi and blood, dispel wind-dampness, relieve *bì* pain.

[Indication] Deficiency in liver and kidney, wind-cold damp *bì*, cold pain in the lumbar and knees, impeded bending and stretching, or numbness, aversion to cold and preference to warmth, pale tongue with white coating, thready and weak pulse.

[Formula Analysis] The lumbar region is the house of kidney and the knee is the house of sinews. Due to the deficiency of both liver and kidney, the wind cold damp pathogens invade the body easily, and linger in the lumbar region and knees. In the formula, a large amount of *dú huó*, acrid, bitter and slightly warm, enters the foot *shaoyin* kidney channel, dispelling wind and overcoming dampness, alleviating *bì* and relieving pain. *Sāng jì shēng* is bitter and neutral, which enters the liver-kidney meridians, tonifying the liver and kidney, strengthening sinews and bones, dispelling wind-damp, *Shennong's Classic of Materia Medica (Shén Nóng Běn Cǎo Jīng*, 神农本草经) (hereinafter referred to as *Běn Jīng*) says, "it treats lumbago", and *Miscellaneous Records of Famous Physicians (Míng Yī Bié Lù*, 名医别录) says "it alleviates *bì*". These two are chief medicines. As deputy medicine, *dù zhòng* is sweet, acrid and warm, enriching and nourishing liver and kidney, strengthening sinews and bones. *Běn Jīng* describes "it treats pain in the lumbar region and spine...consolidates the sinews and bones". *Niú xī* is bitter, sour and neutral, supplementing the kidney and liver, strengthening the lumbar region and knees, and invigorating blood, unblocking joints. *Běn Jīng* says, "it treats cold damp atrophy and *bì*, spasms in the limbs, unable to bend the knees because of pain." *Rén shēn, fú líng* and *gān cǎo* are assistant medicines to boost and reinforce healthy qi, which is the so-called "strengthen the

healthy qi first when you want to dispel the pathogen, the pathogen can be eliminated when the healthy qi is sufficient". *Xì xīn* disperses wind cold in the *shaoyin* channel, then the pathogens will disappear. *Guì xīn* enters the liver and kidney blood level to dispel yin cold. *Qín jiāo* and *fáng fēng* dispel wind and overcome dampness, alleviate impediment and relieve pain. *Dú huó* is the channel conductor of *shaoyin* and also the envoy medicine. The combination of all the medicines reflects the method of treating the root and branch simultaneously; this formula reinforces the healthy qi and dispels pathogen, boosts blood qi and dispels wind-damp, thus the liver and kidney are strong and the pain of *bì* is cured, The intention of the combination is quite thoughtful.

[Clinical Application]   This formula is used to treat deficiency of liver and kidney, root vacuity and branch repletion syndrome caused by wind cold damp *bì*; or insufficienoy in liver and kidney, blood and qi caused by wind cold damp *bì* for a long time. For the patients with severe pain of *bì*, we can add *dān shēn*; for the patients with deficiency of kidney yang, we can add *fù zǐ* and slices of *lù jiǎo*.

Chapter 17

Phlegm-Expelling Formulas

⁓

The formulas consisted of phlegm-dispelling medicines with effects to dispel or dissolve phlegm to treat various diseases caused by phlegm are phlegm-dispelling formulas. It belongs to the dispersion method in the eight methods.

Section 1　Formulas that dries dampness and dissolve phlegm

Dampness-drying and phlegm-dissolving formulas are suitable for damp-phlegm-induced diseases. The cause of damp phlegm is the devitalized spleen yang, which leads to the disturbance of transformation and transportation, and stagnation of water-damp, which leads to coagulation of phlegm. Symptoms include cough with profuse white phlegm, chest oppression, distension in the abdomen, nausea, fatigue, dizziness, palpitation, white moist or white greasy tongue. The commonly used medicines to dry dampness and dispel phlegm are *bàn xià*, *chén pí* to form formulas, such as *Èr Chén Tāng* (Two Matured Substances Decoction, 二陈汤).

Èr Chén Tāng (Two Matured Substances Decoction, 二陈汤)
Formulary of the Pharmacy Service for Benefiting the People in the Taiping Era
(*Tài Píng Huì Mín Hé Jì Jú Fāng*, 太平惠民和剂局方)

[Ingredient]

Bàn Xià (Rhizoma Pinelliae)　washed by hot water for 7 times 5 *liang* (9 g)

Chén Pí (Pericarpium Citri Reticulatae)　5 *liang* (9 g)

Fú Líng (Poria)　3 *liang* (6 g)

Gān Căo (Radix Et Rhizoma Glycyrrhizae)   liquid-fried, one and a half *liang* (3 g)

[Usage]   The original method is by chewing the ingredients, 4 *qian* each time with one cup of water, seven pieces of *shēng jiāng* and one *wū méi*, stew together until six-tenths boiled, filter the mixture and take it warm without a time limitation.

Modern usage: Add three pieces of *shēng jiāng* and one *wū méi*, boil with water, with a proportion referred to the original formula. Or make into pills, grind the first four medicines and make them into pills with *shēng jiāng* soup or water, take 6–9 g each time, twice a day with warm water.

[Action]   Dry dampness and dissolve phlegm, rectify qi and harmonize the middle.

[Indication]   Damp phlegm, cough with profuse white phlegm, chest oppression and distension in the abdomen, nausea and fatigue, dizziness, palpitation, white moist or white greasy tongue, slippery pulse.

[Formula Analysis]   Irregular diets, stomach and spleen disharmony, failure of qi transportation, stagnation of water-damp, leads to coagulation of phlegm. In the formula, *bàn xià* is acrid and warm, which enters the stomach and spleen meridians and is good at drying dampness and dissolving phlegm, directing counterflow downward and arresting vomiting. Inhibited qi leads to coagulation of phlegm, which leads to further stagnation of qi function; thus, we use acrid bitter and warm *chén pí* to rectify qi, dry dampness and dissolve phlegm, normalize qi and eliminate phlegm. The two are chief medicines. The phlegm is generated from dampness, and the dampness can be eliminated if the spleen is healthy; then the phlegm can be dissolved too. Therefore, we use sweet and neutral *fú líng* to fortify the spleen, percolate dampness and dissolve phlegm as deputy medicine. As assistant medicine, *shēng jiāng* is acrid and warm, which eliminates phlegm and lower qi, directs counterflow downward and arrests vomiting, constrains the toxin of *bàn xià*, and also helps *bàn xià* and *chén pí* lower qi and dissolve phlegm. A bit of sour, neutral *wū méi* is added to restrain lung qi and promote fluid production, combining with *bàn xià*, *chén pí*, which is astringent within dissipation, removing phlegm without harming lung qi, drying dampness

without consuming fluids with an effect to bring out the best in each other. As envoy medicine, *gān cǎo* harmonizes all the medicines, and helps *fú líng* supplement the earth and harmonize the middle, leading to a healthy spleen, then the dampness will be removed and phlegm will dissolve. This formula has a strict combination and the effect of drying dampness and dissolving phlegm, rectifying qi and harmonizing the middle. In the formula, the chief medicines, *bàn xià* and *chén pí* have better quality with an older age [prepared for a long time], less dry and dispersing, thus the formula is named "Two Matured [Substances] Decoction".

[Clinical Application] This formula is a fundamental and standard formula for expelling phlegm. The dosage can be added or subtracted according to the disease. It can be widely used in various phlegm syndromes. *Medical Formulas Collected and Analyzed* (*Yī Fāng Jí Jiě*, 医方集解) records "It's common to use two *chén* [matured ingredients]to treat phlegm, for wind phlegm, plus with *dǎn nán xīng, bái fù zǐ, zhú lì*; for cold phlegm, plus with *bàn xià*, juice of *shēng jiāng*; for fire phlegm, *shí gāo, qīng dài* can be added; for damp phlegm, we can add *cāng zhú, bái zhú*; for dry phlegm, we can add *guā lóu, xìng rén*; for food accumulation, add *shān zhā, mài yá* and *shén qū*; for old phlegm, *zhǐ shí, máng xiāo* can be added; for qi phlegm, plus *xiāng fù, zhǐ qiào*; for phlegm in the ribs, inside the skin and outside the membrane, *bái jiè zǐ* is suitable; for the phlegm in the limbs, *zhú lì* should be added".

Section 2   Formulas that clears heat and dissolve phlegm

Heat-clearing and phlegm-dissolving formulas are suitable for heat phlegm-induced disease. The cause of heat phlegm is mainly the heat in the interior burning the fluids into phlegm, or constraint of phlegm generating into the fire. Symptoms include cough with yellow sticky phlegm, which is hard to spit out, yellow greasy coating and slippery rapid pulse, or mania, palpitations due to fright, scrofula. The common bitter and cold heat-clearing medicines are *huáng qín, huáng lián, dà huáng* and phlegm-dissolving medicines are *zhú rú, guā lóu, dǎn nán xīng*, and *méng shí* to form formulas such as *Wēn Dǎn Tāng* (Gallbladder-Warming Decoction, 温胆汤),

Xiǎo Xiàn Xiōng Tāng (Minor Chest-Draining Decoction, 小陷胸汤), *Méng Shí Gǔn Tán Wán* (Chlorite Phlegm-Removing Pill, 礞石滚痰丸), *Xiāo Luǒ Wán* (Scrofula-Dispersing Pill, 消瘰丸) and so on.

Wēn Dǎn Tāng (Gallbladder-Warming Decoction, 温胆汤)
Valuable Prescriptions of Emergency (*Bèi Jí Qiān Jīn Fāng*, 备急千金方)

[Ingredient]
Shēng Jiāng (Rhizoma Zingiberis Recens)　4 *liang* (12 g)

Bàn Xià (Rhizoma Pinelliae)　2 *liang*, washed (6 g)

Chén Pí (Pericarpium Citri Reticulatae)　3 *liang* (9 g)

Zhú Rú (Caulis Bambusae In Taenia)　2 *liang* (6 g)

Zhǐ Shí (Fructus Aurantii Immaturus)　2*liang*, liquid-fried (6 g)

Gān Cǎo (Radix Et Rhizoma Glycyrrhizae)　1 *liang*, liquid-fried (3 g)

[Usage]　Cut the medicines, decoct with 8 *sheng* of water until 2 *sheng* left, filter it and take it three times. Contraindicated: mutton, seaweed, pakchoi seedling and sugar.

Modern usage: Decocted by water.

[Action]　Clear the gallbladder, harmonize the stomach, dissolve dampness and remove phlegm.

[Indication]
1. Insomnia caused by gallbladder deficiency and phlegm heat, with palpitation, bitter mouth and vomiting saliva, greasy tongue coating.

2. Damp heat lingers in the qi level of *sanjiao*, alternative chills and fever, chest oppression and abdominal distension, short and reddish urine, greasy and yellow coating.

[Formula Analysis]　The syndrome of this formula is usually caused by emotional stagnation and qi constraint, which generates phlegm, disorderly qi flow and disharmony in the stomach. In the formula, acrid and warm *bàn xià* harmonizes the stomach and directs counterflow downward, dries dampness, as the chief medicine. *Chén pí* is acrid, bitter and warm, which rectifies qi and harmonizes the

stomach, removes dampness and phlegm. A large amount of acrid and warm *shēng jiāng* removes phlegm and harmonizes stomach, and restrains the toxin of *bàn xià*. These are all deputy medicines. *Zhú rú* is sweet and cold, which clears up phlegm, and relieves depression, clears heat and arrests vomiting. *Zhǐ shí* is bitter and slightly cold, which lowers qi and moves phlegm. It works quickly, so it is used as assistant medicine. A small amout of *gān cǎo* harmonizes all the medicines, acting as envoy medicine. The formula dissolves phlegm without dryness, clear heat without coldness, dispell all the phlegm heat, then the *shaoyang* mild qi of gallbladder would recover naturally; thus it is named "Gallbladder-Warming Decoction".

[Clinical Application]

1. The Gallbladder-Warming Decoction in *Treatise on the Three Categories of Pathogenic Factors and Prescriptions* (*Sān Yīn Jí Yī Bìng Zhèng Fāng Lùn*, 三因极一病证方论[105]) and *Formulas to Aiding the Living* (*Jì Shēng Fāng*, 济生方) are just this formula uplus with *fú líng*, *dà zǎo* that used to treat symptoms such as palpitation and insomnia. In clinical trials, adding *fú líng* is indeed more effective. However, *dà zǎo* is unnecessary because it is too greasy and easily generating phlegm dampness.

2. For patients with heart-gallbladder vacuity temerity, easy to be frighted, many nightmares, or shortness of breath, palpitation and fatigue, or spontaneous sweating, swollen limbs, bland taste, heart deficiency with timidity, fetidness, we can remove *zhú rú* and add *rén shēn*, *shú dì huáng*, *suān zǎo rén*, *yuǎn zhì*, *wǔ wèi zǐ*, *fú líng* and this modification is named "Ten-ingredient Gallbladder-Waring Decoction" from *Effective Formulas from Generations of Physicians* (*Shì Yī Dé Xiào Fāng*, 世医得效方[106]). For patients with vexing heat, we can add *huáng lián*, *fú líng* and this one is named "Huáng Lián Gallbladder-Warming Decoction" in *Medical Formula Verses Collection* (*Yī Fāng Zhèng Zhì Huì Biān Gē Jué*, 医方证治汇编歌诀[107]).

Xiǎo Xiàn Xiōng Tāng (Minor Chest-Draining Decoction, 小陷胸汤)
Treatise on Cold Damage (*Shāng Hán Lùn*, 伤寒论)

[Ingredient]

Huáng Lián (Rhizoma Coptidis)　1 *liang* (3 g)

Bàn Xià (Rhizoma Pinelliae)　half *sheng*, washed (9 g)

Guā Lóu Rén (Semen Trichosanthis)　big one (18 g)

[Usage]　Boil the three medicines with 6 *sheng* of water. Boil the *guā lóu rén* first with 3 *sheng* of water. Filter and add the rest 2 *sheng*. Boil until 2 *sheng* left. Filter again, take it warm for three times.

Modern usage: Decocted by water.

[Action]　Clear heat and clear up phlegm, soothe the chest and dissipate masses.

[Indication]　Heat and phlegm bind under the heart, pain under pressure, yellow slippery or yellow turbid coating, floating and slippery pulse.

[Formula Analysis]　This formula is used to treat inappropriate precipitation of exterior syndrome, inward invasion of pathogenic heat, minor chest bind syndrome caused by heat and phlegm bind under the heart. In the formula, *guā lóu rén* is sweet and cold, which clears heat and removes phlegm, soothes the chest and dissipates masses. Combining with *huáng lián*, which is acrid and bitter medicines promoting descent, clearing phlegm turbidity. This formula is suitable for soothing the chest and dissipating masses. Treats minor chest bind syndrome, attacking but not harsh, removing the bind of heat and phlegm in the chest, just like charged up, thus it's named "Minor Chest-Draining Decoction".

[Clinical Application]　This formula treats the minor chest bind syndrome caused by heat and phlegm binding under the heart. The pattern key points of differentiation are pain below the heart under pressure, yellow and slippery or yellow turbid coating, floating and slippery pulse. For patients with severe pain, we can add *zhǐ qiào*, *jié gěng* to ascend and descend qi function with a better effect.

Méng Shí Gǔn Tán Wán (Chlorite Phlegm-Removing Pill, 礞石滚痰丸)

Life-Nuturing Thesis (*Tài Dìng Yǎng Shēng Zhǔ Lùn*, 泰定养生主论[108])

[Ingredient]

Qīng Méng Shí (Lapis Chloriti)　1 *liang* (30 g)

Chén Xiāng (Lignum Aquilariae Resinatum)　5 *qian* (15 g)

Dà Huáng (Radix Et Rhizoma Rhei)

Huáng Qín (Radix Scutellariae)   8 *liang* each, (250 g)

[Usage]   In the original book, the *qīng méng shí* was shattered and put into the crock with *pò xiāo*, sealed with a mixture of salt and dirt, dried under the sun and calcines as the stone color was like gold, ground and mixed with other medicines and make into water pill...Generally take the formula with a sip of hot water and just for swallowing down, and instantly lie on his back, making pills move downward slowly between the throat and diaphragm...before the patient goes to bed. One should not eat or drink water, or stand up and talk until pills remove the stagnation of phlegm and pathogen in the upper *jiao*, the pills pass the diaphragm and enter the abdomen, then move to attack the pathogen. The patient has to take the pills for two consecutive nights. On second day, the patient who defecates stool with phlegm 3–5 times; then can reduce to 10 pills. For the patients [only defecate] 1–2 times, keep the original dosage. If the defecation is 5–7 times, or just 2–3 times, and the condition is stable, reduce 20 pills. After the first night, if the patient does not have defecation with phlegm, we can add 10 pills in the second night. For the strong [body constitution] patients, we can use hundreds of pills. Mostly the patients lie down after taking the medicine, for the ones with sticky phlegm in the throat, which caused by a counterflow of phlegm qi and attacked by the medicines. After a while, the medicines win and the symptoms disappear. Generally, the first time of defecation in the morning is a normal stool, and the rest is phlegm and pathogen or loose stool in appearance but phlegm and fluids inside...This medicine does not discharge or scrape the large intestine, but it can eliminate the accumulation of phlegm and pathogen flowing down from the stomach and intestines without harming the dregs in the abdomen.

Modern usage: Grind into a fine powder and make into pills with water with the size like *wú tóng zǐ*, 9–12 g each time, take it with warm water before sleep.

[Action]   Direct fire downward and eliminate phlegm.

[Indication]   Excessive hot old phlegm leads to psychosis and mania, or palpitation, coma, cough, panting with thick phlegm, or chest oppression and abdominal distention, or dizziness and tinnitus, constipation, yellow, thick and greasy

coating with slippery strong and rapid pulse.

[Formula Analysis]　Excessive heat old phlegm, accumulated for a long time, is easy to change. In the formula, sweet neutral *qīng méng shí* (30 g) moving down, is good at calming and astringing and eliminating hidden old phlegm as chief medicine. As deputy medicine, *dà huáng* is bitter and cold, which clears up excessive heat to open the pass-way of heat fire moving downward. As assistant medicine, *huáng qín* is bitter and cold, which clears heat and discharges fire, *Miscellaneous Records of Famous Physicians* (*Míng Yī Bié Lù*, 名医别录) says "it treats phlegm heat". A large amount of *dà huáng* and *huáng qín* are used to clear fire to treat phlegm. As envoy medicine, a little bit of acrid bitter warm *chén xiāng* discharges and lowers qi, helps all the medicines attack and eliminate the accumulated phlegm, which is treating phlegm requires disinhibit qi. The combination of the four medicines has the effect to subdue fire and remove phlegm, because of its vigorous power to eliminate excessive heat and stubborn phlegm. After taking the formula, the phlegm rolls down and is dispelled from stool, thus it's named as "Chlorite Phlegm-Removing Pill".

[Clinical Application]　This formula treats diseases caused by excessive heat and old phlegm. All the weird syndromes like psychosis and mania, palpitation, coma, cough, panting with thick phlegm, dizziness and tinnitus, or dry stool, yellow thick and greasy coating, slippery, strong and rapid pulse, which can be used to lower fire and remove phlegm, driving the accumulation of phlegm and other pathogens to go out through the intestines.

Xiāo Luǒ Wán (Scrofula-Dispersing Pill, 消瘰丸)
Medical Revelations (*Yī Xué Xīn Wù*, 医学心悟[109])

[Ingredient]

Xuán Shēn (Radix Scrophulariae)　steamed 4 *liang* (125 g)

Mǔ Lì (Concha Ostreae)　calcined, filed and grinded 4 *liang* (125 g)

Bèi Mǔ (Bulbus Fritillariae Cirrhosae)　remove the core, steamed, 4 *liang* (125 g)

[Usage]　Grind the formula into fine powders and make into pills with honey,

3 *qian* each time, take it with warm water twice a day.

Modern usage: Grind the formula into fine powders and make into pills with honey, 9 g each time, take it with warm water twice a day. Or boil with water, the proportion is adjusted according to the original proportion.

[Action] Clear heat and dissolve phlegm, soften hardness and dissipate masses.

[Indication] Scrofula, phlegm nodule, goiter, dry throat, red tongue and wiry, slippery, slightly rapid pulse.

[Formula Analysis] This formula treats scrofula, phlegm nodule and goiter caused by liver and kidney deficiency, fire and dry blood in the liver channel, burning fluids into phlegm, leading to the coagulation of phlegm and fire. In the formula, as chief medicine: bitter, salty and cold *xuán shēn* enriches yin and lowers fire, dispersing scrofula, phlegm nodule, goiter, *Miscellaneous Records of Famous Physicians* (*Míng Yī Bié Lù*, 名医别录) says "it disperses the nodules below the neck", *The Compendium of Materia of Medica* (*Běn Cǎo Gāng Mù*, 本草纲目) says, "dispersing scrofula is scattering fire". Salty, neutral and slightly cold *mǔ lì* dissolves phlegm, softens hardness and dissipates masses as deputy medicine. *Bèi mǔ* is bitter and cold, which clears heat, dissolves phlegm and dissipates masses as assistant medicine. The combination of these medicines, treating both the root and tip, increases fluids, dissolves phlegm and dissipates masses. Then scrofula, phlegm nodule and goiter can be cured.

[Clinical Application]

1. This formula mainly treats scrofula, phlegm nodule and goiter caused by coagulation of phlegm and heat. For the large and hard masses, we should use *mǔ lì*, sometimes with *hǎi zǎo*, *kūn bù*, *xià kū cǎo* to soften hardness and dissipate masses; for the patients with intense phlegm fire, we should use *bèi mǔ*, sometimes with *guā lóu pí*, *hǎi gé qiào*, *hǎi fú shí* to clear heat, dissolve phlegm and dissipate masses; for the patients with deficiency of yin, we should use more *xuán shēn*, sometimes with *shēng dì*, *mài dōng* to enrich yin and nourish fluids; for the patients with hyperactivity of liver fire, we can add *dān pí*, *shān zhī*, *lián qiào* to clear and discharge the liver fire; for the patients with a constraint of liver qi, we should add *chái hú*, *xiāng fù*, *yù jīn*,

qīng pí to soothe the liver, rectify qi and relieve resolve constraint, or with *Xiāo Yáo Săn* (Free Wanderer Powder).

2. There was calcined *mŭ lì* in the original formula. For decoction, raw *mŭ lì* is better.

Section 3   Formulas that moistens dryness and dissolves phlegm

Dryness-moistening and phlegm-dissolving formulas are suitable for diseases caused by dry phlegm. Dryness harming the lung and burning fluids to phlegm causes the formation of dry phlegm. Symptoms include coughing, hasty breathing, choking, sticky and thick phlegm, not easily expectorated out, dry throat, hoarseness and so on. The common dryness-moistening and phlegm-dissolving formulas like *Bèi Mŭ Guā Lóu* Powder (*Bèi Mŭ Guā Lóu Săn*, 贝母瓜蒌散).

Bèi Mŭ Guā Lóu Săn (Bèi Mŭ Guā Lóu Powder, 贝母瓜蒌散)
Medical Revelations (Yī Xué Xīn Wù, 医学心悟)

[Ingredient]

Bèi Mŭ (Bulbus Fritillariae Cirrhosae)   1 *qian* and 5 *fen* (4.5 g)

Guā Lóu (Fructus Trichosanthis)   1 *qian* (3 g)

Huā Fĕn (Radix Trichosanthis)   8 *fen* (2.4 g)

Fú Líng (Poria)   8 *fen* (2.4 g)

Chén Pí (Pericarpium Citri Reticulatae)   8 *fen* (2.4 g)

Jié Gĕng (Radix Platycodonis)   8 *fen* (2.4 g)

[Usage]   Decocted by water.

Modern usage: Same as original.

[Action]   Moisten lung and clear heat, dissolve phlegm and relieve cough.

[Indication]   Phlegm in the dry lung, dry cough. Hard to spit the phlegm out, dry painful throat with dry tongue and little coating.

[Formula Analysis]   Damp phlegm is mostly generated from the spleen while dry phlegm usually is generated from the lung. In the formula, a large amount of bitter

sweet and slightly cold *bèi mǔ* is used to moisten the lung and clear heat, dissolve phlegm and relieve cough. *Guā lóu* is sweet and cold, which moistens dryness, clears heat and dissolves phlegm as chief medicines with *bèi mǔ*. As deputy medicine, *huā fěn* is sweet and cold, which moistens the lung, dissolves phlegm and relieves cough. As assistant medicines, *fú líng* is sweet and neutral, which can dissolve phlegm-drool; *chén pí* is acrid, bitter and warm, which can rectify qi and dissolve phlegm. As envoy medicine, *jié gěng* is acrid to disperse and bitter to discharge, diffusing the lung and removing phlegm, also as the channel envoy of lung channel. The formula can moisten the lung and clear the qi the heat can be cleared and the phlegm can be removed, which is suitable for the syndrome of dry lung with phlegm.

[Clinical Application] This formula is used to treat dry cough caused by dry heat in the lung channel. If the patient's throat is itchy, then we can add *qián hú*, *niú bàng zǐ* to diffuse the lung and soothe the throat; for the patients with dry and painful throat, we can add *xuán shēn*, *mài dōng* to clear heat and moisten dryness; for those with a hoarse voice and blood in the phlegm, we can remove *chén pí* and add *shā shēn* and *ē jiāo* to nourish the yin and stanch the blood.

Section 4   Formulas that warms and dissolves cold-phlegm

Warming and dissolving cold-phlegm formulas are suitable for the disease of cold phlegm. The cold phlegm is caused by deficiency of spleen and stomach yang and interior fluid retention. The symptoms are manifested as clear spit, cough, chest fullness, cold limbs, white and slippery fur with pale tongue, deep pulse. Acrid and heat medicines like *gān jiāng*, *xì xīn* are usually combined with dissolving phlegm medicines like *fú líng*, *bàn xià*. The representative formula is *Líng Gān Wǔ Wèi Jiāng Xīn Tāng* (Poria Sweet Dew five ingredients Dried Ginger and Asarum Decoction, 苓甘五味姜辛汤).

Líng Gān Wǔ Wèi Jiāng Xīn Tāng (Poria Sweet Dew Schisandrae Dried Ginger and Asarum Decoction, 苓甘五味姜辛汤)
Essentials from the Golden Cabinet (*Jīn Guì Yào Lüè*, 金匮要略)

[Ingredient]

Fú Ling (Poria)   4 *liang* (12 g)

Gān Cǎo (Radix Et Rhizoma Glycyrrhizae)   3 *liang* (9 g)

Gān Jiāng (Rhizoma Zingiberis)   3 *liang* (9 g)

Xì Xīn (Radix Et Rhizoma Asari)   3 *liang* (9 g)

Wǔ Wèi Zǐ (Fructus Schisandrae Chinensis)   half a *sheng* (6 g).

[Usage]   The original formula is stewed with 8 *sheng* of water, until boiled and left with 3 *sheng* water, filtered the decoction. Take the decoction warm for half a liter, three times a day.

Modern usage: Decocted with water.

[Effect]   Warm lung and dissolve fluid retention.

[Indication]   Interior fluid retention, cough, clear spit, more salivary, chest fullness, cold limbs, white and slippery tongue coating, deep and wiry pulse.

[Formula Analysis]   The disease is caused by the exuberance of yin and debilitation of yang as well as internal cold fluid retention. This formula mainly uses sweat and bland *fú líng*, which is, as chief medicine to invigorate the spleen and percolate dampness, remove fluid retention, promote urination. On the one hand, it urinates fluid retention; on the other hand, it invigorates the spleen to prevent phlegm generation. Extreme acrid and heat *gān jiāng* can warm the lung to dissolve cold as well as dry dampness to remove fluid retention. *Xì xīn* is acrid and warm, warming lung and dissolving cold as well as removing phlegm and fluid retention; those two medicines are deputy medicines. Use sour and warm *wǔ wèi zǐ* to astringe the lung and relieve cough to avoid *gān jiāng* and *xì xīn* consume lung qi as assistant medicine; thus, it can disperse qi and astringe lung but not hurt the healthy qi and expel pathogen. *Basic Questions-Discourse on How the Qi in the Depots Follow the Pattern of the Seasons (Sù Wèn-Zàng Qì Fǎ Shí Lùn*, 素问·脏气法时论) says, "the

lung need to be astringed [the treatment of lung disease] requires the immediate use of sour flavor to astringe and supplement and pungent flavor to purge". *Gān cǎo* can warm the center, harmonize all the medicines as envoy medicine. This formula only uses five flavors, but it combines precisely, convergence within dispersion, closeness with opening, accompanied with manifestation and essence. It is a beneficial formula to warm the lung and remove fluid retention.

[Clinical Application]　This formula mainly treats syndromes like internal cold fluid retention, cough, clear phlegm, more salivary, *etc.* According to the [methods of] *Essentials from the Golden Cabinet* (*Jīn Guì Yào Lüè*, 金匮要略), add processed *bàn xià* to dry dampness and dissolve phlegm as well as direct counterflow downward to treat dizziness and vomiting. Add *xìng rén* to diffuse the lung qi and remove fluid retention to eliminate swell. Add *dà huáng* to promote defecation to purge stomach heat manifests in a flushed face.

Section 5　Formulas that dispels wind and dissolves phlegm

Dispelling wind and dissolving phlegm formulas are appropriate for diseases caused by wind and phlegm. Factors of Interior and exterior generate the wind phlegm. External wind-phlegm is caused by external contraction of wind pathogen leading to failure of lung qi to diffuse, with symptoms of fever and aversion to wind, cough with phlegm, *etc.* The internal wind-phlegm is caused by spleen dampness, an internal stirring of liver wind, wind-phlegm disturbing up, with symptoms of dizziness, headache, and even coma *etc.* Usually combine medicines like *jīng jiè*, *zǐ wǎn*, *jú hóng* to diffuse pathogen, stop cough, and dissolve phlegm to treat external wind-phlegm; the representative formula is *Zhǐ Sòu Sǎn* (Cough-Stopping Powder, 止嗽散). Usually add medicines like *tiān má*, *bàn xià*, *bái zhú*, *fú líng* to calm internal wind, dry dampness and dissolve phlegm to treat internal wind phlegm. The representative formula is *Bàn Xià Bái Zhú Tiān Má Tāng* (Pinellia, Atractylodes Macrocephala and Gastrodia Decoction, 半夏白术天麻汤).

Zhǐ Sòu Sǎn (Cough-Stopping Powder, 止嗽散)
Medical Revelations (*Yī Xué Xīn Wù*, 医学心悟)

[Ingredient]

Jié Gěng (Radix Platycodonis)　dry-fried

Jīng Jiè (Herba Schizonepetae)

Zǐ Wǎn (Radix Et Rhizoma Asteris)　steamed

Bǎi Bù (Radix Stemonae)　steamed

Bái Qián (Rhizoma Et Radix Cynanchi Stauntonii)　steamed

Each above 2 *jin* respectively (1000 g)

Gān Cǎo (Radix Et Rhizoma Glycyrrhizae)　dry-fried, 12 *liang* (375 g)

Chén Pí (Pericarpium Citri Reticulatae)　irrigated, without white,1 *jin* (500 g).

[Usage]　This formula is in powder, 3 *qian* every time, drink with water after meal but before sleeping. Drink with ginger juice when attacked by wind-cold.

Modern usage: This formula is in powder, take 9 g every time, twice a day, drink with warm water or ginger juice. It can be decoction, or boiling with water. The dosage is modified according to the proportion of the original formula.

[Action]　Stop cough, dissolve phlegm, release the exterior and diffuse lung.

[Indication]　Wind pathogen invading the lung, coughing, pharyngeal itching, or mild aversion to wind and fever, thin white tongue coating.

[Formula Analysis]　Lung, a tender organ in pair with skin and fur, is easy to catch pathogen. *Zǐ wǎn* is acrid, bitter and warm, directing qi downward, stopping cough, dissolving phlegm as chief medicine. Use sweet, bitter and mild warm *bǎi bù* to moist lung and stop cough as well as use sweet, bitter and mild warm *bái qián* to direct qi downward, stop cough, dissolve phlegm as deputy medicine. *Jīng jiè* is acrid and warm, expelling wind, releasing the exterior and benefiting the pharynx. *Jié gěng* is bitter, acrid and even, diffusing lung and expelling phlegm. *Jú hóng* is acrid, bitter and warm, rectifying qi and dissolving phlegm. Those three are assistant medicines. As envoy medicine, a small amount of *gān cǎo* harmonizes all the medicines and when accompanied with *jié gěng*, it can clear the pharynx as envoy medicine. All the medicines are warm or even, having the main effect of stopping cough and dissolving

phlegm, accompanied by the effects of releasing the exterior and diffusing lung. This formula is appropriate for chronic cough, itchy pharynx. Thus it is called *Zhǐ Sòu Sǎn* (Cough-Stopping Powder).

[Clinic application]   This formula is commonly used to treat external-contraction cough. For severe exterior wind-cold syndrome, *sū yè*, *fáng fēng*, *shēng jiāng* can be used to release the exterior and disperse cold. For symptoms like cough with white phlegm, white greasy tongue, processed *bàn xià*, *fú líng* can be used to dry dampness and dissolve phlegm.

Bàn Xià Bái Zhú Tiān Má Tāng (Pinellia, Atractylodes Macrocephala and Gastrodia Decoction, 半夏白术天麻汤)
Medical Revelations (*Yī Xué Xīn Wù*, 医学心悟)

[Ingredient]

Bàn Xià (Rhizoma Pinelliae)   1 *qian* 5 *fen* (4.5 g)

Tiān Má (Rhizoma Gastrodiae)   1 *qian* (3 g)

Fú Líng (Poria)   1 *qian* (3 g)

Jú Hóng (Exocarpium Citri Rubrum)   1 *qian* (3 g)

Bái Zhú (Rhizoma Atractylodis Macrocephalae)   3 *qian* (9 g)

Gān Cǎo (Radix Et Rhizoma Glycyrrhizae)   5 *fen* (1.5 g).

[Usage]   One piece of ginger, one *dà zǎo*, decocted with water.

Modern usage: Same as the original formula.

[Action]   Invigorate the spleen, dry dampness, dissolve phlegm and calm the wind.

[Indication]   Wind-phlegm disturbing up, dizziness, headache, chest oppression, vomiting, white and greasy tongue coating, wry and slippery pulse.

[Formula Analysis]   The syndrome of this formula is caused by the dampness of the spleen and internal stirring of the liver wind. Use acrid and warm *bàn xià* to dry dampness and dissolve phlegm and use sweet and mild warm *tiān má* to calm internal wind. These two are essential medicines to treat wind phlegm, dizziness and headache. Just as *Treatise on the Spleen and Stomach* (*Pí Wèi Lùn*, 脾胃论) says,

"phlegm syncope and headache of foot *taiyin* cannot be cured unless it is *bàn xià,* blind vision, dizziness and internal wind deficiency cannot be eliminated unless it is *tiān má*". These two are chief medicines. Bitter, sweet and warm *bái zhú* invigorates the spleen and dries dampness as deputy medicines. *Pouch of Pearls* (*Zhēn Zhū Náng,* 珍珠囊) says, "expelling dampness to tonify qi, dissolving phlegm to promote urination". It is compatible with chief medicine to dry dampness, dissolve phlegm, stop the dizziness. *Fú líng* is sweat and mild, invigorating the spleen and percolating dampness as assistant medicine, it helps *bái zhú* to eliminate phlegm. *Jú hóng*, acrid, bitter and warm, dries dampness, regulates qi to eliminate phlegm; *gān cǎo, shēng jiāng, dà zǎo* invigorate the spleen and harmonize the center as envoy. A combination of these medicines invigorates the spleen, drying dampness, dissolving phlegm and calming wind.

[Clinic application]　　This formula is commonly used to treat dizziness, headache and the syndrome of wind-phlegm disturbing up. Add *gōu téng, sāng yè, jú huā, nán xīng* to calm the wind and dissolve phlegm to treat severe dizziness. Use *màn jīng zǐ* to eliminate treat headaches. Add *dǎng shēn* to reinforce qi.

Chapter 18

Worm-Expelling Formulas

The formula comprises medicines that can calm roundworms, expel worms, and treat parasitic diseases in the alimentary tract. These formulas are called calm roundworms and worm-expelling formulas.

Wū Méi Wán (Dark Plum Pill, 乌梅丸)
Treatise on Cold Damage (Shāng Hán Lùn, 伤寒论)

[Ingredient]

Wū Méi (Fructus Mume)   300 pics (500 g)

Xì Xīn (Radix Et Rhizoma Asari)   6 *liang* (180 g)

Gān Jiāng (Rhizoma Zingiberis)   10 *liang* (300 g)

Huáng Lián (Rhizoma Coptidis)   16 *liang* (500 g)

Dāng Guī (Radix Angelicae Sinensis)   4 *liang* (120 g)

Fù Zǐ (Radix Aconiti Lateralis)   prepared without peel 6 *liang* (180 g)

Shǔ Jiāo (Sichuan Pericarpium Zanthoxyli)   sweat, 4 *liang* (120 g)

Guì zhī (Ramulus Cinnamomi)   without peel, 6 *liang* (180 g)

Rén Shēn (Radix Et Rhizoma Ginseng)   6 *liang* (180 g)

Huáng Bǎi (Cortex Phellodendri Chinensis)   6 *liang* (180 g)

[Usage]   The original formula pounds and sieves those herbs respectively, then combine the ten herbs. Soaking the *wū méi* without core in bitter wine (*kǔ jiǔ*, 苦酒①) for a night, steaming it under five buckets of rice, mashing it into mud after the rice is

---

① 苦酒 (*kǔ jiǔ*): vinegar, A liquid containing acetic acid made from rice, wheat, sorghum, wine or distiller grains.

cooked. Pestle all the herbs with honey in a mortar a thousand times. Shaping the pill as big as a Phoenix tree seed. Take ten pills after the meal, three times a day, gradually add to 20 pills. Cold, slippery, stinky food is prohibited.

Modern usage: Soak the *wū méi* in five-tenths vinegar for a night, pound it without core, mix it with other medicines, refine it with honey, and make it into pills. Take 9 g every time by warm water before a meal, two or three times a day. It can also be used as a decoction. The dosage should be reduced according to the proportion of the original formula.

[Action]　Warm the *zang* organs, calm roundworms, relieve the liver and harmonize the stomach.

[Indication]

1. Patient with syncope due to roundworm which happens transiently, frequent abdominal pain, extremely cold limbs, sometimes quiet, sometimes irritable, vomits after eating and usually with roundworms, chronic diarrhea.

2. *Jueyin* syndrome, *xiāo kě* (wasting-thirst), qi rushing up to the heart, pain and heat in the heart, hunger with no desire to eat, vomit roundworms after eating. Purgation can lead to diarrhea without end.

[Formula Analysis]　*Golden Mirror of the Medical Tradition* (*Yī Zōng Jīn Jiàn*, 医宗金鉴) says, "Patient with syncope due to roundworms shows pain and extreme cold limbs." Two reasons lead to the syndrome of syncope due to roundworms. One is that the patient has roundworms inside the body, another is deficiency-cold in the *yangming* stomach and large intestine. Roundworms come up to the diaphragm, thus causing the manifestations of upper heat and lower cold, cold and heat in complexity. This formula mainly use *wū méi*, which is sour and neutral to astringe liver qi, engender fluids to quench thirst, harmonize stomach and clam roundworms. *Shen Nong's Classic of the Materia Medica* (*Shén Nóng Běn Cǎo Jīng*, 神农本草经) says, "*wū méi* governing descending qi, eliminating heat, agitation and fullness". *The Grand Compendium of Materia Medica* (*Běn Cǎo Gāng Mù*, 本草纲目) says that *wū méi* can treat "syncope due to roundworms, vomiting and diarrhea." Thus it can be used to treat the syndrome of *jueyin*, "*xiāo kě* (wasting-thirst), qi rushing up

to the heart, pain and heat in the heart." syncope due to roundworms, used as chief medicine. The effect increases vastly by soaking it in bitter wine (vinegar). *Shǔ jiāo* is acrid and heat, descending qi, warming *zang* organs and expelling roundworms as assistant medicine. *Huáng lián* is bitter and cold, purging roundworms, clearing liver and gallbladder. The match between chief medicine combined with assistant medicine is just as Ke Qi says: "roundworms clam down while encounter with sour, hide while encountering with acrid, descend while encounter with bitterness." Because of deficiency-cold of *zang* organs and dysphoria of roundworms, syncope due to roundworms comes into being. To use a group of acrid and heat medicines, like *xì xīn*, *guì zhī*, *gān jiāng*, *fù zǐ* accompanied with *shǔ jiāo* to warm *zang* organs, expel cold, settle roundworms down in the intestine. *Xì xīn*, *gān jiāng*, which is acrid, can disperse and descend qi into the *jueyin* meridian. Eating acrid [flavor] immediately disperses liver qi (*Basic Questions-Discourse on How the Qi in the Depots Follow the Pattern of the Seasons* (*Sù Wèn-Zàng Qì Fǎ Shí Lùn*, 素问·脏气法时论)) *Gān jiāng*, *fù zǐ* can stimulate stomach yang into *yangming* meridian. *Huáng bǎi* is bitter and cold to help *huáng lián* clear the ministerial fire of the liver and gallbladder, suppress the acrid and heat medicines avoid stimulating ministerial fire and eliminate fluid as assistant medicine. Liver stores the blood. Sweet, acrid, bitter and warm *dāng guī* as assistant medicine can nourish liver blood. This formula mixes cold, heat, bitterness, acidity and sour, so use sweet and warm *rén shēn* to harmonize the center qi. Roundworms become active when it meets sweet, thus adding honey as the paradoxical assistant medicine into honey pill to exert the best pesticide effect. Honey harmonized every medicine as envoy medicine as well. Combine all the medicines to warm *zang* organs, clam roundworms, relieve the liver and harmonize the stomach. The indications include syncope due to roundworms, chronic diarrhea, *jueyin* disease that pertains to cold and heat in complexity and deficiency of qi and blood.

[Clinical Application] This formula is the leading prescription to treat the syncope syndrome due to roundworms and *jueyin* disease of cold and heat in complexity. Mixing cold and heat, harmonizing stomach and liver, calming roundworms and stomach, it is also named "*Wū Méi Ān Huí Wán*, or *Wū Méi Ān Wèi Wán*".

Bù Dài Wán (Cloth Bag Pill, 布袋丸)

Supplement to the Pocket-sized Discussion of Formulas for Children (Bǔ Yào Xiǎo Xiù Zhēn Ér Fāng Lùn, 补要袖珍小儿方论)[110]

[Ingredient]

Yè Míng Shā (Faeces Vespertilionis)　selected 2 liang (60 g)

Wú Yí (Fructus Ulmi Macrocarpae Praeparata)　dry-fried without peel 2 liang (60 g)

Shǐ Jūn Zǐ (Fructus Quisqualis)　mild dry-fried without peel 2 liang (60 g)

Bái Fú Líng (White Poria)　without peel half liang (15 g)

Bái Zhú (Rhizoma Atractylodis Macrocephalae)　with no oil, get rid of Aloe half liang (15 g)

Rén Shēn (Radix Et Rhizoma Ginseng)　get rid of Aloe half liang (15 g)

Gān Cǎo (Radix Et Rhizoma Glycyrrhizae)　half liang (15 g)

Lú Huì (Aloe)　grind half liang (15 g)

[Usage]　The original formula is powdery, decocted, drowned, steamed and made into pills shaped as a pellet, one pill at a time. Put it in a raw silk bag, then decocted with lean meat about 2 liang, hung at the windward area for a day after meat cooked, then let children eat meat and soup. Decocting the herbs with the above method, abandoned until the formula's effect is exhausted.

Modern usage: Grind all the herbs to powder at the original ratio, 6–9 g a time, put it in a cloth bag, decocted with lean meat 30–60 g, take out the bag when meat ripe, then let children eat meat and decoction before a meal.

[Action]　Kill parasites, eliminate malnutrition, invigorate qi and strengthen the spleen.

[Indication]　Parasites, and malnutrition in children, yellowish complexion, abdominal distension, emaciation, blurred vision, pale tongue, thin and weak pulse.

[Formula Analysis]　Children with an unclean diet will accumulate parasites that damage the spleen and stomach, consume qi and blood, lead to chronic malnutrition. Without killing the parasites, the pathogens will not be eliminated, without tonifying the deficiency, the health qi will not be restored. This formula

mainly uses acrid and cold *yè míng shā* to treat chancre and improve eyesight, treat malnutrition. *Wú yí* is acrid, bitter and warm, while *shǐ jūn zǐ* is sweet and warm; these three herbs are chief medicines to eliminate malnutrition and kill parasites. Use bitter and cold *lú huì* to help chief medicine eliminate malnutrition, kill parasites, and expel parasites by purgation as deputy medicine. A small amount of *rén shēn*, *bái zhú*, *bái fú líng*, and *gān cǎo* can supplement qi and fortify the spleen as assistant medicines. *Gān cǎo* also can harmonize all the medicines, as the envoy medicine. The original formula is decocted with lean pork meat, which can gain muscle and moisturize skin. It is a subtle formula to expel parasites and eliminate malnutrition without damaging health qi by treating with both attack and supplementation. Because of decocting those medicines in a raw silk bag, we name it *Bù Dài Wán* (Cloth Bag Pill).

[Clinical Application] This formula can kill parasites and eliminate malnutrition and supplement qi and fortify the spleen. It is appropriate for kids with parasites and malnutrition, as well as deficiency of spleen and stomach qi.

Féi Ér Wán (Childhood-Malnutrition Rectifying Pill, 肥儿丸)
Formulary of the Pharmacy Service for Benefiting the People in the Taiping Era (*Tài Píng Huì Mín Hé Jì Jú Fāng*, 太平惠民和剂局方)

[Ingredient]
Shén Qū (Massa Medicata Fermentata)   dry-fried, 10 *liang* (300 g)

Huáng Lián (Rhizoma Coptidis)   without fibre, 10 *liang* (300 g)

Ròu Dòu Kòu (Semen Myristicae)   roasting drugs wrapped in flour paste, 5 *liang* (150 g)

Shǐ Jūn Zǐ (Fructus Quisqualis)   without peel, 5 *liang* (150 g)

Mài Yá (Fructus Hordei Germinatus)   dry-fried, 5 *liang* (150 g)

Bīng Láng (Semen Arecae)   filing without fire then drying under sunshine (150 g)

Mù Xiāng   2 *liang* (60 g)

[Usage] The original formula is grinding the herbs and concentrating to millet-size pills with porcine bile. The average dosage is 30 pills and can be adjusted

according to age. Take the pills with hot water before meals.

Modern usage: Fine grinding and making pills with porcine bile. Each pill weighs 3 g. Take two pills each for those over three years old, one pill for two-year-olds, and half a pill for those under one year old. Melting the pills with warm water and drinking it on an empty stomach.

[Action]   Kill worms, disperse accumulation, clear heat and strengthen the spleen.

[Indication]   Infantile malnutrition with accumulation, dyspepsia, weak body with yellow complexion, halitosis with fever, yellow greasy coating.

[Formula Analysis]   The symptom of worm accumulation and malnutrition is caused by dyspepsia and lead to internal heat. *Shǐ jūn zǐ* is sweet and warm, kills worms and eliminates infantile malnutrition; *bīng láng* is bitter, acrid and warm, kills worms and disperses accumulation; these two are chief medicines. *Shén qū* and *mài yá* are good at promoting digestion; *huáng lián* are good at clearing constraint-heat as deputy medicines, *ròu dòu kòu* is added to strengthen the spleen and promote digestion, *mù xiāng* is added to move qi and remove food stagnation; then porcine bile is added together with *huáng lián* to clear constraint-heat. This formula not only contributes to dispelling worms and accumulation, but also promotes spleen and clears heat which keeps the infant healthy so-called Childhood-Malnutrition Rectifying Pill.

[Clinical Application]   This formula is commonly used to kill kinds of worms, especially ascaris and tapeworms. If the manifestation is without constraint-heat, remove *huáng lián* and use [flour] paste to make pills instead of porcine bile. For patients with spleen deficiency, we can add *dǎng shēn*, *bái zhú* and *fú líng*. For those also with constipation, we can add *dà huáng* and *zhǐ shí* after the worms are killed, tonify the spleen and the stomach to regain the healthy qi.

Annotation

[1] *Treatise on Cold Damage* (*Shāng Hán Lùn*, 伤寒论): A classic work of Chinese medicine written by Zhang Zhong-jing (张仲景) in the Eastern Han dynasty, it is a monograph on the treatment of exogenous diseases, with 12 volumes. Today there are 10 volumes and 22 chapters left. In the process of spreading, Zhang Zhong-jing's original book was compiled by later generations into *Treatise on Cold Damage* caused by exogenous febrile diseases. The other part mainly discussed miscellaneous diseases in internal medicine, which was named *Essentials from the Golden Cabinet* (*Jīn Guì Yào Lüè*, 金匮要略).

[2] *Shen Nong's Classic of the Materia Medica* (*Shén Nóng Běn Cǎo Jīng*, 神农本草经): Also known as *Ben Cao Jing* or *Ben Jing*, written under the name of "*Shen Nong*" in the Han dynasty, it is one of the four classic works of Traditional Chinese medicine and the earliest extant works of Traditional Chinese medicine.

[3] *Golden Mirror of the Medical Tradition* (*Yī Zōng Jīn Jiàn*, 医宗金鉴): It is a large medical series written by Wu Qian and his colleagues in the Imperial Hospital organized by the Qing government and completed in 1742 AD. It consists of 90 volumes. The book collected from the Spring and Autumn period, the Warring States, Qin and Han Dynasties, down to the Ming and Qing dynasties the essence of all previous dynasties medical books.

[4] *Concise Supplementary Exposition on Cold Damage* (*Shāng Hán Míng Lǐ Lùn*, 伤寒明理论) It is a book of typhoid fever in Chinese medicine compiled by Cheng Wu-ji, a famous medical scientist in Song [宋] and Jin [金] dynasties.

[5] Wang Shu-he (210–280): Medical scientist of the Jin [晋] dynasty, whose given name was Xi, was born in Gaoping (today's Shandong area). In the history of the development of Traditional Chinese Medicine, he made two important contributions, one is to sort out *Treatise on Cold Damage* and the other is to write and compile the *Mai Jing*.

[6] Li Shi-zhen (1518–1593): style name Dongbi, he was known as *Bin Hu Shan Ren* in his later years and was a famous medical scholar in the Ming [明] dynasty. *The Grand Compendium of Materia Medica* (*Běn Cǎo Gāng Mù*, 本草纲目), a 1.92-million-character masterpiece, was honored as the "Holy medicine" by later generations. He has written many works, such as *Study on The Eight Extra-Meridians* and *[Li] Bin-hu's Teachings on Pulse Diagnosis* (*Bīn Hú Mài Xué*, 濒湖脉学).

[7] Wang Xu-gao (1798–1862): first name: Tai Lin, courtesy name: Yi Xing, pseudonym: Tui Si Ju Shi, born in Wuxi, Jiangsu. At first, he was engaged in surgery. Later, he specialized in miscellaneous diseases in internal medicine, and paid more attention to warm-heat diseases. Wang's representative academic work is Xi Xi Library Night Talk record. Many of them were lost, and only 30 methods of liver treatment were left.

[8] *Emergency Formulas to Keep Up One's Sleeve* (*Zhǒu Hòu Bèi Jí Fāng*, 肘后备急方), 8 volumes, 70 chapters, written by Ge Hong in the Eastern Jin [晋] Dynasty. [It is the] Ancient Chinese medicine formula works, [known as the] China's first clinical first aid manual.

[9] *Formulary of the Pharmacy Service for Benefiting the People in the Taiping Era* (*Tài Píng Huì Mín Hé Jì Jú Fāng*, 太平惠民和剂局方) compiled by *Tài Píng Huì Mín Hé Jì Jú* [Medicine Preparation Bureau] in the Song [宋] dynasty, it is the world's first standard of patent medicine compiled under the official auspices.

[10] *Systematic Differentiation of Warm Diseases* (*Wēn Bìng Tiáo Biàn*, 温病条辨): Wu Tang (Ju Tong), Qing [清] dynasty. On the basis of the achievements of many scholars of warm disease in the Qing dynasty, [Wu Tang] made out the general theory of warm diseases[febrile disease], this book further established a system which completely independent of cold damage system, and established a three-jiao syndrome differentiation program, which is known as a landmark work of the theory of warm diseases in the Qing dynasty.

[11] *Craft of Medicines and Patterns for Children* (*Xiǎo Ér Yào Zhèng Zhí Jué*, 小儿药证直诀), the Northern Song dynasty, Yan Zhong-Xiao (闫孝忠), the follower of Qian Yi, collected the teacher's clinical experiences and make it become the

monographs of traditional Chinese medicine pediatrics.

[12] Yu Jia-Yan (1585–1670): Yu Chang, styled Jia Yan, was a famous medical scientist in late Ming and early Qing dynasties. Together with Zhang Lu-yu, Wu Qian, known as the early three famous doctors.

[13] *Revised Popular Guide to the Discussion of Cold Damage* (*Chòng Dìng Tōng Sú Shāng Hán Lùn*, 重订通俗伤寒论): the Original work made by Yu Gen-chu, a famous Shaoxing doctor in the Qing dynasty; later, He Xiu-shan composed and He Lia-chen emendated; and in the modern times, Cao Bing-zhang and Xu Rong-zhai revised and formed the last version. It is a treatise on exogenous febrile disease, which is a collection of all ages' long and full of laws and remedies.

[14] *The Grand Compendium of Materia Medica* (*Běn Cǎo Gāng Mù*, 本草纲目) Li Shi-zhen of Ming dynasty (Dong Bi), Volume 52. It took nearly 30 years for the author to compile and collect 1892 kinds of drugs, with more than 1000 pictures attached, to elucidate the natures and taste, main treatment, medication rules, place of origin, morphology, collection, processing, formula compatibility, *etc.*, with more than 10,000 attached formulas. It is a collection of great achievements of Pharmacy in China before the 16th century, and is praised as the Encyclopedia of China by foreign scholars.

[15] *Classical Formulas* (*Xiǎo Pǐn Fāng*, 小品方), 12 Volume, written by Chen Yan-zhi in the Eastern Jin dynasty. The original book is lost, the anonymous prose can be found in the *Arcane Essentials from the Imperial Library* (*Wài Tái Mì Yào*, 外台秘要); *Collected prescriptions from Clinical Experiences* (*Yī Xīn Fāng*, 医心方).

[16] *Plain Question* (*Su Wen*, 素问): Namely, *Huang Di Nei Jing-Plain Question*, 9 volumes, 81 chapters. With *Huang Di Nei Jing-Ling shu* (Also known *Lingshu*) is a companion volume.

[17] *Essentials from the Golden Cabinet* (*Jīn Guì Yào Lüè*, 金匮要略): It is part of miscellaneous diseases in *Treatise on Febrile and Miscellaneous Diseases* (*Shāng Hán Zá Bìng Lùn*, 伤寒杂病论), which was written by Zhang Zhong-jing, a famous medical scientist in The Eastern Han[汉] dynasty of China. It is also the earliest existing book dealing with miscellaneous diseases in China. mainly include medical miscellaneous diseases, surgical and gynecological diseases, emergency death, dietary

taboos, *etc.* It is honored as "*The Ancestor of Fang Shu*" by later generations.

[18] *Medicine Notes of Xian Xing Zhai* (*Xiān Xǐng Zhāi Yī Xué Guǎng Bǐ Jì*, 先醒斋医学广笔记), 4 volumes, written by Miao Xi-yong in Ming Dynasty.

[19] *Discussion of Medical Prescription* (*Yī Fāng Lùn*, 医方论), written by Fei Bo-xiong in the Qing dynasty, published in 1865 AD.

[20] *Essential Teachings of [Zhu] Dan Xi* (*Dān Xī Xīn Fǎ*, 丹溪心法), A comprehensive medical book written by Zhu Zhen-heng in the Yuan[元] Dynasty and edited by Cheng Chong in the Ming dynasty, 5 volumes, published in 1481. This book is not written by Zhu himself, but compiled by his students according to his academic experiences and general words.

[21] *Indispensable Tools for Pattern Treatment* (*Zhèng Zhì Zhǔn Shéng*, 证治准绳),The book was compiled by Wang Ken-tang, a famous medical scientist in the Ming dynasty, and published in 1602 A.D. The law of syndrome management is described in detail, because of its six contents, so it is named "*Indispensable Tools for Pattern Treatment*", and it is also called "*Criterion of Syndrome Management of Six Subjects*" and "*Criterion of Six Subjects*".

[22] Liu He-jian (about 1110–1200): Liu Wan-su, styled name: Shouzhen, was born in Hejian (now Hejian County, Hebei Province), hence later known as Liu He-jian. He was the founder of the "Cold and Cool School", one of the famous "four medical schools" in the history of Chinese medicine.

[23] *Six Volume of Cold Damage* (*Shāng Hán Liù Shū*, 伤寒六书), also named (*Táo Shì Shānghán Quán Shū*, 陶氏伤寒全书), 6 volumes, compiled by Tao hua (Jie an), published in 1445 AD, it made up by *Shang Han Suo Yan, Shang Han Jia Mi De Ben, Shang Han Sha Che Chui Fa, Shang Han Yi Ti Jin, Shang Han Jie Wang, Shang Han Ming Li Xu Lun*, those six books.

[24] Ke Qin (1662–1735), style name: Yun Bo, pseudonym: Si Feng, come from Cixi county, Zhejiang province, the *Shang Han* scientist of Qing dynasty, His *Syndrome Named by Formulas* and *Syndromes Classification Based on Formulas* were quite practical in clinical practice and had great influence on the later studies of *Treatise on Cold Damage*.

[25] Wang Ang (1615–1694): a doctor in the early Qing dynasty, style name: Ren An, used name: Heng. Come from Xiuning County, Anhui province, was a famous doctor in Xin An Medical School. He is also the author of *Su Wen Ling Shu Class Compacts Annotation* (*Su Wen Ling Shu Lei Zhuan Yue Zhu*), *Medical Formulas Collected And Analyzed* (*Yi Fang Ji Jie*), *Essentials of The Materia Medica* (*Ben Cao Bei Yao*), *Versified Prescriptions* (*Tang Tou Ge Jue*)and so on.

[26] *Revised Guide to the Discussion of Cold Damage* (*Tōng Sú Shāng Hán Lùn*, 通俗伤寒论), Written by Yu Gen-chu in the Qing dynasty, 12 Volume. This book is a combination of ancient and modern related works, combined with personal experiences of clinical syndrome, carried on an in-depth elaboration on Cold Damage syndrome treatment of the law.

[27] *Complete Works of Jingyue* (*Jǐng Yuè Quán Shū*, 景岳全书), In the late Ming dynasty, Zhang Jing-yue collected his own academic thoughts, and compiled a summary of various clinical disciplines and formulasof acupuncture and moxibustion. The book is rich in content, including theory, herbal, formula, clinical diseases, is a comprehensive and systematic clinical reference book.

[28] Liu Cao-chuang: A physician of the Ming dynasty, born in Changzhou (now Suzhou county, Jiangsu province). The head of the ten talents of Jing Tai.

[29] *Miscellaneous Records of Famous Physicians* (*Míng Yī Bié Lù*, 名医别录) (abbreviated as *Beilu*), written by anonymous (i. W. Tao), published in late Han dynasty, Pharmaceutical Works, 3 volumes. It is the Qin and Han dynasties' doctors add some more functions and application of herbs based on the book *Shen Nong's Classic of the Materia Medica* (*Shén Nóng Běn Cǎo Jīng*), and additional recording 365 new drugs.

[30] *Pouch of Pearls* (*Zhēn Zhū Náng*, 珍珠囊). A book of Traditional Chinese medicine (TCM) written by Zhang Yuansu in the Jin Dynasty (about 1234 AD).

[31] *Continuous Formulas to Aid the Living* (*Jì Shēng Xù Fāng*, 济生续方): A TCM book o written by Yan Yaohe in the Song Dynasty, with 8 volumes and 1 volume of adscription, published around 1267.

[32] Wang Mian-zhi (1923–2009) : tenured professor and doctoral supervisor

of Beijing University of Chinese Medicine, the first master of Traditional Chinese medicine, a famous Chinese medical scientist in China, and one of the founders of modern Traditional Chinese medicine Formulaology.

[33] Zhang Jing-yue (1563–1640): his name was Jie Bin, styled name: Hui Qing, pseudonym: Jing Yue, alias Tong Yi Zi. He was also known as "Zhang Shuidi" for his good use of *shu di huang*. He was born in Shanyin, Shaoxing (now Shaoxing, Zhejiang). The outstanding medical scientist of Ming Dynasty, was the representative of the Warm-recuperation school.

[34] *Complete Collection of Patterns and Treatments in External Medicine* (*Wài Kē Zhèng Zhì Quán Shēng Jí*, 外科证治全生集): Written by Wang Hong-xu (Styled name: Wei de) of Qing dynasty, published in 1740 AD. [the book is] surgical works. This book is written by Wangs Based on 40 years of clinical practice experiences.

[35] *Truth-Seeking Herbal Foundation* (*Běn Cǎo Qiú Zhēn*, 本草求真): Compiled by Huang Gong-xiu (pseudonym: Jin Fang) in the Qing dynasty, published in 1769 AD, 12 volumes, [in other addition say] 10 volumes. This book contains 520 kinds of herbs, [and] divided into two parts, the part one recorded very detailed information of the drug form, taste, function, indications and contraindications, the part two is divided into three parts: *zang-fu* disease syndrome main herbs, six pathogenic diseases syndrome, and the total meaning of herbs.

[36] Ye Tian-shi (1666–1745), Ye Gui, alias: Xiang yan, pseudonym: Nan Yang Xian Shen. He was born in Wuxian, Jiangsu (now Suzhou, Jiangsu), and was a famous medical scientist in the Qing dynasty. He was also one of the four great masters who research on febrile diseases.

[37] *Valuable Prescriptions of Emergency* (*Bèi Jí Qiān Jīn Yào Fāng*, 备急千金要方): Also known as *Qian Jin Yao Fang* and *Qian Jin Fang*, it was written by Sun Si-miao in the Tang dynasty in 652. AD. It consists of 30 volumes and is a comprehensive clinical work. The collection of diagnosis and treatment experience before the Tang Dynasty has a great impact on later medical scholars, and is regarded as the earliest Chinese clinical encyclopedia.

[38] *Arcane Essentials from the Imperial Library* (*Wài Tái Mì Yào*, 外台秘

要): Volume 38.40 is a comprehensive medical book compiled by Wang Tao of tang Dynasty from many medical works before Tang dynasty.

[39] *Achievements Regarding Epidemic Rashes* (*Yì Zhěn Yì Dé*, 疫疹一得): Written in 1794 AD by Yu Shi-yu in the Qing dynasty, 2 volumes, focuses on the diagnosis and treatment of epidemic diseases.

[40] *Dong-Yuan's Tried and Tested Formulas* (*Dōng Yuán Shì Xiào Fāng*, 东垣试效方): a prescription type Chinese medicine literature wrote by Li Gao in Jin dynasty, 9 volumes, completed in 1266 AD. A wide range of diseases involved in the book, but it focuses on the syndrome of spleen and stomach, reflecting the characteristics of the school of spleen and stomach.

[41] *Fine Formulas for Women with Annotations and Commentary* (*Jiào Zhù Fù Rén Liáng Fāng*, 校注妇人良方): Edited and annotated by Xue Ji (style name: Li-chai), a famous medical scientist in the Ming dynasty, on the basis of Chen Zi-ming's "*Fine Formulas for Women*" in the Song dynasty. The book consists of 24 volumes.

[42] Yue Mei-Zhong (1900–1982): Famous medical scientist, clinician, educator, and founder of postgraduate education in Chinese medicine. Put forward the principle of combining special disease, special formula, special medicine and syndrome differentiation together, make good use of the formula to treat serious diseases.

[43] Yoshinori Otsuka (1900–1980): Japanese physician who studied Chinese medicine. In September 1972, the Japanese Medical Doctors Association awarded him the "Highest Merit Award" for his outstanding contribution to the development of Hanfang medicine.

[44] *Medical Formulas Collected and Analyzed* (*Yī Fāng Jí Jiě*, 医方集解): written in 1682 AD by Wang Ang, a famous doctor in The Qing dynasty, who collected ancient and modern famous formulas and compiled them with great care. The book is divided into 3 volumes, including more than 700 ancient and modern commonly used clinical formulas in the form of main body and supplements, among which includes 388 formulas.

[45] *Secrets from the Orchid Chamber* (*Lán Shì Mì Cáng*, 兰室秘藏): Compiled by Li Gao of the Yuan dynasty, published in 1276 AD, 3 volumes. The book is divided

into 21 sections, including internal, external, gynecological and pediatric clinical departments. This book is one of Li Dong-yuan's representative works.

[46] *Collection of Writings on the Mechanisms of Disease, Suitability of Qi, and the Safeguarding of Life as Discussed in Basic Questions* (*Sù Wèn-Bìng Jī Qì Yí Bǎo Mìng Jí*, 素问·病机气宜保命集): Written by Liu Wan-yu in the Jin dynasty in 1186 AD, it is a comprehensive medical book, consisting of 3 volumes, which summarizes the author's lifelong medical theories and clinical experience in his later years.

[47] *Miscellaneous Writings of Famous Physicians of the Ming Dynasty* (*Míng Yī Zá Zhù*, 明医杂著): The book was written by Wang Lun in the Ming dynasty in 1502 AD, explained by Xue Ji and published in 1549 AD. [it is a] Comprehensive medical book, 6 volumes.

[48] *Direct Investigation of Cold Damage* (*Shāng Hán Zhí Gé*, 伤寒直格): Written by Liu Wan-yu in the Jin dynasty and edited by Ge Yong in 1186 AD, the book was completed in 3 volumes (originally 6 volumes). The book only 17009 words, from the perspective of fever syndrome treatment play the significance of cold damage disease..

[49] *A chapter of Warp and Woof of Warm-febrile Diseases* (*Wēn Rè Jīng Wěi*, 温热经纬): edited by Wang Shi-xiong (Meng Ying) in the Qing dynasty (1852 AD), 5 volumes, is a general theory of febrile diseases [warm disease]. This book "takes the principles from Xuan Qi [Huang Di Nei Jing] Zhongjing as the warp, and the standpoints of Ye Xue [Ye Tianshi and Xue Ji] as the woof", so it using "The warp and woof" to name book.

[50] Wu Ju-tong (1758–1836): first name was Tang, courtesy name was Pei Heng, pseudonym: Ju Tong. He was born in Huaiyin, Jiangsu province. the outstanding physician in the Qing dynasty and the founder of the *Shan Yang Medical School*.

[51] *Summarized Dissemination of the Classic of Materia Medica* (*Běn Cǎo Jīng Shū*, 本草经疏): Also known as *the Commentary on Shen Nong's Classic of the Materia Medica* (*Shén Nóng Běn Cǎo Jīng Shū*), written by Miao Xi-yong in Ming dynasty, 30 volumes, [it is a]pharmaceutical works.

[52] Su Gong: Su Jing, A Chinese pharmacologist in the Tang dynasty, who was

renamed Su Gong or Su Jian in the Song dynasty because he avoided zhao Ji [the emperor of Song dynasty]'s first name. He was born in Huaiyang, Chenzhou (now Huaiyang County, Henan Province). Presided over the compilation of the world's first officially promulgated by the state pharmacopoeia *"New herbal revision"* (*Xīn Xiū Běn Cǎo*, 新修本草) (also known as *"Tang Ben Cao"*).

[53] *Extensive Aiding Formula Collection* (*Guǎng Jì Fāng*, 广济方): Compiled in the period of Emperor Xuan Zong of Tang dynasty. The book includes more than 60 kinds of diseases in internal, external and gynecological departments, and 104 were collected.

[54] *Encountering the Sources of the Classic of Materia Medica* (*Běn Jīng Féng Yuán*, 本经逢原): This Book is written by Zhang Lu, a famous doctor in the Qing dynasty. It was published in 1695 and consists of four volumes.

[55] *Ji Feng Formulas of Universal Benefit* (*Jī FēngPǔ Jì Fāng*, 鸡峰普济方): written by Zhang Rui in the Southern Song dynasty (1133 AD), Works of Formula, 30 volumes.

[56] Huang Gong-xiu (1720–1817): styled name: Jinfang, born in Tangyin Junshan, Yihuang County, Jiangxi Province, was a famous medical scientist in the Qing dynasty and a imperial physician in the Emperor Qianlong Era.

[57] Zhang Bing-cheng (age of birth and death not specified): A physician in the Qing dynasty, styled name: Zhaojia, born in Wujin County, Jiangsu Province.

[58] *Treatise on the Spleen And Stomach* (*Pí Wèi Lùn*, 脾胃论), Written in 1249 AD, in 3 volumes, it is a representative work of Li Dong-yuan's theory of creating the Spleen and stomach.

[59] Li Dong-yuan (1180–1251): first name: Gao, styled name: mingzhi, pseudonym: Dong Yuan Lao Ren, born in Zhending (now Zhengding, Hebei). He was one of the "four masters of Jin and Yuan dynasties" in the history of Chinese medicine and the founder of the *"theory of spleen and stomach"* in Traditional Chinese medicine.

[60] *Clarifying Doubts about Damage from Internal and External Causes* (*Nèi Wài Shāng Biàn Huò Lùn*, 内外伤辨惑论), 3 volumes, written by Li Dong-yuan in 1247 AD. The book mainly discusses the etiology, symptoms, pulse condition,

treatment and other problems of internal injury and external infection.

[61] *Essentials of The Materia Medica* (*Běn Cǎo Bèi Yào*, 本草备要): Works on Traditional Chinese Medicine written by Wang Ang in 1694 AD in the Qing dynasty, 8 volumes. This book can be regarded as a clinical medicine manual and a medical guide book.

[62] *Formulas to Aid the Living* (*Jì Shēng Fāng*, 济生方): also named (*Yan Shi Jì Shēng Fāng*), Written by Yan Yao-he (styled name: Zi li) in the Southern Song dynasty, the book was written in 1253 AD and consists of 10 volumes.

[63] *Categorized Essentials for Normalizing the Structure* (*Zhèng Tǐ Lèi Yào*, 正体类要), Written by Xue Ji in the Ming dynasty in 1529 AD, 2 volumes. This book mainly discusses the experiences of treating common soft tissue injury, and there are medical cases report after each disease.

[64] *Supplement to Important Formulas Worth a Thousand Gold Pieces* (*Qiān Jīn Yì Fāng*, 千金翼方): compiled by Sun Si-miao, a medical scientist in the Tang dynasty, published in 682 AD, 30 volumes. The author collected nearly 30 years of experience in his late years to make up for the shortcomings of his earlier masterpiece, *Important Formulas Worth a Thousand Gold Pieces* (*Qiān Jīn Yào Fāng*, 千金要方), so it is named Yi [supplement] Fang.

[65] Qian Yi (about 1032–1113), courtesy name: Zhongyang and born in Dongping, was a famous pediatrician in The Song dynasty. He was also known as "the Saint of pediatrics" and "the father of pediatrics".

[66] Zhu Dan-xi (1281–1358): courtesy name: Yanxiu, a famous medical scientist of the Yuan[元] dynasty, was born in Yiwu of Wuzhou (now Yiwu in Jinhua, Zhejiang province) and the founder of the "Zi yin [Nourishing Yin] School". With Liu Wan-cu, Zhang Cong-zheng, Li Dong-yuan and listed as the "four masters of Jin and Yuan [dynasties]".

[67] *Supplement to 'Classified Case Records of Famous Physicians'* (*Xù Míng Yī Lèi Àn*, 续名医类案): edited by Wei Zhi-xiu (Yu Huang) in the Qing dynasty, originally 60 volumes, but reedited by Wang Meng-ying into 36 volumes. 345 Branches, collected the case of the famous doctor of past dynasties before Qing

dynasty, include clinical each branch, especially the discussion on warm-heat disease is more outstanding, certain medical record has Wang Meng-ying note.

[68] Wei Yu-huang (age of birth and death not specified): pseudonym: Liuzhou, a medical expert in the Qing dynasty, born in Hangzhou, Zhejiang.

[69] *Analogous Medical Prescriptions Collection* (*Yī Fāng Lèi Jù*, 医方类聚). Written in 1443 AD, by Kim Limun et al., Korea, the original issue is 365 volumes. It is a collection of 152 famous Chinese medical books from the Tang, Song, Yuan and early Ming Dynasties, as well as a Korean medical book, *Summary of Imperial Doctors*, totaling 153 books. The comprehensive works of medical formulas before the Chinese Ming dynasty

[70] *The Original Prescription Collection* (*Jiū Yuán Fāng*, 究原方): a formula for clinical Examination written by Zhang Song, a medical expert in the Southern Song dynasty, has been lost.

[71] *Extension of the Materia Medica* (*Běn Cǎo Yǎn Yì*, 本草衍义): written by Kou Zong-shi in the northern Song dynasty, published in 1116 AD, 20 volumes.

[72] Wang Jin-san (birth year Japan): the famous doctor in Qing dynasty.

[73] *Summary of Internal Medicine* (*Nèi Kē Zhāi Yào*, 内科摘要): Written by Xue Ji in the Ming dynasty in 1529 AD, 2 volumes. This book is a record of Xue's experience in diagnosing and treating miscellaneous diseases in clinic, which is selected from *Xue's medical case*.

[74] *Essays on Medicine Esteeming the Chinese and Respecting the Western* (*Yī Xué Zhōng Zhōng Cān Xī Lù*, 医学衷中参西录): written by zhang Xi-chun, a famous modern doctor, This book is a summary of the author's many years of experience in clinical practice and his understanding of China and the western medicine.

[75] *Fu Qing-Zhu's Women's Disorders* (*Fù Qīng Zhǔ Nǚ Kē*, 傅青主女科): Written by Fu Shan (Qing dynasty), published in 1827 AD, Works on gynecology, 2 volumes.

[76] *New Compilation of Materia Medica* (*Běn Cǎo Cóng Xīn*, 本草从新): Written by Wu Yi-luo in the Qing dynasty in 1757, 18 volumes, was widely circulated in the Qing Dynasty.

[77] *Effective Use of Established Formulas* (*Chéng Fāng Qiè Yòng*, 成方切用): Written by Wu Yi-luo in the Qing dynasty, With the aim of "Medicine[practice] is precious, Herbs[using] is appropriate", 1102 ancient and modern medical *Formula*s are included, which is another famous works on Formulas after *Investigations of Medical Formulas* (*Yī Fāng Kǎo*, 医方考) in Ming dynasty and *Medical Formulas Collected and Analyzed* (*Yī Fāng Jí Jiě*, 医方集解) in the Qing dynasty.

[78] *The Classic of Difficult Issues* (*Nàn Jīng*, 难经): There are many different views on the authors and the completion date. It is generally believed that its completion is no later than that of the Eastern Han dynasty, and its contents may have something to do with the People of Qin Yue-Ren (Bian Que). "Difficult" is the meaning of "question[verb]", or "difficult and complicated" solution. The "*Jing*" refers to the *Neijing,* so the name of this book is questioning on the *Neijing*. The author puts forward his own difficulties and doubts [of *Neijing*], and then explains them one by one. Some of the problems have been elaborated. The book is divided into 81 difficulties [chapters], the functional form of the human heart, diagnosis pulse, acupuncture, and many other problems discussed one by one.

[79] *Secret Formulas of the Yang Family* (*Yáng Shì Jiā Cáng Fāng*, 杨氏家藏方): edited by Yang Tan, styled name: Zi Jing, Southern Song dynasty, formulas collection book, 20 volumes, 1178 AD.

[80] *Materia Medica of Sichuan* (*Shǔ Běn Cǎo*, 蜀本草): This book is a supplement to "Bencao" by Meng Chang and Han Bai-sheng, the master of shu in the later five dynasties, especially the explanation of the drug graphics, more detailed in the previous Ben Cao. 20 volumes.

[81] Zhang Xi-chun (1860–1933), courtesy name Shoufu, was born in Yanshan County, Hebei Province. He was one of the representatives of the integration school of traditional Chinese and western medicine, a medical master in modern Chinese medicine.

[82] *Formulas from the Discussion Illuminating the Yellow Emperor's Basic Questions* (*Huáng Dì Sù Wèn Xuān Míng Lùn Fāng*, 黄帝素问宣明论方): also known as *Xuan Ming Lun Fang*, written by Liu Wanyu in the Jin dynasty, in 1172 AD, 15

volumes. It is a work of great clinical value. In the Jin and Yuan dynasties, it prevailed in the north and formed a confrontation with *Formulary of the Pharmacy Service for Benefiting the People in the Taiping Era (He Ji Ju Fang)* of the Southern Song dynasty. Later generations called it "The South Ju [bureau] and the North Xuan[*Xuan Ming Lun Fang*]".

[83] *Precepts for Physicians (Yī Mén Fǎ Lǜ, 医门法律)*: written by Yu Chang (Jia Yan) of the Qing dynasty, 6 volumes. Classified by wind, cold, heat, wet, dry, fire six pathogens and miscellaneous syndromes. Each group is divided into three parts: theory, Law and Precept. "Theory" is the general theory of disease, "Law" is the principle of treatment, "Precept" is to point out the doctor's fault in treatment.

[84] *Jade Key to the Secluded Chamber (Chòng Lóu Yù Yào, 重楼玉钥)*: Written by Zheng Mei-jian (style name:Hong Gang) in the Qing dynasty during the Reign of Emperor Qianlong and supplemented by his son Cheng Cheng-han, it was first published in 1838 AD. Laryngology works, 2 volumes.

[85] Zhang Yuan-su (1131–1234): style name: Jie Gu was born in Jin-bi Yi Shui (now Yi County, Hebei province) and was the founder of the School of Yi Shui. He focus on the Zang-fu syndrome differentiation and the theory of nourishing the stomach qi, has an important impact on Li Gao who create a "Nourishing Earth" as the characteristics of the system of spleen and stomach theory, and eventually become the most prominent theoretical characteristics of "Yi Shui School".

[86] *Confucians' Duties to Their Parents (Rú Mén Shì Qīn, 儒门事亲)*: compiled by Zhang Cong-zheng of the Jin dynasty, 15 volumes, which were completed in 1228 AD. Adhering to Zhang's idea, "Confucian scholars know the truth, and those who care for their relatives should know the doctor", it was named "*Confucians' Duties to Their Parents*".

[87] *Simple Book of Formulas (Yì Jiǎn Fāng, 易简方)*: Written by Wang Shuo in the Song dynasty, published in the late 12th century, Works on Medical formulas, 1 volume.

[88] *Multitude of Marvelous Formulas for Sustaining Life (Shè Shēng Zhòng Miào Fāng, 摄生众妙方)*: Series of Zhang Shi-che in the Ming dynasty, published in 1550 AD, 11 Volume, works on medical formulas.

[89] *Comprehensive Medicine According to Master Han* (*Hán Shì Yī Tōng*, 韩氏医通): Written by Han Mao in the Ming dynasty in 1522 AD, 2 volumes, comprehensive medical book.

[90] *Symptom, Cause, Pulse, and Treatment* (*Zhèng Yīn Mài Zhì*, 症因脉治): written by Qin Jing-ming in the Ming dynasty, supplement by Qin Huang-shi in the Qing dynasty, published in 1706 AD, 4 volumes.

[91] *Correction of Errors in Medical Works* (*Yī Lín Gǎi Cuò*, 医林改错): written by Wang Qing-ren in the Qing dynasty, published in 1830 AD. The book is divided into upper and lower volumes, which records Wang's theory of qi and blood viscera, correction of viscera errors in ancient medical books, and differentiation and treatment of miscellaneous diseases, especially syndrome differentiation and treatment of qi deficiency and blood stasis.

[92] Wang Qing-ren (1768–1831): Styled great minister, born in Zhili Yutian (now Part of Hebei province), was a medical scientist in the Qing dynasty.

[93] *Illumination of Medicine* (*Yī Xué Fā Míng*, 医学发明): written by Li Dong-yuan in the Yuan dynasty and published by his disciple Luo Qian-fu in 1315 AD. Each article is titled with the arguments of the scriptures and its source, such as *the Needle scriptures, The Plain Question, and the Classic of Difficulties*. Then, it explores the source, demonstrates the meaning of the scriptures, and gives full play to more than 70 formulas. It always refers to the topic of warming up the spleen and stomach. This book fully embodies the achievements of Dongyuan's theory.

[94] *Ri Hua-zi Master Medica* (*Rì Huá Zǐ Běn Cǎo*, 日华子诸家本草): abbreviated as "*Rihua Zi Materia Medica*" or "*Rihua Materia Medica*", the date and author of the work are unknown. [This book]Rich in content and practical, is an important document for the study of traditional Chinese medicine and the history of five generations of pharmacy.

[95] *Supplement to 'The Materia Medica'* (*Běn Cǎo Shí Yí*, 本草拾遗): A Bencao collection compiled by Chen Zang-qi in the Tang dynasty in 739 AD, 10 volumes. Chen Zang-qi mainly collected the missing herbs in the book, which supplemented the *New herbal revision*.

[96] *Treatise on Blood Syndromes* (*Xuè Zhèng Lùn*, 血证论), written by Tang Zong-hai in the Qing dynasty and completed in 1884 AD, 8 volumes, is the first monograph on the treatment of blood syndrome in China.

[97] *Divine Book of Ten Medicine Formulas* (*Shí Yào Shén Shū*, 十药神书): Written by Ge Ke-jiu in the Yuan Dynasty, published in 1348 AD. This book contains ten experienced formulas for the treatment of vomiting blood due to Consumption, which are arranged in the order of A, B, C and D [the ten Heavenly Stems]. practical and effective.

[98] *Formulas of Universal Benefit from My Practice* (*Pǔ Jì Běn Shì Fāng*, 普济本事方): written by Xu Shu-wei in the Song dynasty, published in about 1132 AD, 10 volumes. This book is a collection of Xu's experience, with medical records, and the facts.

[99] *Treatise on Seasonal epidemic disease* (*Shí Bìng Lùn*, 时病论): written by Lei Feng (style name: Shaoyi) in the Qing dynasty in 1882 AD, is the first treatise on the epidemic.

[100] *Correct Transmission of Medicine* (*Yī Xué Zhèng Zhuàn*, 医学正传): Yu Tuan of the Ming dynasty inherited his grandfather's medical profession and affected by Zhu Dan-xi. After 40 years of studying the ancient medical books such as The *Plain Question* and The *Classic of Difficulties*, he compiled the book in 1515 AD by referring to the doctors in previous dynasties and combining his own clinical experience.

[101] *Convenient Reader of Established Formulas* (*Chéng Fāng Biàn Dú*, 成方便读): Written by Zhang Bing-cheng in Qing dynasty, published in 1904 AD. This book is a compilation of more than 290 commonly used in ancient and modern times.

[102] *Treasury Classic* (*Huá Shì Zhōng Zàng Jīng*, 华氏中藏经): a comprehensive clinical book, 3 volumes. According to legend, it was written by Hua Tuo. The exact date of the book is unknown. This book put forward a syndrome differentiation method based on the combination of complexion, color, pulse and syndrome, centered on the pulse syndrome is proposed to describe the cold, heat, deficiency and excess of the five *zang-fu* organs.

[103] *Sign of Herbs* (*Yào Zhēng*, 药征): written by Yoshimasu Todo, Japan, in

1771 AD, 3 volumes. This book is a work of his lifelong research on the law of herbs use in Treatise on Cold Damage.

[104] *Effective Medical Formulas Arranged by Category by Master Zhu* (*Lèi Biān Zhū Shì Jí Yàn Fāng*, 类编朱氏集验方): written by Zhu Zuo in the Song dynasty, published in 1266 AD. This book collects more than 1000 formulas and folk formula commonly used by medical experts in the Song Dynasty.

[105] *Treatise on the Three Catergories of Pathogenic Factors and Prescriptions* (*Sān Yīn Jí Yī Bìng Zhèng Fāng Lùn*, 三因极一病证方论): written by Chen Yan in the Southern Song dynasty, published in 1174 AD. 18 volumes, divided into 180 Branches, collected more than 1050 receipts.

[106] *Effective Formulas from Generations of Physicians* (*Shì Yī Dé Xiào Fāng*, 世医得效方): Compiled by Wei Yi-lin in Yuan dynasty, 19 Volumes. With "according to the ancient recipe, participate with the family tradition[experiences]", hence the name, it is the experienced medical prescription from Five families of *Wei*.

[107] *Medical Formula Verses Collection* (*Yī Fāng Zhèng Zhì Huì Biān Gē Jué*, 医方证治汇编歌诀): a book of traditional Chinese medicine compiled by Wang Tai-Lin in the Qing dynasty. It was written in 1897 AD, and is one of the *Six Kinds of Wang Xu-gao's Medical Books*.

[108] *Life-Nuturing Thesis* (*Tài Dìng Yǎng Shēng Zhǔ Lùn*, 泰定养生主论): Written by Wang Yao (style name: Zhong-yang) in the Yuan dynasty, edition year is unknown, 19 volumes, monograph of health preserving.

[109] *Medical Revelations* (*Yī Xué Xīn Wù*, 医学心悟): Written by Cheng Guo-peng (style name: Zhong Ling) in the Qing dynasty, written in 1732 AD, 5 volumes. The eight principles, the eight methods, set the formula depend on the syndrome, the continuous analysis of syndrome differentiation are summarized, which are mostly the revelations of clinical experience. *Ten Laws of Surgery* are attached in the end.

[110] *Supplement to the Pocket-Sized Discussion of Formulas for Children* (*Bǔ Yào Xiǎo Xiù Zhēn Ér Fāng Lùn*, 补要袖珍小儿方论): Supplied by Zhuang Ying-qi's Prescription in the Ming dynasty, corrected by Zhu Da-nian and Meng Ji-kong, published in 1574 AD. It is the Pediatric literature, 10 volumes.